Conceptual Foundations *of* Occupational Therapy

THIRD EDITION

Gary Kielhofner, DrPH, OTR/L, FAOTA
Professor and Wade/Meyer Chair
Department of Occupational Therapy
College of Applied Health Sciences
University of Illinois at Chicago
and
Visiting Professor
London South Bank University

 F. A. DAVIS COMPANY • Philadelphia

F. A. Davis Company
1915 Arch Street
Philadelphia, PA 19103
www.fadavis.com

Printed in the United States of America

Last digit indicates print number: 10 9 8 7 6 5 4

Publisher: Margaret Biblis
Manager, Creative Development: Susan Rhyner
Associate Developmental Editor: Michelle Clarke
Design Manager: Joan Wendt

As new scientific information becomes available through basic and clinical research, recommended treatments and drug therapies undergo changes. The author(s) and publisher have done everything possible to make this book accurate, up to date, and in accord with accepted standards at the time of publication. The author(s), editors, and publisher are not responsible for errors or omissions or for consequences from application of the book, and make no warranty, expressed or implied, in regard to the contents of the book. Any practice described in this book should be applied by the reader in accordance with professional standards of care used in regard to the unique circumstances that may apply in each situation. The reader is advised always to check product information (package inserts) for changes and new information regarding dose and contraindications before administering any drug. Caution is especially urged when using new or infrequently ordered drugs.

Library of Congress Cataloging-in-Publication Data

Kielhofner, Gary, 1949-
Conceptual foundations of occupational therapy / Gary Kielhofner.— 3rd ed.
  p. cm.
Includes bibliographical references and index.
  ISBN 10: 0-8036-1137-4 (hardcover : alk. paper) ISBN 13: 978-0-8036-1137-5
  1. Occupational therapy. I. Title.
  RM735.K54 2004
  615.8'515—dc22

2003019517

For Beatrice D. Wade and Robert K. Bing

In memory and gratitude for the legacies they have left. Ms. Wade founded and led the University of Illinois at Chicago (UIC) Occupational Therapy Department. Dr. Bing, UIC alumnus, was an historian, scholar, and leader of the profession. Both were mentors who influenced the views in this volume.

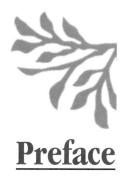

Preface

Throughout the writing of this book, both this and the first two editions, I was constantly reminded of my own personal journey in occupational therapy. Thirty years ago I first entered an occupational therapy clinic as an aide, fulfilling the alternative service obligation of a conscientious objector. What originally promised to be a 2-year detour from a career in clinical psychology turned out to be an introduction to my life work. I was drawn to the combination of helping and practical action in occupational therapy, which seemed so much more cogent than the predominantly talk-oriented approaches used in psychology. At the end of a year, I matriculated into an occupational therapy program with the support of a supervisor who allowed a flexible work schedule to accommodate my classes.

The educational program was my first big disappointment in occupational therapy. Almost all I had seen in the clinics impressed me. But in the classroom I (along with my classmates) found a disconcerting lack of coherence. It was not so much that the specific facts and concepts offered in classes were not useful enough in and of themselves. Rather, it seemed that, although I was beginning to understand human anatomy, how the unconscious worked, and the intricacies of neuromuscular physiology, and although I had acquired a number of practical skills,

something more basic was missing. Simply put, it seemed that I was not really learning about occupational therapy, that all the important knowledge in the curriculum came from other fields. The occupational therapy content was elusive at best. There was only a vague hope offered by several professors that everything would "come together" in clinical internships. I often wondered why the best was saved for last.

My misgivings were reinforced upon attending the American Occupational Therapy Association annual conference, where a number of presentations focused on the problem of identity in occupational therapy. It seemed as though members of the field shared a collective identity crisis. We all were, or were becoming, occupational therapists, but no one seemed altogether sure of what that meant. At that same conference, I was encouraged by a number of presentations in which therapists were proposing conceptual ways to explain occupational therapy on its own terms instead of resorting to other disciplines' theoretical constructs. This effort was particularly notable in the work of Dr. Mary Reilly and her students and colleagues at the University of Southern California (USC). The experience had an impact on me. I dropped out of my occupational therapy program at the end of the first year and began again at USC. There I had the opportunity to participate in the exciting enterprise of developing a more comprehensive conceptualization of the nature of occupational therapy.

As a result of this experience and my desire for a clearer conceptual articulation of occupational therapy, I begin writing immediately as a new therapist. In the beginning years, I presented my ideas as constituting, variously, a conceptual framework, a model, and a paradigm. It would be nice to say that I had some clear ideas at the outset about what these different terms meant, or, more to the point, that I had a clearly formulated idea about how knowledge gets generated and organized in a profession. However, that was not the case. Rather, I have struggled throughout my professional life with the problem of how we might properly think about the range of knowledge within occupational therapy. And I have pondered related questions about which knowledge is relevant, irrelevant, and most important. A tendency to be opinionated on the topic has provided me with a wealth of good, critical feedback, both in conversation and in the literature. Increasingly, I realize the debt I owe to those who cared enough about what I said to disagree with me.

This third edition represents my current thinking on the knowledge base of occupational therapy—my best attempt to decipher what exists and to speculate about what could and should be. In attempting to mirror the ideas and themes manifest in occupational therapy, I have interjected the perspective of my own grasp of these elements and a particular ideological position developed through a personal history of experiences in the field. In the end, that will be both the strength and weakness of the arguments contained herein.

What I hope resonates with most readers is my concern that the conceptual foundations of the field must be in the service of practice. I have been heartened over the years by the realization in the field that we cannot neglect the "occupation" in occupational therapy. I am equally dismayed that some seem to be leaving behind or forgetting the "therapy" in occupational therapy. In the end, I hope to have achieved some kind of balance in this text.

Because I like to recognize order in the world, there is an admitted tendency in this text to perceive a systematic structure in the knowledge base where others might legitimately disagree, recognizing a more disorderly reality. However, I believe that my approach provides a valuable way of thinking about occupational therapy knowledge. It allows comparison of different ideas and concepts, and it recognizes the fact that we use knowledge in different ways and for different purposes. Thus, I offer it as one of a number of ways to view occupational therapy knowledge—a way that I hope will prove useful for those entering into occupational therapy and for those in the field who wish to step back and take a new look at their profession.

Part of the purpose of this text is rhetorical; that is, to persuade the reader to take a different view of occupational therapy. Nevertheless, the book will have best served the reader if it becomes a springboard for further serious thought about the field's knowledge and how it is used in practice. Similarly, the book will have best served the field if it stimulates further dialogue and critical thought about the nature of occupational therapy and the nature of the knowledge that defines and explains it. Finally, I look forward to critical feedback to help my own thoughts to continue to evolve.

Gary Kielhofner

Acknowledgments

The arguments in this book have been in the making for some time. Along the way, more people than I can recall have influenced the three editions of this text. I am grateful to them all, although my thanks here is oriented to those who had a direct impact on this third edition.

Kirsty Forsyth, Lynn Summerfield-Mann, and Renee Taylor each had a major role in shaping my thinking about the relationship between knowledge production and practice. Their insights resonate in several parts of this text, and their feedback on my arguments was most helpful.

I am indebted to the following graduate students at the University of Illinois at Chicago, who did research papers on important historical figures in the field: Eynat Shevil, Anna Blazevic, Jessica Carr, Michelle Query, Melissa Ross, Orit Schwartz, Emily K. Simpson, Wendy Roberts, and Chaula Badiani. Their papers provided excellent background information that was used in creating the brief biographies in Chapter 3. Additionally, Susan Anthony provided critical information on her ancestor Herbert Hall.

I am grateful to Amy Paul-Ward and Dr. David Mitchell for providing helpful discussion and criticism of the disability studies chapter. Jeff Hall provided the excellent visual renditions of the concepts put forth in this book.

My research assistants, Judith Abelelenda, Lisa Jacobson, and Shilpa Desphande, made invaluable contributions to organizing the text, photographs, and other visual elements of this book. Jessica Keller arrived as a new research assistant and took over responsibility for many aspects of this text early in its production. Her organizational skills, thoughtful input, and constant gentle reminders have contributed more than I can say.

F. A. Davis has always believed in and supported this volume and its predecessor, Health Through Occupation. Dating back to the first edition, Jean-François Vilain and Lynn Borders Caldwell of F. A. Davis provided unfailing support of the project. I will always be grateful for their faith in me, their patience, and their persistence. As I produced this third edition, Margaret Biblis, Michelle Clarke, and Susan Rhyner have provided guidance, enthusiasm, and moral support that made producing this volume a pleasure.

The images in this edition have been an important addition to this book. Riva Lehrer's support of our concept for the opening of the disabilities studies chapter is much appreciated, and her work is much admired. The staff and clients at the University of Illinois Medical Center at Chicago contributed countless hours in order to provide meaningful images of occupational therapy, thanks to Sarah Skinner, Kathy Preissner, Michael Littleton, Supriya Sen, Joan Bourgeois, Stephanie Krieger, and Jennifer Steiner. In addition, other wonderful photos were collected from around the world and were the contributions of: Carmen Gloria de la Heras and Reencuentros, Sue Parkinson and Carter's Café at the Bolsover Community Mental Health team, Genevieve Pepin and Julie Godin at Université Laval, Cheyenne Smythe and the Connections Clubhouse, Karen Rebeiro and Northeast Mental Health Centre, Mary Binderman and the American Occupational Therapy Association, Inc. Archives, Junko Hayashi and Takatoshi Ono, Franciscan Communities Home Care, Helen Hayes Hospital, United Kingdom Center for Outcomes Research and Education, Bror Karlsson and Banzai, Frank Kronenberg, and Chicago activists and Disability Scholars Sharon Snyder, Mike Ervin, and Sharon Lamp.

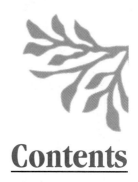

Contents

CHAPTER 4

SECTION TWO

CHAPTER 5

CHAPTER 6

CHAPTER 7

CHAPTER 8

SECTION THREE

CHAPTER 14

CHAPTER 15

CHAPTER 16

CHAPTER 17

SECTION FOUR

CHAPTER 18

CHAPTER 19

Section One

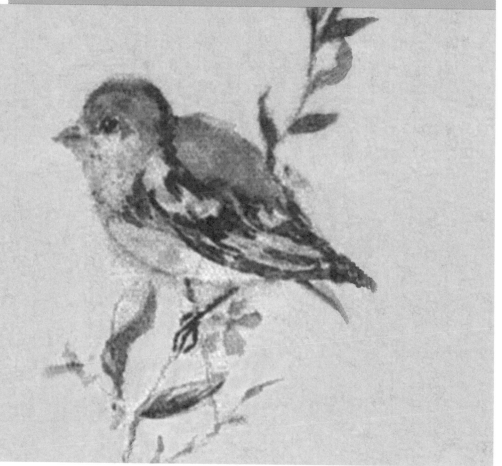

Chapter 1

Introduction

Early in this century, Susan Tracy, one of the founders of occupational therapy in North America, sent a greeting card to another occupational therapist, Jennie K. Allen. The front of the card bore a finely executed watercolor of a bluebird perched on a blooming tree branch. On the reverse side of the card, Tracy wrote, "Done without help by a patient sent from the [psychiatrist] tagged 'not able to concentrate *at all!*" As she offered no further elaboration, Tracy apparently expected Allen straightaway to grasp the significance of the story she was relating.

When I first encountered this card, it occurred to me that I had heard other versions of this story told by occupational therapists. For example, Chin-Kai Lin, a therapist from Taiwan, told me the story of a woman with a severe head injury. Her face, distorted from facial nerve palsy and the weight of her dark future, seemed fixed in a permanent frown. One day, Chin-Kai convinced the client to join in with a traditional Chinese choir. As the client began to sing an ancient sacred poem, her face slowly lifted, transforming into a cheerful smile. That the same kind of story remains alive in the lore of occupational therapy across time and culture suggests that it evokes something that occupational therapists recognize as deeply important about their practice.

Ultimately, Tracy's and Chin-Kai's stories, along with others of the same genre, are about the power of the field's therapeutic tool, occupation, to evoke capacity. These narratives typically contrast a client's performance in therapy with how the client was judged capable of performing by others or with the client's prior performance. The stories tell how non-apparent capacities, motives, or feelings are summoned by occupations.

More than 15 years ago, Nelson (1988) published a theoretical paper in which he introduced the concept of occupational form. The concept postulated that occupations (water-coloring being one of an endless number of such occupations) have a shape or form. This occupational form consists of the context, the objects used, the social definition and meaning of the thing to be done, and the ways of doing it that are known within a society or culture. Occupational form, Nelson and others now hypothesize, can exert an important influence on people, eliciting and shaping performance and experience. Research by occupational therapists has provided some support for this hypothesis. For example, studies have shown that varying the occupational form can change how persons move their bodies, how much effort they use, what they experience, and even the degree of impairment they exhibit (LaMore & Nelson, 1993; Mathiowetz, 1994; Wu, Trombly, & Lin, 1994; Yoder, Nelson, & Smith, 1989). Colleagues and I have developed and tested assessments that incorporate information on the influence of occupational forms on a person's functions (de las Heras, Geist, Kielhofner, & Li, 2002) .We have also studied the interaction between a person's outlook on life and occupational forms used in therapy (Helfrich & Kielhofner, 1994; Kielhofner & Barrett, 1998).

Tracy's and Chin-Kai's stories, the theoretical concept of occupational form, the research into how occupational forms influence performance and experience, and the incorporation of this concept into a practical assessment are all aspects of occupational therapy's conceptual foundations. That is, they all represent part of the perspective, knowledge, and practical tools that make up the profession. Assumptions, values, theory, and research, along with practice viewpoints, strategies, and tools, are part of the conceptual foundations of the field.

> **Assumptions, values, theory, and research, along with practice viewpoints, strategies, and tools, are part of the conceptual foundations of the field.**

Together they make up part of a complex unfolding conversation about the nature and practice of occupational therapy. Oral traditions, including stories about occupational therapy's impact on clients, perpetuate certain views of the nature of occupational therapy. The introduction of theoretical concepts in publications provides better understanding of phenomena that are part of the practice in the field. The development of practical tools increases the technical expertise with which occupational therapists can complete their work. These very different ways of considering or enacting occupational therapy give substance, depth, clarity, validity, and practicality to some aspect of occupational therapy. Each gives voice to a particular matter of concern.

Unfortunately, these voices are not always integrated into a coherent whole. That is, practical knowledge and perspectives, theoretical concepts, and research findings each have a way of leading a separate existence in the field. Therefore, one of the most compelling challenges to the conceptual foundations of the field is to find ways of bringing these elements together. One of the major themes of this text will be how the field can better interrelate these disparate components of our conceptual foundations.

🌿 Occupational Therapy Practice

Occupational therapy practice takes on many forms as seen on page 5. An occupational therapist in Zimbabwe working with a boy in a Bulawayo hospital uses a loom as a meaningful occupation to regain hand strength and dexterity after injury. In Stockholm, an occupational therapist monitors an archery rehabilitation program that helps clients with recent spinal cord injuries build a sense of personal capacity and interest while developing upper extremity strength and control. Street children from Guatemala participate in a public performance organized by a community-based therapist, giving them the opportunity to explore meaningful roles and appropriate social interaction. In an outpatient psychiatric day center in Japan, clients with cognitive and emotional impairments participate in and practice formalized skills in a traditional tea ceremony supervised by an occupational therapist. A therapist in the United States

goes to the convent home of a retired nun who experienced a cerebrovascular accident to coach her in adaptive dressing techniques.

In all these circumstances, occupational therapists provide services to persons whose impairments interfere with satisfying participation in their everyday occupations. Whether by helping a boy regain hand function in a culturally relevant activity, assisting clients to learn and develop skill, supporting children to exercise their capacity and creativity, teaching adults to engage in a traditional ceremony, or coaching an elderly person to maintain independence in dressing, all these occupational therapists were enabling persons to occupy themselves in keeping with their desires and circumstances.

These occupational therapists have specialized knowledge about such things as:

◆ The importance of play to development
◆ How limited ability for movement in activities can be augmented by specialized equipment and environmental modifications that can maximize function
◆ The importance and consequence of a person's beliefs about personal ability and interest in doing things
◆ How to identify which activities are most critical to a person's rebuilding a life following a traumatic event

These therapists also have a conviction in common, that being meaningfully occupied is fundamental to well-being. They share a philosophical orientation that emphasizes respect for the unique desires and abilities of the individual. These occupational therapists deliver their services in different cultures and health care systems, yet there is a striking similarity in their outlook and practices. Despite different languages, cultures, sociopolitical systems, and local circumstances, occupational therapy always remains essentially the same.

That these occupational therapists share common views about what is important for

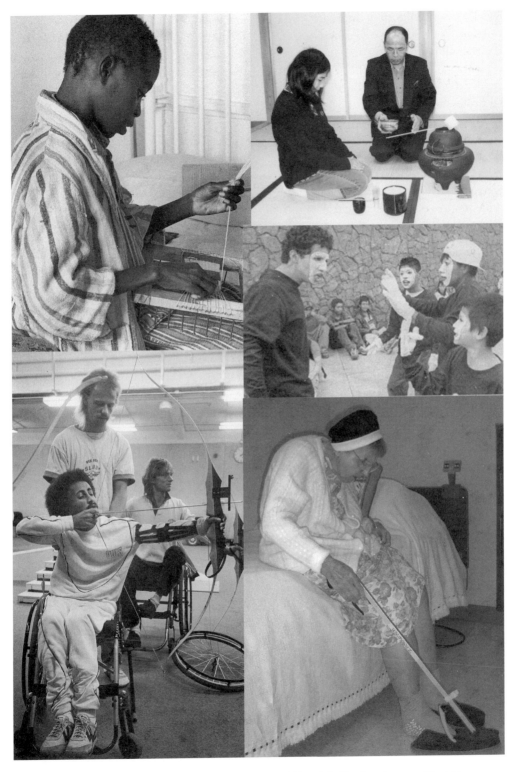

Occupational therapy (clockwise from top left) in Africa, Asia, the Americas, and Europe.
(Photos courtesy of Bror Karlsson/Banzai Archive or Frank Kronenberg.)

their clients and that they approach diverse problems along similar lines suggests that they have all partaken in some kind of common dialogue. One cannot but conclude that some kind of collective discourse has shaped their professional views and abilities. Another way of framing this is to say that they share identity and competence.

Identity and Competence

Together, identity and competence give a unique stamp to any professional group. They are what members of a field such as occupational therapy hold in common. They are what bind the members together.

Identity refers to both that which distinguishes a person and to the way that person sees things. For example, when persons refer to themselves as conservative or liberal, they are saying something about who they are and about a set of beliefs and perspectives they hold. Identity thus refers to a recognizable characteristic or aspect of a person and, at the same time, to the person's outlook. This is no less true of professional identity. It is professional identity that allows therapists to have a consistent view of the nature and meaning of their work and to present themselves to others as a particular type of professional.

Professional identity enables one to say, in effect, "As an occupational therapist, this is my perspective; these are things I consider important; these are the kinds of problems I address, and this is how I try to solve them." Moreover, this professional identity helps to make the collective field of occupational therapy a particular kind of profession (i.e., one that emphasizes or focuses on certain things, solves certain kinds of problems, and uses particular kinds of methods to solve those problems). This identity allows other professionals and laypersons to know something about what occupational therapists are and what they do.

One reason, then, that occupational therapists throughout the world appear quite similar is that they share a common professional identity. They have an understanding of the nature and purpose of their profession, and they share certain perspectives that, in their totality, are unique to occupational therapists. This shared understanding of occupational therapy and this outlook bind the world community of occupational therapists into a single professional community. In this sense, the profession transcends the national organizations, the unique educational institutions, and the particular variations of the profession in each country or culture.

Competence is the knowledge and abilities that therapists bring to bear on a particular problem of a specific client. Competence involves being able to identify and understand certain problems that clients face. It also involves knowing how to address those problems (e.g., how to employ appropriate strategies, techniques, equipment, and other resources in the course of therapy to solve problems effectively).

In the same way that identity gives therapists worldwide a similar character and outlook, shared competence enables therapists worldwide to offer similar kinds of services in a variety of circumstances.

The Relationship of Conceptual Foundations to Identity and Competence

The central thesis of this book is that the identity and competence of the individual therapist come from the shared conceptual foundations of the field. As already noted, I use the term "conceptual foundations" to refer to the collection of beliefs, assumptions, values, concepts, and techniques that make up the collective knowledge and know-how of the field.

These conceptual foundations are shaped by writing, practice, teaching, discussion, theorizing, research, and story-telling. The conceptual foundations of a field are represented in books and articles, and they are developed and advanced through research. Just as importantly, these conceptual foundations find expression and are tested and refined through how therapists practice, think about their actions, and talk or write about their work. Every occupational therapist, thus, participates in the conceptual foundations of the field. Each therapist, in his or her own way, receives and carries the messages of the conceptual foundations.

In framing the argument this way, I am proposing a particular viewpoint on how theory, ideology, reasoning, and action should interact in the field. For example, more than a few questions have been raised about the role that the conceptual has in the everyday practice of therapists. Some writers (Mattingly & Fleming, 1994; Schon, 1983) have emphasized that therapists practice in ways that go beyond what theory can specify. Many practitioners bemoan that theory does not always keep pace with the changing demands of practice environments or speak to all the situations and problems encountered in practice. Consequently, in place of using theory to guide their practice, therapists often rely on experience and common sense. On the other hand, theorists and educators sometimes observe that practitioners do not keep pace with changes in theory or make use of research. Each of these claims has some validity. Concepts sometimes fail to inform practice, and practice sometimes falls short of what theory and research would indicate.

Nevertheless, practice and theory have the potential to augment each other. Therapists who consciously and reflectively work from a theoretical perspective gain more from their experience. Practical experience can deepen our understanding of theory and lead to new lines of theory development and research. When conceptual and practical concerns become interrelated parts of a common dialogue about occupational therapy, the field is advanced more readily. This, then, is why I assert that discussion, writing, clinical decision making, and research should be interactive parts of the field's conceptual foundations.

The Plan of This Book

This book aims to explain and describe the conceptual foundations of occupational therapy. I begin by proposing a way to think about the conceptual foundations of occupational therapy. This view builds on the viewpoints I have already introduced and considers both what the profession is doing and could do to advance its knowledge and practice.

Trying to understand occupational therapy's conceptual foundations is a bit like trying to follow multiple conversations at an extended gathering of people. New themes sprout up out of a line of talking, some discussions die off, and others branch into separate lines of conversation. How and in what directions the talk goes depends on who is talking and responding, on the unique unfolding of a topic, and on what themes capture interest. When one examines the conceptual foundations of any field, it can be hard to see an explicit order in them. In part, sorting out elements of the field's conceptual foundations is difficult because, as knowledge develops, it does not neatly line up any more than the multiple conversations of a large group of people.

This lack of apparent coherence points out that some means of ordering the knowledge would be useful. To understand and use the field's knowledge, one must have a way of seeing how all its parts are related. One of the goals of this book, then, is to find and, to an extent, impart some order. Hence, in this text I present conceptual foundations of the field in a way that should allow the reader to identify, understand, compare, and critique the field's knowledge in all its manifestations.

Specifically, I will consider how the various beliefs, assumptions, values, theories, research findings, and know-how make up the conceptual foundations that are related to each other. I will also explore how all the elements that make up the conceptual foundation of the field have come into existence and have changed over time. Along with this, I will consider what kinds of processes (e.g., public discussion, theory development, research, application of ideas in practice) maintain and change the conceptual foundations of the field. Finally, I will examine the current content of the conceptual foundations of occupational therapy, focusing on what kind of identity and competence they provide for occupational therapists.

The organization of this text is as follows. In Chapter 2 of Section One, I outline a particular way of viewing the knowledge organization of occupational therapy, relating this organization to the concepts of identify and competence. Briefly stated, this chapter proposes that occupational therapy's conceptual foundations consist of three concentric layers of knowledge. At the inner core is a paradigm that provides the field and individual therapists with a sense of identity and a unique perspective. Surrounding this inner core is a band of conceptual practice models. These models provide the knowledge that gives occupational therapists their unique competence. The models incorporate theory that explains different phenomena occupational therapists address in practice; they also provide rationales, guidelines, and tools for doing therapy. The outermost layer is related knowledge. This knowledge is not unique to occupational therapy, but it supports therapists' competence because it provides information necessary to specific areas of practice. Hence, it is taught, written about, and used as part of occupational therapy's conceptual foundations.

In Chapter 3, I analyze the history of development of the innermost layer of occupational therapy's conceptual foundations, the paradigm. This history traces the emergence of occupational therapy knowledge as the profession developed in the 20th century. Chapter 4 is devoted to a discussion of the field's contemporary paradigm. It examines the knowledge that provides occupational therapy with its current identity and outlook.

Chapter 5 begins Section Two by discussing in more detail what a conceptual model of practice is and how I identified the field's current models. The subsequent chapters present these conceptual models of practice. Each of these chapters uses the same format for presenting and critiquing the models. This should enable readers to compare and contrast models and ultimately to decide how to interrelate and use models together in practice. At the end of each chapter, I provide a list of the model's major concepts and their definitions. These chapters are designed to introduce the reader to the conceptual models of practice, and they allow the models to be readily compared. However, my discussion of the models is general and, therefore, insufficient to provide the reader enough depth of knowledge to understand detailed theory and practical elements of each model. Hence, readers who wish to learn a particular model in depth should refer to the references at the end of each chapter and make use of these original sources. The final chapter of Section Two considers the state of model development as a whole, considering the relationship of models to the paradigm and anticipating model development in the future.

Section Three is devoted to discussion of related knowledge used by occupational therapists. Chapter 14 considers how related knowledge is chosen and used by therapists. Chapters 15 through 17 discuss three major bodies of related knowledge as examples. These chapters discuss the medical model, disability studies, and intrapersonal and interpersonal concepts.

The concluding Section Four reflects on the conceptual foundations as a whole and looks toward the future of knowledge development and practice in occupational therapy. Chapter 18 considers how the conceptual foundations (models and the paradigm) influence the identity and competence of occupational therapists. This chapter brings the discussion full circle to the view of the conceptual foundations that I outlined earlier. Finally, Chapter 19 considers the arguments of this book in relationship to other viewpoints concerning the conceptual foundations of occupational therapy. This concluding chapter should serve to contextualize what I have argued.

Overall, the book should provide the reader a broad overview of the conceptual foundations of occupational therapy. From this perspective, the reader should be able to see the field as a whole and recognize how the various parts of occupational therapy's conceptual foundations fit together. Additionally, the book should give a perspective on how the conceptual foundations have developed and where they might be headed in the future.

My hope is that each reader will finish the book with a more complete grasp of occupational therapy and with a sense of how to participate in the conceptual foundations of occupational therapy. And, above all, I want readers to recognize that each new article they read in the profession's journal, each new concept they encounter in occupational therapy textbooks, each new technique or tool to which they are introduced, and every new clinical story told by another therapist represents a continuation and unfolding of the conceptual foundations of occupational therapy.

References

de las Heras, CG, Geist, R, Kielhofner, G & Li, Y. (2002). The Volitional Questionnaire (VQ) (Version 4.0). Model of Human Occupation Clearinghouse, Department of Occupational Therapy, College of Applied Health Sciences, University of Illinois at Chicago.

Helfrich, C & Kielhofner, G. (1994). Volitional narratives and the meaning of therapy. American Journal of Occupational Therapy, 48, 319-326.

Kielhofner, G & Barrett, L. (1998). Meaning and misunderstanding in occupational forms: A study of therapeutic goal-setting. American Journal of Occupational Therapy, 52, 345-353.

LaMore, KL & Nelson, DL. (1993). The effects of options on performance of an art project in adults with mental disabilities. American Journal of Occupational Therapy, 47, 397-401.

Mathiowetz, V. (1994). Informational support and functional motor performance. Paper presented at the American Occupational Therapy Association National Conference, Boston.

Mattingly, C & Fleming, M. (1994). Clinical Reasoning: Forms of Inquiry in a Therapeutic Practice. Philadelphia: F.A. Davis.

Nelson, D. (1988). Occupation: Form and performance. American Journal of Occupational Therapy, 42, 633-641.

Schon, D. (1983). The Reflective Practitioner: How Professions Think in Action. New York: Basic Books.

Wu, CY, Trombly, C & Lin, KC. (1994). The relationship between occupational form and occupational performance: A kinematic perspective. American Journal of Occupational Therapy, 48, 679-687.

Yoder, RM, Nelson, DL & Smith, DA. (1989). Added purpose versus rote exercise in female nursing home residents. American Journal of Occupational Therapy, 43, 581-586.

Chapter 2

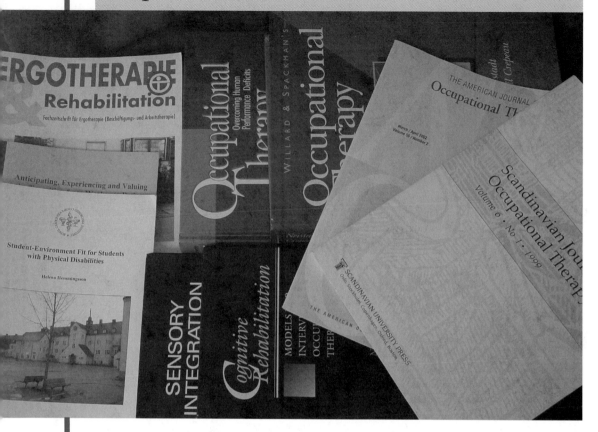

The Organization and Use of Knowledge

This chapter proposes a way to view the conceptual foundations of occupational therapy. This view is influenced by the ideas of authors concerned with knowledge development in other fields as well as by contributors to the knowledge base of occupational therapy. In formulating this view of the field's conceptual foundations, my first goal was to create a valid characterization of how persons are viewing and going about the work of building these foundations. My second goal was to find coherence among the current collection of concepts, frameworks, and techniques in occupational therapy.

Sometimes it seemed that these two goals were not compatible. In looking for purposes, processes, and patterns in occupational therapy literature, one finds that authors have used different terms to refer to the knowledge they are discussing, developing, or applying. They describe their work as "theory," "science," "conceptual frameworks," "frames of reference," and so on. This is not merely a matter of semantics. Persons genuinely differ in how they think about occupational therapy's conceptual foundations.[1]

I have sought to construct a useful way of thinking about occupational therapy's conceptual foundations and to use it as a means of organizing and interpreting existing knowledge. This way of viewing the conceptual foundations is partly descriptive (i.e., it explains how knowledge has developed) and partly prescriptive (i.e., it suggests how knowledge development might profitably proceed in the future). Arguably, my schema creates a partial fiction, identifying more coherence than may be available in the literature or intended by the authors. In defense of this approach, it allows for a necessary comparison and synthesis of a wide range of occupational therapy ideas.

The Relationship of Knowledge to Practice

In the previous chapter I argued that occupational therapy's conceptual foundations must involve a discourse between theory, research, and practice. Others in occupational therapy have also discussed the relationship of theory to practice. I will consider their viewpoints in order to contrast and clarify the point of view taken in this text.

Mosey (1992) distinguishes between theory that provides explanation of phenomena and the application of theory in practice. Arguing that occupational therapy's role is limited to theory application, she sees the work of developing and validating theory as belonging to academic disciplines (fields such as biology, sociology, physics, and philosophy) whose concern is with basic knowledge and not application.

Another perspective is represented in the movement to create an occupational science. When originally proposed, occupational science was defined as "the study of the human as an occupational being" (Clark et al., 1991, p. 306). It was planned as a new discipline, separate from but nevertheless supporting occupational therapy. Envisioned to be more like biology or sociology, it embraced the idea of developing knowledge without immediate concerns for applicability.[2] Nonetheless, occupational science was envisioned as being useful for practice because the insights about occupation it generated would be useful to practitioners.

Neither Mosey nor the proponents of occupational science propose theory development and practice as integrated activities of the profession. That is, Mosey argues that the work of occupational therapy involves only the application of knowledge, and proponents of occupational science propose developing a basic science separate from practice. In what follows I will propose an alternative to both these approaches.

---

[1] I have not made an attempt to address all these different views on knowledge development. However, in this chapter I acknowledge differences of opinion that are important for the present argument. Furthermore, in Chapter 19, I will compare the viewpoint I take in this book with two important alternative views of knowledge development on occupational therapy.

[2] Some writers have argued that occupational science embraces applied work as well (Clark, 1993; Zemke & Clark, 1996). Such inclusiveness not withstanding, the primary emphasis of occupational science remains generating knowledge about occupation and the idea that practice will benefit from such knowledge.

A Scholarship of Practice

Distinctions between basic and applied science reflect an outmoded view of how knowledge should develop. These distinctions are grounded, first of all, in a view that "intellectual progress must be decisively dissociated from human or social progress, the former being progress in knowledge, the latter being progress toward a good social world" (Maxwell, 1992, p. 209). This distinction has traditionally been made in the interest of allowing scholarship to reveal truth without the encumbrance or bias of practical concerns. The distinction between basic and applied scholarship has also led to a hierarchical relationship in which the pure or basic sciences have traditionally been accorded a place of higher status while applied work has occupied a lesser position.

My view is influenced by the argument that the separation of theory development and solving practical problems is irrational and results in much theory of questionable practical value, while many pressing human problems remain unsolved (Maxwell, 1992). As a consequence, traditional theory is an "utterly removed elite activity" that is "head-driven, not world-driven" (MacKinnon, 1991, p. 22).

The idea of a science separate from practice implied in both Mosey's argument and the occupational science perspective presupposes that science holds a privileged position of shaping what should go on in practice. As MacKinnon (1991) argues, such a perspective assumes "a relationship between theory and practice that places theory prior to practice, both methodologically and normatively, as if theory is a terrain unto itself" (p. 13). This viewpoint of how knowledge relates to practice, known as "technical rationality" (Schon, 1983), assumes that knowledge generated by basic science will naturally lead to applications of that knowledge. Stated another way, it assumes that practice consists of the application of theory and research that reveals the workings of nature (Higgs & Titchen, 2001; Schon, 1983). This viewpoint implies that professional knowledge is a "hierarchy in which 'general principles' occupy the highest level and 'concrete problem solving' the lowest" (Schon, 1983, p. 24). As shown in Figure 2–1, technical rationality assumes that it is the work of theorists and researchers to discover knowledge. Then the implications of that knowledge for application or practice are derived. Finally, the practitioner must figure out how to apply those principles in practice.

However, this view of how science informs application has been criticized as unrealistic because the structure and kind of knowledge that guide decision making in practice is different from those generated to simply explain phenomena (Barnett, 1997; Higgs & Titchen, 2001; MacKinnon, 1991; Schon, 1983). Occupational therapy writers have highlighted this difference, distinguishing between knowing about something and knowing how to con-

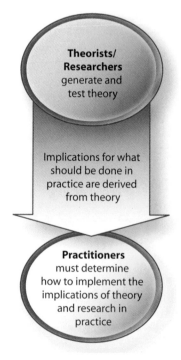

Figure 2-1. The hierarchical model of technical rationality.

duct practice (Mattingly & Fleming, 1994; McColl, Law, & Stewart 1993). This is an important distinction; simply knowing about something is not the same as knowing how to use that knowledge. Indeed, as Schon argues (1983), theory and related research designed to explain phenomena often fall short of the complexity that persons must deal with in solving problems related to those phenomena.

To remedy the gap between theory and practice, contemporary authors have proposed a rethinking of the nature and purpose of science and scholarship, proposing that instead of simply pursuing truth, science and scholarship should proceed in the interest of solving real problems (MacKinnon, 1991; Maxwell, 1992; Barnett, 1997). Such a perspective calls for a shift in science from simply knowing *about* something to focusing instead on knowing *how to do* something. In this way, knowledge generation is linked to its use. This scholarship of application requires replacing the old hierarchy of basic-over-applied research with dialogue between knowledge and its application.

> **The idea of a division of labor in which academic disciplines or researchers/theorists create and test theory and therapists practice the profession only perpetuates an unnecessary and unproductive division of theory and application.**

When these ideas are applied to occupational therapy, it means that the generation of theory and subsequent research and practice should not be undertaken as separate activities with the former shaping the latter. Rather, as shown in Figure 2–2, there should be an interaction between generating theory and research on the one hand and developing practice on the other. This concept, referred to as a scholarship of practice (Hammel et al., 2002; Kielhofner, 2002), calls for researchers and theorists in the field to work with practitioners to generate the field's theory and research and to advance practice. This means that what needs explaining in the profession and how it gets explained should arise out of the conditions of practice (Dickoff, James, & Wiedenbach, 1968).

Consequently, it is not advisable to separate the search for knowledge in the field from the search for better ways to practice. The idea of a division of labor in which academic disciplines or researchers/theorists create and test theory and therapists practice the profession only perpetuates an unnecessary and unproductive division of theory and

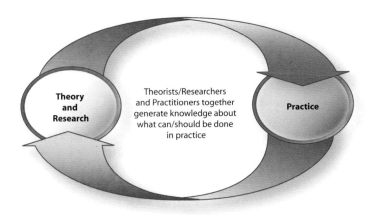

Figure 2-2. A scholarship of practice.

application. Pursuing a basic science or relegating occupational therapy science to the mere application of preexisting knowledge only serves to accentuate the divide between theoretical explanation and practice. Instead, in this text I underscore the need for organizing and developing knowledge in ways that link theoretical explanation and practice.

Hence, the view I take is calculated to bring into bold relief the challenge of uniting theory and action in the profession. This viewpoint hinges on three assumptions:

1. Theory development and theory application are both responsibilities of the profession.
2. The gap often found between theoretical explanation and practical action is, to a large extent, a function of how knowledge is developed and organized.
3. When knowledge is developed and organized as part of a dialogue between explanation and practical problem-solving, the gap between theory and practice can be eliminated.

These three beliefs have guided my attempts to unravel and describe the conceptual foundations of occupational therapy. I have sought to avoid unnecessary distinctions and separations between basic or applied work and between the theoretical and the practical in occupational therapy, emphasizing instead their interaction and interdependence. Theory provides ways of understanding necessary to practice. Practice points to what we should know and, by applying theory to real life, enriches our understanding and development of theory. The theoretical and practical can and should be interwoven.

> **Theory provides ways of understanding necessary to practice. Practice points to what we should know and, by applying theory to real life, enriches our understanding and development of theory.**

 # Conceptual Foundations as Concentric Layers of Knowledge

Chapter 1 argued that occupational therapy's conceptual foundations address professional identity and competence. Identity has to do with the nature of the service that occupational therapy provides and the outlook that therapists employ. Competence refers to what a therapist knows how to do in providing service. Consequently, practice requires both knowledge that provides a general outlook or vision of practice as well as knowledge that provides tools for practice.

To the extent that identity and competence are the two fundamental practical problems that a field must address, knowledge development should proceed along lines that address these problems. In occupational therapy, knowledge development resonates with these two issues.

First, occupational therapists generate knowledge aimed at defining and identifying what occupational therapy is and at providing therapists with a unique way of seeing their work. A second type of knowledge gives occupational therapists guidance in knowing how to understand specific client problems and what to do about them. Members of the field have generated these two types of knowledge to make sense of what occupational therapists do.

In addition to these two areas of knowledge, occupational therapists need a range of knowledge to provide necessary background for different areas of practice. Such knowledge is not generated in occupational therapy but is incorporated into the conceptual foundations

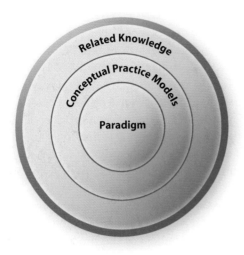

Figure 2-3. Concentric layers of knowledge in the conceptual foundations.

as adjunctive or related knowledge. Therefore, as shown in Figure 2–3, the conceptual foundations of occupational therapy can be envisioned as three concentric layers of knowledge:

◆ An innermost core, or paradigm
◆ A surrounding band of conceptual practice models
◆ An outer sphere of related knowledge

I refer to the paradigm as the innermost core because it most directly addresses the identity and outlook of the field. Surrounding the paradigm, several conceptual practice models articulate diverse concepts that are being generated, tested, and applied in practice. It is through these models that the field's theoretical concepts are developed and its therapeutic approaches are laid out. Conceptual practice models articulate theory that provides a theoretical and empirical rationale for therapy and guides therapists in practice. The related knowledge of the field is a collection of concepts, facts, and techniques from other fields that are used in occupational therapy practice. Unlike the paradigm and the models, this layer of knowledge is not unique to occupational therapy. Rather, it is gathered into the field because of its relevance to the kind of work done by therapists. Like every field, occupational therapy uses related knowledge to support and fill in gaps between its own unique knowledge (i.e., its paradigm and models) and the demands of practice for knowledge. Table 2–1 summarizes the characteristics of these three layers of knowledge. In the following sections I discuss each layer in more detail.

The Paradigm

The concept of the professional paradigm proposed here builds on the original work of

TABLE 2-1. CHARACTERISTICS OF THE LAYERS OF KNOWLEDGE		
Layer	**Content**	**Purpose**
Paradigm	Broad assumptions and perspectives	• Unify the field • Define the nature and purpose of occupational therapy
Conceptual Practice Models	Diverse concepts organized into unique occupational therapy theory	• Develop theory • Provide rationale for and guide practice
Related Knowledge	Concepts, facts, and techniques borrowed from other disciplines	• Supplement unique knowledge of the field • Applied in practice

Kuhn (1970) and on that of others who have critiqued and applied his ideas. In his examination of how knowledge developed in the physical sciences, Kuhn observed that members of a discipline are bound together by a shared vision. Further, he argued that this collective vision was a set of perspectives, ideas, and values that constitute a unique perspective shared by members of the discipline. These perspectives, ideas, and values create a context for the work of the discipline. Kuhn referred to this common vision as its paradigm.

In this book, we will use the concept of paradigm in two interrelated ways. First, it is a conceptual perspective, made up of fundamentals articulated in the literature and discussed by those seeking to define the nature and purpose of the field. Second, it is the cultural core of the discipline.

Tornebohm (1985, 1986) argues that a paradigm is reflected in that with which members of the profession are concerned and in how they view the phenomena with which they are concerned. He also argues that the paradigm defines the profession for its members and presents ideals about how to practice. Thus, he notes that the paradigm proposes a conceptual perspective that incorporates a definition of practice, a viewpoint that characterizes practice, and ideals about how practice should occur.

Macintyre (1980) argues that to share a professional culture is to have common beliefs and perspectives that both make sense of and guide or regulate professional action. As the culture of the profession, the paradigm allows therapists to understand, in a very broad way, what they are doing when they practice. That is, it provides them with an understanding of the nature of their work, its primary concerns and methods, and its values. These elements of the paradigm provide the profession a viewpoint and a self-image. In short, the paradigm provides professional identity.

Elements of the Profession's Paradigm

The perspectives of Kuhn (1970), Macintyre (1980), and Tornebohm (1985, 1986) are useful for considering, in a general way what a paradigm is. However, it is also necessary to think about the elements that make up a paradigm. Consequently, it is important to consider occupational therapy as a profession, asking: what does its paradigm consist of, and why?

Inasmuch as the paradigm functions as an integrating culture, it contains core themes or ideas that members of the profession see as their basic concerns. I refer to this element of the paradigm as core constructs. Secondly, because the paradigm must provide a particular outlook or perspective, it also needs to contain a way of seeing those things with which members of the profession are concerned. This aspect of the paradigm I call the focal viewpoint. Lastly, any integrating culture provides ideas and a vision of what matters most to members of the group. Therefore, the paradigm's third element is the values of the profession. Hence, as shown in Figure 2–4, the paradigm of occupational therapy is made up of its core constructs, focal viewpoint, and values.

Core Constructs As a practice profession, occupational therapy must address essential questions about the service it provides:

◆ What human need does the service address?
◆ What kinds of problems does it solve?
◆ How does it solve those problems (i.e., what is the nature of its service)?

These are the questions to which the core constructs of the paradigm are addressed. By identifying the aspect of human well-being for which occupational therapists take responsibility, the kinds of problems they solve, and the methods they

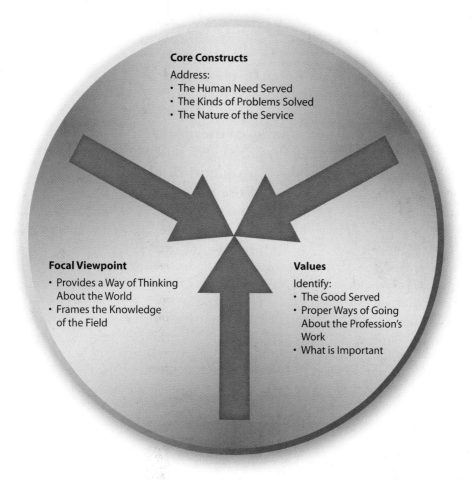

Figure 2–4. Elements of the paradigm.

use to solve those problems, the field defines itself. These three elements are explicated in a collection of themes or ideas that together are the field's core constructs.[3]

To illustrate the idea of core constructs, let us consider the profession of medicine. Physicians address the human need for biological well-being and survival. These medical practitioners solve problems (diseases and traumas) that threaten survival and well-being. They do this by repairing damage and by slowing, minimizing, or eradicating disease. Knowledge of what is normal (e.g., blood pressure, temperature, physiology) provides a picture of how the body works. The problems medicine addresses are disturbances to this normal state of affairs. Medicine defines and categorizes these problems through a diagnostic system. Moreover, physicians seek to resolve these problems

---

[3] The concept of core constructs refers to those constructs that are global to the field as a whole and therefore part of the paradigm. These are different than the concepts that are used as part of the theoretical arguments within models of practice. Core constructs do influence the kinds of concepts that appear in the theoretical arguments of models of practice, but they transcend these specific models and represent a more universal way of thinking in the field. In fact, when similar concepts are found in several models of practice, it is likely that these concepts reflect or derive from a core construct in the paradigm.

through therapies that include medication and surgery.

For medicine, this vision of its practice is articulated through such core constructs as disease, diagnosis, and medication. Not everything that physicians do fits neatly into such core constructs, but they do give medicine a general identity. In later chapters, we will look to occupational therapy, asking what themes and ideas make up its core constructs. These themes and ideas are distinct from those of medicine and help to differentiate occupational therapy from medicine. For example, whereas medicine focuses on disease and diagnosis, occupational therapy focuses on how persons' occupational lives are disrupted by disease and other factors. Such differences of perspective are essential elements of the paradigm of each profession that give it a distinct identity.

Focal Viewpoint Professions require more than concepts to identify what human need they address and what they do. Because they develop and use knowledge, they need a viewpoint that organizes their knowledge and gives them a way of thinking about the phenomena they address in theory and practice. Medicine's viewpoint sees the body as a complex machine made up of parts and processes (Leder, 1990; Toombs, 1993). Medicine is predicated on being able to see inside this human machine; this is made possible by such things as physical examinations, x-rays, laboratory tests, and biopsies.

Also basic to medicine's viewpoint is the idea of laws of causation. Medicine sees the body as made up of component parts that operate according to discoverable laws. Understanding diseases or traumas means understanding how they cause disruptions to

> **By identifying the aspect of human well-being for which occupational therapists take responsibility, the kinds of problems they solve, and the methods they use to solve those problems, the field defines itself.**

normal structure and function. This concept of causation also guides medicine's use of biochemical and other physical interventions to cause changes that counter the effects of disease or trauma. Thus, medicine is made sense of by a viewpoint that (a) emphasizes the machine-like nature of the human body, (b) looks for the causal links between structures and functions in the body, (c) understands the causes of conditions that threaten the body, and (d) applies treatments designed to cause a restoration of order.

In contrast to medicine, occupational therapy's viewpoint is oriented to understanding complex connections between the person and the environment and how these are influenced by impairments that restrict performance. Hence, for example, occupational therapists seek to restore order in the relationship between the person and the environment despite permanent impairments of the body or mind.

Professional paradigms all contain this focal viewpoint, which frames the situation, identifying what the specific facts of a field will mean. The focal viewpoint allows the profession to attend to and interpret the world in its own way. This viewpoint also influences what kind of knowledge the field will consider relevant to its work. For example, medicine is not centrally interested in the concept of culture because culture is not considered to figure strongly in the causation or treatment of disease. Occupational therapy, on the other hand, must consider culture as an essential element of the environment in which the person functions.

Values Finally, because professions are engaged in practical action they require ideas about the good they serve and about proper ways of going about what they do. Hence, each profession has its own unique values that emphasize what is important from its point of view. In medicine the preservation of life operates as an important value. Physicians see their work as fundamentally good because it preserves and extends life. In occupational therapy, the quality of life as attained in one's everyday participation in occupations is the central consideration.

Expression of the Field's Paradigm

As Kuhn (1970) points out, paradigms are largely implicit. They are often taught and reinforced through the use of exemplars in which the paradigm is illustrated in a particularly salient way. Exemplars are succinct demonstrations of how the work of the discipline could and should be done. Stories about practice in occupational therapy, which reveal something essential to occupational therapy, are exemplars that illustrate the field's paradigm.

Recall the example of Susan Tracy's story about the psychiatric client who was able to produce a fine watercolor despite the physician's judgment that he could not concentrate. This story illustrated how occupational therapy's paradigm was different from that of medicine. Tracy's story suggested a different view of the client. Moreover, the story did not tell about how something was done to modify the client from within. Rather, it suggested that when environmental circumstances are right, behavior could be elicited from the client. It emphasized getting the client to do something rather than what could be done to the client. In this story are implied certain core concepts, a viewpoint, and values, as we will see in the next chapter. Stories about practice always mirror some aspect of the paradigm.

Of course, the paradigm is articulated and exemplified in other ways as well. Theoretical articles, books, and professional presentations that introduce or expand the core constructs or focal viewpoint of the field are important contributions to the paradigm. Official documents and professional publications that outline, discuss, and debate values of occupational therapy are significant expressions of the field's integrating values. Moreover, the paradigm is taught, reinforced, and reshaped in education and in practice as persons learn about, experience, and put into action the identity and perspective of occupational therapy.

The Paradigm: Summary

The paradigm of a field functions as a conceptual perspective and as a culture. It consists of core constructs, a viewpoint, and values. These elements of a paradigm are what define and give coherence or wholeness to the entire profession and thus unify the field.[4] Together, the elements reveal what the

---

[4] Discussions of occupational therapy's conceptual foundations have sparked an ongoing debate over the relative merits of unity versus diversity in the body of knowledge. I have argued, along with others, that occupational therapy requires a unified body of unique knowledge for its own coherence and to sustain societal support (Fleming, 1987; West, 1984; Wiemer, 1979). Additionally, proponents of a unified body of knowledge point to the needs to articulate an identity for the field, to unite practice across specialty areas, and to facilitate cumulative knowledge development in the field (Christiansen, 1981; Kielhofner & Gillette, 1979; West, 1984).

In contrast to these arguments, others have raised concern that a unified theory of occupational therapy would be too confining, block creativity, and negate ideas that did not fit neatly within it (Labovitz & Miller, 1986; Mosey, 1985). This counterargument asserts that the field cannot afford to become too single-minded or narrow in its orientation.

Consequently, there appears to be a conflict between the need to achieve a coherent and unified conceptual foundation and the need to maintain openness, creativity, and originality. I do not believe, however, that this conflict is real. Both diversity and unification can and must be accommodated in the conceptual foundations of a practice profession. In fact, the two tendencies—one toward unification and the other toward diversification—can be complementary forces that keep each other in check as the knowledge base develops. That is, the field's conceptual foundation must consist of both a defining, unifying core and a surrounding, related collection of diverse knowledge.

discipline takes to be its fundamental nature and purpose and how the paradigm envisions the phenomena it addresses in practice and what it considers important in practice.

The core constructs are interrelated themes that underlie the entire field. They can be found in the literature of the field and in what members fundamentally know and believe about the field and about their practice. These concepts articulate what human need occupational therapy serves, what problems it addresses, and how it solves these problems. The focal viewpoint of the field is the commonly shared view of the phenomena with which members of the field are interested. It is how therapists collectively envision that aspect of the world with which they are concerned. It serves as a "map of the territory" that provides therapists a perspective on how their universe of concern is put together. The integrating values are the deeply held convictions of the discipline concerning the values of the profession and how it should carry out its business. These values identify why practice matters and what ought to be done in practice. Members of the profession contribute to, assimilate, and give expression to the paradigm in their action. The paradigm, in turn, gives members a distinctive professional identity. In this sense, the paradigm is a culture through which members, individually and collectively, make sense of their profession.

> **Members of the profession contribute to, assimilate, and give expression to the paradigm in their action. The paradigm, in turn, gives members a distinctive professional identity.**

Conceptual Practice Models

Although the paradigm provides a common understanding of what it means to be an occupational therapist, it does not provide specific details of how to engage in practice. The conceptual practice models, which make up the second layer of knowledge in the conceptual foundations of occupational therapy, provide this more detailed knowledge.

A conceptual practice model presents and organizes theory used by therapists in their work. In occupational therapy, each model addresses some specific phenomenon or area of human function. For example, one model addresses the biomechanics (i.e., structures and functions of the musculoskeletal system) underlying movement. Other models address such phenomena as sensory processing, perception and cognition, and motivation. Each model explains an area of functioning and specifies the interventions pertaining to particular kinds of problems in that area. Because each model focuses on specific areas, the field requires more than one model to address occupational therapy's range of concerns.

Components of a Conceptual Practice Model

Models can be thought of as having the following components:

◆ An interdisciplinary conceptual base
◆ Theory about the organization and function of the area of concern
◆ Problems or challenges in the area of concern
◆ Therapeutic intervention designed to preserve and/or change the organization and function of the phenomena with which the model is concerned
◆ Technology for application (e.g., assessment protocols, instruments, and therapeutic methods)
◆ Empirical scrutiny of the model (i.e., research that tests theoretical arguments

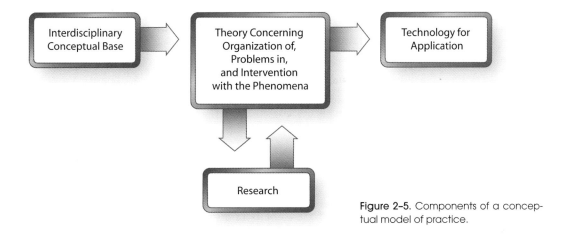

Figure 2–5. Components of a conceptual model of practice.

and demonstrates how the model works in practice)

As shown in Figure 2–5, these components are parts of a dynamic and ongoing process of knowledge development.

Let us examine in more detail how this process occurs. Authors of conceptual practice models build on knowledge from other disciplines as well as from concepts inside the field. For example, sensory integration (discussed in Chapter 12) is a conceptual practice model concerned with the brain's processing of sensory information for motor action; the model builds on knowledge from neurology and neuropsychology and on sensorimotor treatment concepts developed in occupational therapy. The model of human occupation (see Chapter 10) synthesizes knowledge from systems theory, psychology, social psychology, sociology, and anthropology, while building on previous occupational therapy knowledge, to explain the motivation for and patterning of occupation. The interdisciplinary foundation on which a model is built includes theories and the research supporting those theories.

The authors of conceptual practice models create theory to explain the organization and function of some aspect of occupation on which the model focuses. Similarly, the models provide theoretical arguments about problems or challenges. Finally, they provide theoretical explanations of how therapy can be used to maintain or alter function. The theory in conceptual practice models is the primary theoretical activity of occupational therapy. A mature conceptual practice model organizes concepts from within and outside the field into unique theory that reflects the paradigm of the profession. In this way, models are much more than mere structures to guide application of theory.[5] The theory in each model gives logic and coherence to the practice applications that the model provides.

---

[5] Although this definition of models of practice shares attributes of Mosey's (1981) frames of reference, a critical difference is that the models express theory unique to occupational therapy (Leder, 1990). Mosey views frames of reference as organizing theoretical concepts for practice. In many cases, a frame of reference (e.g., the developmental, acquisitional, and analytical object relations frames of reference) borrows a theory from another discipline and applies it to occupational therapy practice without formulating unique occupational therapy theory. Such a frame of reference does not qualify as a model of practice (as defined here). I consider such a frame of reference as related knowledge. This point is elaborated in Chapter 14.

As a model develops, its technology for practical application is constantly expanded and refined. Theorists and practitioners working within the model create assessments, accumulate case examples, write guidelines or protocols for application, and develop programs based on the model. Dissemination of these practical applications in journals, textbooks, and presentations make the model more useful in practice. Similarly, problems and insights encountered in practice may lead to changes in the model.

Research allows empirical scrutiny of the practice model. Studies test the accuracy of the theoretical arguments as they relate to the phenomena they seek to explain. Research also produces descriptive data helpful in elaborating the theory. Further, research tests the effectiveness of the technology for application based on the theory. Practice models provide a context for both applied and basic research. Basic research examines the model's theoretical arguments about organization and dysfunction. Applied research tests arguments about preservation and change and the usefulness of practical applications. The two types of research are complementary, and both are necessary.

The number and relevance of applications that the practice model offers influence how widely it is adopted in the field, but only empirical support of the model will ensure its survival. Practitioners understandably concern themselves with how readily a practice model will provide them useful guidelines for application. Eventually, however, when pressed to justify or demonstrate the effectiveness of services, occupational therapy must offer empirical support for the truth and utility of its conceptual practice models.

> **The models provide special professional lenses through which the therapist sees the client, develops plans, and solves problems.**

As I noted earlier, each conceptual practice model represents a dynamic process in which knowledge is developed and used through theorizing, application, empirical scrutiny, and revision (see Fig. 2–3). The theory of the model provides explanations of phenomena with which it is concerned; these explanations can be verified, falsified, or refined through research. The theory also explains and directs practical application. Basic and applied research provide feedback to the model, allowing theory to be corrected and elaborated as scientific evidence is accumulated. Similarly, applications in practice can provide critical feedback leading to changes and elaborations of the theory. This dynamic process of input from the interdisciplinary base and the feedback loops from practice and research are necessary to keep a model vital. Finally, the theoretical and empirical work done within the model may make contributions to the interdisciplinary areas from which the model's underlying concepts came.

The conceptual practice models are part of the know-how of members of the field. When therapists use the field's knowledge, they engage in an active process of reasoning using conceptual practice models. The models provide special professional lenses through which the therapist sees the client, develops plans, and solves problems.

Related Knowledge

Although conceptual models provide much of the knowledge for doing practice, therapists routinely need additional knowledge. For instance, practice may require the use of some concepts and skills not unique to occupational therapy and not contained in occupational therapy's conceptual practice models. For example, all helping professions involve a therapeutic use of self. Consequently, therapists may employ, as related knowledge, theory and techniques concerning therapeutic use of self. Related knowledge may also include information that belongs to another profession that is also useful and necessary to occupational therapy practice. For example, medicine's knowledge of disease processes is critical to occupational therapy practice even though occupational therapy is very different from medicine. Another example, from the field of psychology, is the theory of behavior modification, whose principles and techniques are sometimes useful in occupational therapy practice. In these instances, occupational therapists use related knowledge to supplement the knowledge that defines and guides the main elements of occupational therapy practice. Another example of related knowledge is growing literature in the interdisciplinary field of disability studies (e.g., Albrecht, Seelman, & Bury, 2001; Longmore, 1995; Oliver, 1996; Scotch, 1988; Shapiro, 1994). Disability studies scholars emphasize understanding disability from the perspective of persons who have disabilities. They argue that many of the problems faced by persons with disabilities can more properly be located in the environment—in everything from physical barriers to stigmatizing attitudes to outright discrimination. Ideas from disability studies have many lessons to teach occupational therapists and therefore constitute important related knowledge. Related knowledge is also used in research, administration, politics, and other activities of the field (e.g., knowledge about how to conduct scientific inquiry and information about the workings of the health care system).

Related knowledge is necessary to support practice, research, and other activities of the field. Although theorists and other writers use such knowledge in discussing occupational therapy concerns, it is not knowledge developed by the field. Related knowledge is not unique to occupational therapy. It is important that the field distinguish between the related knowledge it employs and its own unique knowledge.

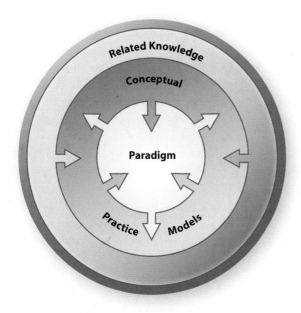

Figure 2-6. Dynamics of the knowledge base.

✿ Dynamics of Conceptual Foundations

The paradigm, conceptual practice models, and related knowledge together constitute the conceptual foundations of occupational therapy. The paradigm and the models of practice constitute the field's unique knowledge.

The relationship between the paradigm and the models is one of mutual influence (Fig. 2–6). The paradigm is a global vision, and the models are practical bodies of knowledge designed to implement that vision in practice. The core constructs, focal viewpoint, and integrating values of the paradigm are part of the perspective of those who develop and refine conceptual practice models. Additionally, as new models are developed and used, they may challenge and shape the paradigm. Experience in developing and using practice models may point to ways that the paradigm might be questioned, refined, and/or elaborated.

Although the paradigm is the most stable element of a discipline, its elements may change gradually over time as it is elaborated and modified. Occasionally, paradigm change involves a radical transformation, which Kuhn (1970) called revolution. This occurs when the core constructs, viewpoint, and values undergo a major redefinition. Such overall paradigm change means a transformation in the deep culture of the profession—that is, changes in the beliefs, perspectives, and values of members of the profession. In the following chapter, I will discuss how such radical transformation has been part of the history of occupational therapy.

On the other hand, conceptual models of practice constantly change. Application of the model in practice and research provide feedback that results in constant alteration of the model. Models need to change more rapidly than the paradigm in order to respond to changing client populations, changing health care delivery circumstances, research findings, and other practical demands emanating from therapeutic work.

The paradigm allows the field to maintain stability in the midst of this change. That is, the field can sustain its most important character while developing new concepts and extending its technology. New knowledge can develop, and ideas can change within the larger, more stable culture of the paradigm. In this way, the paradigm and models together moderate change in the discipline. The core culture of the field is relatively constant while its models are always changing.

✿ Conclusion

In this chapter, I argued that the field's conceptual foundations are reflected in three different types of knowledge relevant to occupational therapy, each used for a different purpose. The occupational therapy paradigm is the fundamental vision of the field. It constitutes a professional culture that is revealed in the assumptions, viewpoints, and values that members of the profession share. Conceptual practice models lay out theory and guide practice. The paradigm is a force for unity, whereas the various models, which address a range of phenomena, provide diversity. The paradigm and models influence each other. The paradigm provides stability and constancy; it changes much more slowly than the models, which are constantly revised as information from research and practice becomes available. Related knowledge supplements the field's unique paradigmatic and model-based knowledge.

In the next chapter, I will chronicle the history of the field's paradigm development, thereby telling the story of the profession from its beginnings. Chapter 4 looks at the field's contemporary paradigm. Subsequent chapters explain and critique several conceptual models of practice. The organization of knowledge described in this chapter will be used as a framework throughout these discussions.

References

Albrecht, GL, Seelman, KD & Bury, M. (eds.). (2001). Handbook of Disability Studies. Thousand Oaks, CA: Sage Publications.

Barnett, R. (1997). Higher Occupational Education: A Critical Business. The Society for Research into Higher Education. UK: Open University Press.

Christiansen, C. (1981). Toward resolution of crisis: Research requisites in occupational therapy. Occupational Therapy Journal of Research, 1, 115–124.

Clark, F. (1993). Occupation embedded in a real life: Interweaving occupational science and occupational therapy. American Journal of Occupational Therapy, 47(12), 1067–1078.

Clark, FA, Parham, D, Carlson, ME, et al. (1991). Occupational science: Academic innovation in the service of occupational therapy's future. American Journal of Occupational Therapy, 45(4), 300–310.

Dickoff, J, James, P & Wiedenbach, E. (1968). Theory in a practice discipline. Nursing Research, 17, 415–435.

Fleming, MN et al. (1987). Occupational Therapy: Directions for the Future. Rockville, MD: American Occupational Therapy Association.

Hammel, J, Finlayson, M, Kielhofner, G, et al. (2002). Educating scholars of practice: An approach to preparing tomorrow's researchers. Occupational Therapy in Health Care, 15(1/2), 157–176.

Higgs, J & Titchen, A. (eds.). (2001). Practice Knowledge and Expertise in the Health Professions. London: Butterworth Heinemann.

Kielhofner, G. (2002). Knowledge development in occupational therapy: Directions for the new millennium. Keynote address at the World Federation of Occupational Therapy Conference, Stockholm, Sweden.

Kielhofner, G & Gillette, N. (1979). The impact of specialization on the professionalization or the survival of occupational therapy. American Journal of Occupational Therapy, 33(1), 20–28.

Kuhn, T. (1970). The structure of scientific revolutions (2nd ed.). Chicago: University of Chicago Press.

Labovitz, DR & Miller, RJ. (1986). Commentary: Organization of knowledge in occupational therapy: A proposal and a survey of the literature. Occupational Therapy Journal of Research, 6, 85–92.

Leder, D. (1990). The Absent Body. Chicago: University of Chicago Press.

Longmore, PK. (1995). The second phase: From disability rights to disability culture. The Disability Rag and Resource, Sept/Oct, 4–11.

Macintyre, A. (1980). Epistemological crises, dramatic narrative, and the philosophy science. In Gutting, G. (ed.). Paradigms and revolutions; appraisals and applications of Thomas Kuhn's philosophy of science (pp 54–74). South Bend, IN: University of Notre Dame Press.

MacKinnon, C. (1991). From practice to theory, or what is a white woman anyway? Yale Journal of Law and Feminism, 4 (13), 13–22.

Mattingly, C & Fleming, MH. (1994). Clinical Reasoning: Forms of Inquiry in a Therapeutic Practice. Philadelphia: F.A. Davis.

Maxwell, N. (1992). What kind of inquiry can best help us create a good world? Science, Technology, and Human Values, 17, 205–227.

McColl, MA, Law, M & Stewart, D. (1993). Theoretical Basis of Occupational Therapy. Thorofare, NJ: Slack, Inc.

Mosey, AC. (1981). Occupational Therapy: Configuration of a Profession. New York: Raven Press.

Mosey, AC. (1985). A monistic or a pluralistic approach to professional identity. American Journal of Occupational Therapy, 39(8), 504–509.

Mosey, AC. (1992). Applied Scientific Inquiry in Health Professions. Rockville, MD: American Occupational Therapy Association.

Oliver, M. (1996). Understanding Disability: From Theory to Practice. London: St. Martin's Press.

Schon, DA. (1983). The Reflective Practitioner: How Professionals Think in Action. New York: Basic Books.

Scotch, R. (1988). Disability as a basis for a social movement: Advocacy and the politics of definition. Journal of Social Issues, 44(1), 159–172.

Shapiro, J. (1994) No Pity: People With Disabilities Forging a New Civil Rights Movement. New York: Times Books.

Toombs, SK (1993). The Meaning of Illness: A Phenomenological Account of the Different Perspectives of Physician and Patient. Boston: Kluwer Academic Publishers.

Tornebohm, H. (1985). Reflections on practice-oriented research. Goteborg, Sweden: University of Goteborg.

Tornebohm, H. (1986). Caring, Knowing and Paradigms. Goteborg, Sweden: University of Goteborg.

West, W. (1984). A reaffirmed philosophy and practice of occupational therapy for the 1980's. American Journal of Occupational Therapy, 38(1), 15–23.

Wiemer, R. (1979). Traditional and nontraditional practice arenas. In Occupational Therapy: 2001, pp. 42–53 [monograph]. Rockville, MD: American Occupational Therapy Association.

Zemke, P & Clark, F. (eds.). (1996). Occupational Science: The Evolving Discipline. Philadelphia: F.A. Davis.

Chapter 3

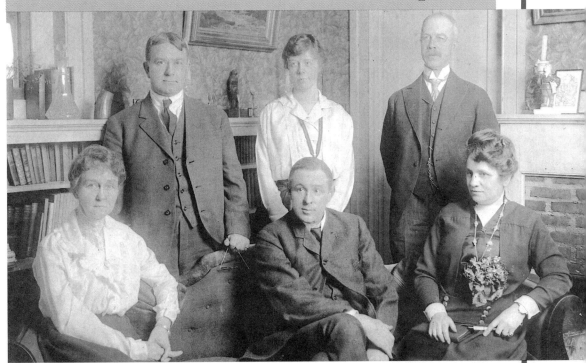

The Development of Occupational Therapy Knowledge

In 1917 a small group of individuals gathered to form the National Association for the Promotion of Occupational Therapy. This event is generally viewed as the formal beginning of occupational therapy in North America. In fact, this meeting was preceded by other significant accomplishments. Occupational therapy services were being offered in hospitals and other settings. Training of occupational therapists had already begun. Several books and numerous articles about occupational therapy had been written. It was this development of practice and the formal sharing of knowledge about practice that earmarked the emergence of the profession. A single unifying idea brought together people from diverse professional backgrounds who were the first occupational therapists. This idea was articulated in many ways in the field's early literature and expressed in its practice. A 1915 book titled *The Work of Our Hands* neatly set forth the early occupational therapy vision:

When [the client] gets down to honest work with her hands she makes discoveries. She finds her way along new pathways. She learns something of the dignity and satisfaction of work and gets an altogether simpler and more wholesome notion of living. This in itself is good, but better still, the open mind is apt to see new visions, new hope and faith. There is something about simple, effective work with the hands that makes [humans] . . . creators in a very real sense, makes them kin with the great creative forces of the world. From such a basis of dignity and simplicity anything is possible. Many a poor starved nature becomes rich and full. All this is aside from the actual physical gains that may come from new muscular activities. (Hall & Buck, 1915, pp. 57–58)

The occupational therapy vision and its realization in early practice gave an important

HERBERT JAMES HALL

Born in 1870 in New Hampshire, Herbert James Hall graduated from Harvard Medical School in 1895 as a general practitioner. He began a private general practice in Marblehead, Massachusetts, but soon developed an interest in the problems of persons with various forms of mental illness. In 1904 Hall and craftswoman Jessie Luther began a sanatorium called Handcraft Shops. In 1905 Hall obtained a grant from Harvard to study the therapeutic use of occupation (Peloquin, 1990; Presidents of the AOTA, 1967). This grant built on Hall's work with persons who had neurasthenia, which Hall believed resulted in part from improper or misguided habits related to the overstrain of modern life (Creighton, 1993; Hall, 1915; Quiroga, 1995). Through his research, Hall intended to demonstrate that physical, mental, and moral health could be restored and maintained through occupation (i.e., involvement in a healthy pattern of activity) (Quiroga, 1995).

In 1912, Hall moved his sanatorium to Devereux Mansion at Marblehead and continued to apply his principles developed from earlier research and collaboration with occupational therapists (Presidents of the AOTA, 1967; Quiroga, 1995). This sanatorium used arts and crafts as its primary therapeutic approach. Hall favored artistic crafts such as hand weaving, pottery making, and cement working for therapeutic use (Hall & Buck, 1915; Hall & Buck, 1916). Hall considered crafts to present the just-right level of physical and mental stimulation to engage patients, allowing them to avoid the idleness and isolation, while preventing discouragement (Quiroga, 1995).

Hall believed that neither rest nor strenuous work was effective in relieving the symptoms of mental illnesses such as neurasthenia. He used progressively demanding occupations to eventually achieve a routine of alternating periods of work, play, and rest (Creighton, 1993; Hall & Buck, 1916; Quiroga, 1995). He developed a classification system for the crafts, grading them based on the demands of the task. Patients were advanced as they demonstrated improvements in attention span, coordination, and mastery of the craft (Creighton, 1993). This use of progressive and graded manual occupation allowed Hall's patients to improve their mental conditions gradually without becoming frustrated or bored in the process. Hall also espoused the idea that occupation was a useful tool in diverting a patient's thoughts away from illness. He also proposed that patients experienced the success of creation through crafts that eventually replaced their sense of failure (Quiroga, 1995). These concepts of grading tasks, balancing routines, and diversion became central themes in early occupational therapy.

Hall published three occupational therapy books, two with coauthor and teacher-craftswoman Mertice M. C. Buck. He created the editorial department of occupational therapy and rehabilitation in the journal *Modern Hospital* as a vehicle for promoting the profession (Presidents of the AOTA, 1967). Hall organized the Boston School of Occupational Therapy in 1918 (Hall & Buck, 1915; Hall & Buck, 1916; Presidents of the AOTA, 1967; Quiroga, 1995).

In 1921 Hall was elected to serve as the president of the National Society for the Promotion of Occupational Therapy, which was renamed during his term as the American Occupational Therapy Association (AOTA). In 1923 Hall died of a long illness at the age of 53 (Quiroga, 1995).

In addition to his tireless advancement of occupational therapy as a scientific practice and as a profession, Hall contributed greatly to the knowledge base and theoretical ideas of the field's first paradigm of occupation. He helped to legitimize the field of occupational therapy in the 1920s, promoting its use outside of traditional mental hospitals.

identity to the fledgling profession. They reflected a new and unique way of viewing and dealing with the problems of persons whose capacities were impaired. Furthermore, they allowed the field to define itself as a useful service and thereby find a place in the health care system. What occupational therapy had achieved was the construction of its first paradigm.

This chapter explores the evolution of occupational therapy's paradigms. In so doing, it tells the story of the emergence and shifts of mainstream ideas of occupational therapy theory and practice. As we will see, this is a story of shifting identity.

Paradigm Development

The members of emerging fields do not set out to create paradigms. Rather, they seek to put into operation a fundamental idea, to explain the worth of what they are doing, to gain support, and to impart to others what they know how to do. Nonetheless, paradigm construction is what results when people accomplish the aforementioned tasks.

From his examination of physical science, Kuhn (1970) concluded that paradigms develop in identifiable stages (Fig. 3–1, see p. 30). During a preparadigm period, the initial ideas that instigate the formation of a field first emerge. The paradigm is later formed as members of a discipline articulate and subscribe to a common set of ideas.

Over time, paradigms may change. According to Kuhn (1970), the transition from one paradigm to another involves an intermediate state of crisis wherein discipline members reject the guiding principles of the old paradigm. Rejection of a paradigm can occur for such reasons as criticism by powerful outsiders or the inability of the paradigm to deal with new problems in the field. Because the paradigm is a field's basic culture and conceptual viewpoint, members find it unsettling to abandon the ways of thinking and doing that the paradigm provides. In everyday language, we might say that a paradigm shift represents a change of both mind and heart. This is why the transition is referred to as a crisis.

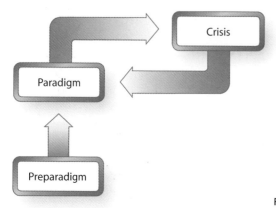

Figure 3-1. Stages of paradigm development.

Crisis terminates when a new paradigm is articulated and accepted. When the paradigm changes, the world that is out there to be acted on appears fundamentally different to practitioners. Importantly, paradigm shifts in a profession alter the sense of identity and the vision of practice that members share. Kuhn (1970) calls this conceptual shift "revolution," a term intended to convey the dramatic conceptual restructuring that takes place. As we will see, occupational therapy has had its own revolutions.

Kuhn's thesis concerning paradigm change challenges the idea that science or knowledge develops slowly and incrementally and new facts are added to the stockpile of already existing knowledge. Rather, a field can and does go through periods of radical change in its most fundamental views. When this happens, the field must reinterpret previous knowledge. This means that what members of a field thought was the correct and proper way to see and do things is recognized as somehow flawed. The change from an old to a new paradigm requires members of the field to make a leap of faith, undergoing, as it were, conversion to a new point of view. MacIntyre (1980) points out that this change from an old to a new viewpoint is narratively structured; that is, when members of a discipline abandon one fundamental way of seeing things for

another, it is because they understand how it was possible to have seen the world in the old way and, at the same time, see the new way as superior. Consequently, to understand the sequence of paradigms in a field, one must grasp the story of the profession's changing views of its nature, purpose, practical concerns, and values. Occupational therapy's history of changing paradigms is, then, the basic story of the profession. Within the story of its paradigm development, the identity of occupational therapy may be found. Hence, this history traces the essence of occupational therapy.

 The Moral Treatment Preparadigm

In the 18th and 19th centuries there arose, first in Europe and then in North America, an approach to the care of mentally ill persons referred to as moral treatment. This approach was inspired by the humanitarian philosophy of the Enlightenment (Magaro, Gripp, & McDowell, 1978). A central premise of moral treatment was that participation in the various tasks and events of everyday life could restore persons to more healthy and satisfying functioning. Occupational therapy's most important roots are found in moral treatment (Bing,

1981; Bockoven, 1972; Dunton, 1915; Licht, 1948). Early occupational therapists derived their fundamental concepts from the moral treatment writings, and the early practice of occupational therapy reflects its therapeutic concepts and practices. We can consider moral treatment the preparadigm of occupational therapy.

Proponents of moral treatment believed that people became mentally ill because they succumbed to external pressures by adopting faulty habits of living that disengaged them from the mainstream of life. Moreover, they believed society had an obligation to help those with mental illness return to a satisfying life pattern. The treatment approach was predicated on the assumptions that the mentally ill person retained a measure of self-command and that improvement depended largely on the person's own conduct. Thus, "employment in various occupations was expected as a way for the patient to maintain control over his or her disorder" (Bing, 1981, p. 504). Moral treatment was an environmental therapy. Physical, temporal, and social environments were engineered to correct the person's faulty habits of living, which were believed to be a central factor in mental illness. Participation in such occupations as education, daily living tasks, work, and play was used to restore persons to healthy habits of living (Bockoven, 1972).

In the mid-19th century converging forces led to the end of moral treatment in the United States. Rapid population growth abetted by large waves of immigration led to overcrowding in state hospitals. Social Darwinism and its "survival of the fittest" outlook, coupled with prejudice toward those in mental hospitals, eroded the social commitment to treat mentally ill persons. As state hospitals became congested and underfunded, moral treatment gave way to a custodial model in which people were primarily warehoused (Bockoven, 1972; Magaro, Gripp, & McDowell, 1978).

> A central premise of moral treatment was that participation in the various tasks and events of everyday life could restore persons to more healthy and satisfying functioning.

 The Paradigm of Occupation

At the beginning of the 20th century a diverse group of people (e.g., physicians, nurses, architects, craftspeople) began to reapply principles of moral treatment in several areas of caring for ill and disabled persons. They generated a new therapy that came to be known as occupational therapy. As these early leaders developed and described the principles of using occupation to influence recovery from illness and adjustment to disability, they generated the elements that made up the first paradigm.

Recall from the previous chapter that the paradigm consists of core constructs, a focal viewpoint, and integrating values. The core constructs reflect the basic themes of the field. The focal viewpoint is the way in which members of the field conceptualize the phenomena with which they are concerned. The integrating values specify what is important in practice. Together, these elements form the basic conceptual perspective and professional culture that give identity to the field and that bind members together into a shared vision of their work.

The first four decades of occupational therapy literature show a significant degree of consensus concerning the core constructs, focal viewpoint, and integrating values of the field. Writers articulated a paradigm of

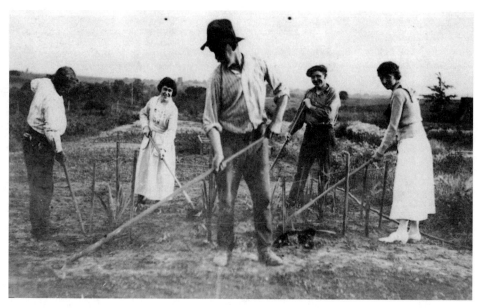

In early occupational therapy, clients in psychiatric hospitals engaged in productive outdoor occupations such as gardening and foresting.

occupation that guided practice and formed a divergent group of people into a new discipline.

Core Constructs

Writing in the inaugural issue of the field's formal journal, *Archives of Occupational Therapy*, Meyer (1922) articulated a core construct that concerned the role of occupation in human life:

Our conception of man is that of an organism that maintains and balances itself in the world of reality and actuality by being in active life and active use, i.e., using and living and acting its time in harmony with its own nature and the nature about it. It is the use that we make of ourselves that gives the ultimate stamp to our every organ. (p. 5)

This construct identified the need of humans to be occupied. Furthermore, it pointed out that participation in occupations shaped human minds and bodies.

Meyer and William Rush Dunton, Jr another physician and early leader of the profession, articulated a second construct that asserted that occupation consists of an alternation between modes of existing, thinking, and acting (Dunton, 1919; Meyer, 1922). Early leaders postulated that a balance between creativity, leisurely diversion, aesthetic interests, celebration, and serious work was central to health (Dunton, 1919; Kidner, 1930; Meyer, 1922). Consequently, healthy living was seen to depend on and to be reflected in the habits that organized the everyday use of time (Meyer, 1922). Habits controlled the basic rhythm and balance of life. These habits were, in turn, maintained through ongoing engagement in everyday occupations.

A third construct asserted that the mind and body were inextricably linked. The concept of mind-body unity was interwoven with the observation that occupation was a particularly powerful force in maintaining well-being; that is, while individuals employed their bodies in occupations, their

ADOLF MEYER

Adolf Meyer was a critical figure in the development of American psychiatry and occupational therapy. He received an M.D. in his native Switzerland, focusing in the area of neurology. After emigrating to Chicago in 1892, he began working as a pathologist for the Kankakee State Hospital in Illinois. Influenced by his mother's mental illness, Meyer developed a growing interest in psychiatric problems (Lidz, 1985). He went on to work in New England at such places as Cornell Medical College and Clark College in Massachusetts. At Johns Hopkins University he became director of its Henry Phipps Psychiatric Clinic and there collaborated with Eleanor Clarke Slagle to develop occupational therapy services.

Although he met Freud and Jung and generally supported psychoanalysis, Meyer was skeptical about some of its tenets (Quen & Carlson, 1978). Freud's emphasis on the unconscious conflicted with Meyer's concept of commonsense psychiatry. Meyer emphasized the connections of mind and body and of thinking to action. In contrast to Freud's emphasis on delving into clients' past, Meyer focused on clients' present state through interview and observation and on cultivating a healthy pattern of living (Lidz, 1985).

Meyer also challenged the view that mental disorders were due solely to brain abnormalities. He emphasized the role of the environment and stressed that a person's feelings could affect the body just as much as the body affected feelings. Meyer saw psychiatric disorders as patterns of behavior, action, and feeling that depended on a person's constitution and life experiences (Meyer, 1931). Rather than focusing on psychopathology, Meyer emphasized what could be changed in the client such as habit patterns, problem solving, and negative patterns of thinking (Lidz, 1985). Meyer also emphasized the importance of each client's unique life story and how it reflected personal attitudes, behavior, and life situation (Winters, 1951). He recommended depicting life stories as charts that summarized the life pattern over time (Meyer, 1931). Meyer argued that a large component of mental illness had to do with the development of faulty habits; he emphasized assisting clients by helping them recognize and change these habits (Kielhofner & Burke, 1977). He argued that an important part of the care of a person with mental illness was to "support development of a regime of work, rest, play, and socialization" (Meyer, 1931, p. 170). Meyer also emphasized that clients need to do work that is meaningful to them (Winters, 1952). Meyer's ideas significantly shaped early occupational therapy.

attention was also directed to the creative and practical dimensions of the task at hand. Thus, the body's capacities and mind's morale and will were maintained by engagement in occupations that provided a sense of interest, value, accomplishment, and challenge (Dunton, 1919; Meyer, 1922). Morale, a concept borrowed from the moral treatment era, referred to the ability to see the present and future with a sense of interest and commitment. Will referred to the ability to make decisions based on a clear sense of value and desire (Barton, 1919; Training of Teachers of Occupational Therapy, 1918). Occupation created a synergy of body and mind that maintained the integrity of each.

A fourth construct concerned what occurred when participation in occupation was interrupted. Because it is human nature to be engaged in occupation and because

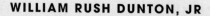

WILLIAM RUSH DUNTON, JR

William Rush Dunton, Jr, was born in 1868 in the Philadelphia area of Chestnut Hill. He was named after his uncle and came from a long line of early influential Americans (Licht, 1967). After earning a degree in medicine at the University of Pennsylvania, he began working in Maryland at Sheppard Asylum, a private hospital for the mentally ill (Bing, 1967). Dunton's extensive reading in psychiatry led him to the work of Tuke, the moral treatment writer and founder of the York Retreat in England, as well as to the writings of his ancestor Benjamin Rush, the father of American psychiatry and early proponent of moral treatment. Exposure to moral treatment principles provided Dunton a foundation for leading the development of early occupational therapy. In 1912 he was appointed the director of occupation at the Sheppard Asylum and thereafter devoted a major portion of his time and energy to understanding occupation as a therapeutic agent.

In 1915, Dunton published *Occupational Therapy: A Manual for Nurses* and in 1919 a second book, *Reconstruction Therapy*, which outlined basic principles of occupational therapy. Dunton was the first to conceive of and originally use the term "occupational therapy" (Bing, 1967). He became one of the original founders of the National Society for the Promotion of Occupational Therapy in 1917 and a year later was elected president (Licht, 1967).

Dunton later opened a small private hospital, Harlem Lodge, where he developed occupational therapy as a key element of treatment. In 1939 he left clinical work to concentrate more on editing *Occupational Therapy and Rehabilitation*, the profession's first journal. In 1950 he collaborated with Sidney Licht to publish *Occupational Therapy: Principles and Practice*, which reintroduced many moral treatment writings to the field (Dunton & Licht, 1950).

In sum, Dunton was an important influence in the early development of the field. He introduced moral treatment principles that served as an important basis for the emerging profession. He developed early principles and approaches to practice. He was a founder and leader of the national association. Finally, he contributed to the early literature of the field through his own writing and his editorial leadership of the field's first journal.

occupation maintains mind and body, "enforced idleness … [could] do damage to the mind and to the body of the ill person" (Slagle & Robeson, 1941, p. 18). Idleness (or lack of occupation) resulted in demoralization, breakdown of habits, and physical deterioration with the concomitant loss of ability to perform daily life occupations (Hass, 1944; Weiss, 1969). The following statement exemplifies this view:

In every functional disturbance, in addition to disorders of the central nervous system, there is a mental reaction. Pain, anemia, impairment of circulation, and sense impressions and emotions, such as anxiety and depression, are all communicated to the brain … In ennui the tonicity of the muscles is affected so that they actually contract less strongly and develop less force. In melancholia the general physique, and especially the heart, is acted on … Morbid introspection produces a particularly vicious cycle of thinking, since continued attention focused on any particular part of the

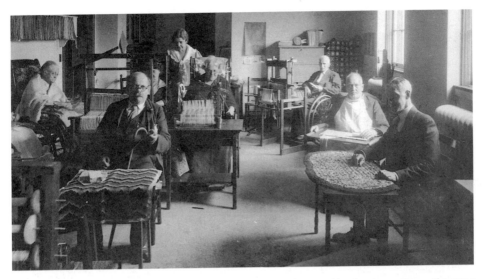

The therapeutic occupations of weaving and sewing were often used to develop a sense of competence and productivity.

body may actually increase its morbid condition. (Training of Teachers for Occupational Therapy, 1918, p. 35)

As the statement illustrates, the negative effects of idleness infiltrate both body and mind, with each magnifying the problem in the other.

A final construct asserted that, since occupation maintained the body and mind, it was particularly suited as a therapeutic tool for regenerating lost function. Occupation was recognized as a successful organizing force because it required an exercise of function in which mind and body were united (Dunton, 1919; Kidner, 1930; Training of Teachers for Occupational Therapy, 1918). Occupation was thought to provide a diversion from physical and psychic pain that encouraged the individual to use his or her mental and physical capacities. The following statement by Slagle and Robeson (1941) illustrates this view:

Let our minds be engaged with the spirit of fun and competitive play and leave our muscles, nerves and organs to carry

on their functions without conscious thought—then our physical exercise will be correspondingly more beneficial and we can readily picture the effect exerted on the mood of the sullen, morose patient by the genial glow which suffuses the body following active exercise. (p. 53)

Focal Viewpoint

The focal viewpoint of early occupational therapy centered on three phenomena and their interrelationships: mind, body, and environment. The mind was the pivotal area of concern. Motivating the person, influencing attitudes and morale, and eliciting physical activity through mental engagement were primary themes. In her discussion of how to motivate people, Tracy (1912) typifies discussions of the time:

It is easier to find something that he can do than to find something he will do. One needs to be resourceful, with a large variety of appeals, for it goes without saying that even in health what

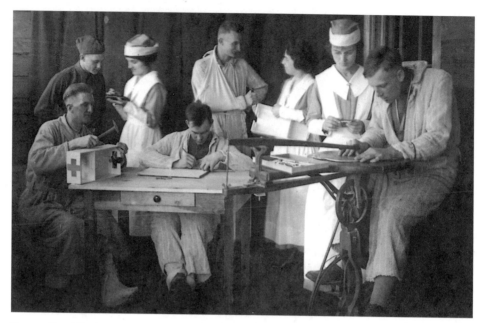

Occupational therapy was an important component of the rehabilitation of injured soldiers during World War I, supporting recovery from psychological and physical trauma.

ELEANOR CLARKE SLAGLE

Eleanor Clarke Slagle was born circa 1871 in New York. There she attended a private academy and high school, where she studied music. Her interest in disability-related services likely grew from her experiences as a family caregiver to her father who returned from the Civil War impaired from a gunshot wound, her brother who had tuberculosis and problems with substance abuse, and her nephew who contracted polio and later experienced emotional problems (Quiroga, 1995).

In 1911, Slagle enrolled at Hull House in the Chicago School of Civics and Philanthropy in a course of amusements and occupation. This course had been influenced by the work of Adolf Meyer, who had developed an occupational therapy program at the nearby Kankakee State Hospital. Slagle deplored the prevailing negative social attitudes toward those with disabilities and took an active interest in how state institutions treated persons with mental illness. After completing her Hull House training, Slagle began organizing similar training programs in Michigan and New York mental health facilities, later returning to Chicago's Hull House as a faculty member (Schultz & Hast, 2001).

Next, Slagle joined Adolf Meyer at Johns Hopkins Hospital in Baltimore, where she created and directed a department of occupational therapy. In 1915, she returned to Chicago and served as director of the Henry B. Favill School of Occupations at Hull House and as director of Occupational Therapy for Illinois state mental hospitals (Schultz & Hast, 2001).

Building on Meyer's idea that disorganized habits characterized mental illness, Slagle developed programs of habit and moral training. These programs, which were designed for patients with chronic and severe mental illness, included a 24-hour regimen of self-care, occupational classes, walks, meals in small groups, recreational activity, and physical exercise (Loomis, 1992). Slagle was later appointed by the governor of Illinois to be general superintendent of occupational therapy for the Illinois Department of Public Welfare. In this role, she supervised occupational therapy services throughout state institutions (Schultz & Hast, 2001). In 1922, Slagle became director of occupational therapy for the New York State Department of Mental Hygiene, where she continued promoting habit training in education. She held this position until her death in 1942.

At the outbreak of World War I, Slagle was asked by the Chicago Red Cross chapter to direct a 6-week training course for volunteers in occupational therapy (reconstruction aides) to meet the urgent demands of returning injured and battle-fatigued soldiers. Slagle, along with William Rush Dunton, approached the American Armed Services with their evidence on occupational therapy's positive effect on rehabilitation of soldiers. Eventually, the US Surgeon General appointed Slagle a consultant to the US Army for the training of reconstruction aides. In 6 months, Slagle toured up to 20 military hospitals and directed the training of 4,000 therapists (Schultz & Hast, 2001).

In 1917, Slagle joined other early leaders in Clifton Springs, New York, to form the National Society for the Promotion of Occupational Therapy. Slagle was elected the Society's first vice-president and served in this post in 1919. She became president in 1920 (Schultz & Hast, 2001). As Executive Secretary for the American Occupational Therapy Association (formerly the National Society for the Promotion of Occupational Therapy), Slagle was instrumental in forming the Association's theoretical underpinnings and designing standards for occupational therapy educational and treatment programs. In 1933, she published the *Syllabus for Training of Nurses in Occupational Therapy*, and in the mid-1930s she worked with the American Medical Association to develop guidelines for the accreditation of occupational therapy programs as well as a system for registering trained practitioners.

In sum, Slagle's influence on occupational therapy was at multiple levels. She helped shape the concepts of the first paradigm. She developed new approaches to practice, especially habit training. She tirelessly promoted occupational therapy in state institutions and the military. Finally, she was one of the most influential leaders in developing the professional association and mechanisms for ensuring quality education and credentialing of occupational therapists.

appeals to one person will not to another. The difference is even more marked among the insane. Appeals may be made through praise, competition, rewards; to the sense of the beautiful or to the useful; through affection for relatives, home needs, gifts to friends, or more diffuse altruism, as helping other patients, making preparations for special entertainments, such as Christmas gifts and decorations, or work for children .... (pp. 157–158)

To early occupational therapists, motivation was seen not only as a problem of how to engage the person in therapeutic occupations but also as a necessary component of recovery. For example, there was the caveat, "Remember that restoration of physical capacity without the will to do is a futile thing. Good medical practice demands healing of the mind as well as of body or organ..." (Slagle & Robeson, 1941, p. 29). Therefore, the aim of therapy was to

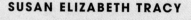

SUSAN ELIZABETH TRACY

Susan Elizabeth Tracy was born in 1878 in Massachusetts and died in 1928. She studied nursing at Massachusetts Homeopathic Hospital, graduating in 1898. There she observed that patients who engaged in activity during hospitalization fared better than those who were idle (Licht, 1967). Consequently, when Tracy went to work as a private nurse, she began using occupation in treatment (Parsons, 1917).

After studying hospital economics and manual arts in 1905, she became administrator of the training school for nurses at the Adams Nervine Asylum in Jamaica Plain, Massachusetts (Barrows, 1917; Licht, 1967).

Tracy originally held occupation classes for patients in her own home. After construction of a new facility with specialized occupational therapy space, she began including student nurses in the occupation classes. Soon the nursing course in occupation extended to be year-round (Barrows, 1917).

In 1912 Tracy decided to devote her life to occupational therapy (Cameron, 1917). She began her own Experiment Station for the Study of Invalid Occupations in Jamaica Plain. There she instructed patients and public health and graduate nurses (Quiroga, 1995). Tracy's courses are considered the first systematic instruction in occupational therapy.

Although invited, Tracy was unable to join the 1917 meeting in which founders gathered to sign the certificate of incorporation of the National Society for Promotion of Occupational Therapy. Nonetheless, Tracy was listed as an incorporator and elected as an officer to the Board of Management (Dunton, 1917).

Tracy's first book, *Studies in Invalid Occupation,* was published in 1910, becoming the first American book on occupational therapy (Licht, 1967; Tracy, 1912). It was used widely as a textbook in the field until around 1940 (Quiroga, 1995). Tracy emphasized the importance of engaging patients properly in occupations by correctly matching activities to interests and by grading occupations to the capacities. She emphasized that therapeutic occupation needed to "possess a certain dignity" (Tracy, 1912, p. 14) and hold meaning for the patient.

In sum, Tracy contributed to the founding of occupational therapy and development of the professional association. She developed some of the first education of practitioners. She contributed to the development of concepts and practice.

… create a wholesome interest in something outside the patient's morbid interest in himself and his symptoms … [and] to prepare his mental attitude so that he may adjust himself to normal demands and environment after the hospital discharge. (Training of Teachers for Occupational Therapy, 1918, p. 50)

The human body was viewed as a dynamic entity, integrated into the larger pattern of everyday occupation:

Our body is not merely so many pounds of flesh and bone figuring as a machine, with an abstract mind or soul added to it. It is throughout a live organism pulsating with its rhythm of rest and activity…. (Meyer, 1922, p. 10)

This focus meant that the therapist tried to

understand not only how the body was used in various tasks but also how it required regular rhythms of work, rest, recreation, and sleep. When the body was compromised through illness or injury, the immediate concern was to prevent further degeneration by engaging the body in occupations in whatever way possible.

Engaging a person who had impairments of capacity in occupations required creativity. Tasks had to be adapted so that the person could use remaining capacities to perform. Kidner (1930) outlined the principle that tasks had to be graded according to individuals' capacity throughout the course of therapy.

Like the proponents of moral treatment, early occupational therapists believed that the environment was an important element of the therapeutic process. They recognized that the environment included (1) social attitudes concerning involvement in occupations (e.g., the ideas of craftsmanship and sportsmanship; the value of work) and (2) occupations in which persons participated in ordinary life. Occupational therapy was viewed as a carefully structured environment in which people could explore potentials and learn about effective and satisfying ways to participate in everyday life. To this end, the social and task environments were carefully managed.

Therapists sought to provide a facilitating environment in the hospital. Natural rhythms of time use were seen as essential to the regeneration of habits in persons (Meyer, 1922; Slagle, 1922; Slagle & Robeson, 1941). Moreover, the occupational therapy environment, in order to be therapeutic, required the presence of creative and challenging opportunities and of persons (usually therapists) who demonstrated interest and a high level of competency in these occupations:

> Much importance was placed on the occupation room, wherein opportunity was provided for various forms of interesting and useful work. Weaving rugs and finer fabrics, basket work, book binding and clay modeling were employed at the start. Fortunately there

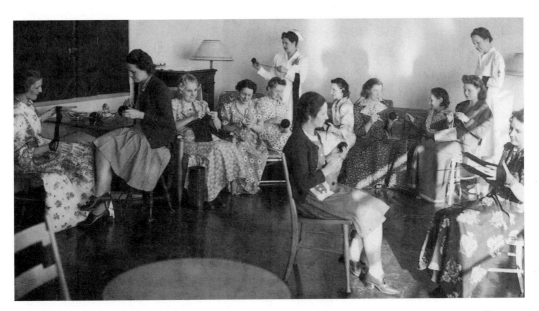

Occupational therapy groups provide an opportunity to socialize while engaging in creative occupations.

THOMAS B. KIDNER

Born in England in 1866, Thomas Bessell Kidner studied architecture and building construction at the Merchant Venturer's College in Bristol and London. He specialized in designing hospitals and other rehabilitation institutions. In 1900, he moved to Canada, going on to hold several positions; in 1915 he was appointed Vocational Secretary of the Canadian Military Hospitals Commission. Because of his experience in developing vocational rehabilitation for Canadian soldiers, in 1918 the Canadian government lent Kidner to the United States to become a special advisor to the Surgeon General of the Army on the vocational rehabilitation of disabled veterans (obituary, 1932, 321). In the following years, until his death in 1932, Kidner held various governmental and private positions in the United States as a consultant on planning, building, and organizing hospitals and other rehabilitation institutions for persons with tuberculosis and various other disabilities. He was on the staff of the Surgeon General, worked with the Public Health Service and the Veteran Bureau, and served from 1919 to 1926 as the Secretary of the National Tuberculosis Association. He played a major role in the early development of occupational therapy as a profession and a field of therapeutic practice.

Kidner's relationship with occupational therapy in the United States began in March 1917 when George E. Barton invited him to serve as one of the founders of the National Society for the Promotion of Occupational Therapy. At Consolation House he became one of the six incorporators of the association and was elected a member of the Association Board; he later served as President of the American Occupational Therapy Association (AOTA) from 1922 to 1928 (Licht, 1967, p. 272; Quiroga, 1995, p. 122). He remained on the AOTA Board of Management until his death in 1932 (obituary, 1932, 321).

During and after his terms as president of AOTA, Kidner sought to establish occupational therapy as a valuable and effective approach to rehabilitation (Kidner, 1925, p. 407). He promoted specialized education and development of a national registry for qualified occupational therapists (Kidner, 1924a).

In his 1930 book, Kidner outlined his vision for the scope and structure of occupational therapy in various in- and outpatient settings, including mental hospitals, general hospitals, orthopedic cases, pediatrics, long convalescence, and community based curative workshops. He wrote numerous publications that discussed the therapeutic nature of occupations and the structure and methods of occupational therapy in rehabilitation. In one he notes:

Occupational Therapy provides a means of conserving and bringing into play whatever remains to the sick and injured of capacity for healthy functioning. The patient is aided in mobilizing his physical, mental and spiritual resources for overcoming his disability. The tedium and consequent depression occasioned by the enforced idleness of illness are relieved, suffering is diminished, the care and management of the patient present fewer difficulties, convalescence is hastened, and the danger of relapses, invalidism and dependency is reduced. (Kidner, 1930, p. 40)

For this reason, he argued that engagement in occupations played a central role in rehabilitation (Kidner, 1922, p. 365).

Kidner proposed "surveying" patients to find out what they used to do before their illness or injury and what they hoped to do in the future so that the occupations used in their treatment would combine considerations of therapeutic value with the value of interest (Kidner, 1924b). He later elaborated that therapists should consider factors such as the patient's personality, attributes of tasks, and physical and environmental conditions of work settings when they determine individualized treatment plans (Kidner, 1924b, p. 178).

Kidner also discussed the methods for engaging patients in curative occupations and emphasized the overriding principle of gradualism (grading tasks in terms of the level of participation they require and their physical demands). Kidner suggested that occupational therapists begin with bedside habit training, progress patients to participation in simple occupations for diversion in the ward (e.g., reading or crafts), and then introduce them to the curative occupational therapy workshop (Kidner, 1930).

In sum, Kidner played a major role in defining the scope, organization, and characteristics of occupational therapy services in the profession's formative years. He sought to expand occupational therapy's areas of practice and define the specific and unique nature of its services. Finally, he contributed to developing an approach to occupational therapy in the rehabilitation of individuals requiring long convalescence from illness or injury.

was secured an excellent leader, trained in teaching, conversant with the work taken up and interested in it. The room was open at definite hours each day, but at other times those who wished could work without the presence of the teacher if their condition permitted... The atmosphere of interested activity

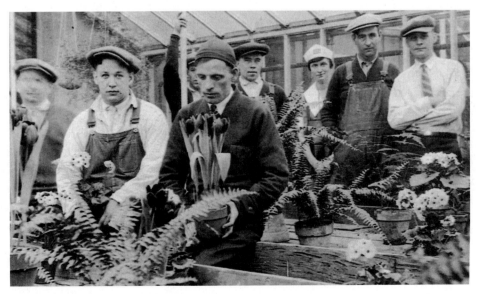

Occupational therapy clients developed a sense of responsibility and utility while working in a greenhouse, caring for plants.

prevailed. The work became the source of new purposes, of changed avenues of thought and of stimulated ambitions. (Fuller, 1912, p. 7)

In some cases the environment was highly regulated in an effort to imprint an orderly pattern of living on highly disorganized persons—that is, to develop healthy habits. Such habit-training programs for severely mentally ill persons employed highly organized schedules of everyday occupation.

The environment was also seen as a context for meeting a variety of needs. Simple games, music, and a colorful atmosphere were used to stimulate the senses of regressed individuals. As persons progressed, therapists directed them toward more demanding occupations that emphasized sportsmanship and craftsmanship (Dunton, 1922; Hass, 1944). Industrial therapy, the final phase of therapy, prepared people for the world of work (Bryan, 1936; Marsh, 1932). Individuals worked in various hospital industries (e.g.,

laundry, building and grounds maintenance, kitchen) engaging in real-life tasks under conditions that mirrored work outside the institution.

In sum, therapists saw the individual as a whole person (body and mind) in interaction with life tasks in the environment. Although the therapists realized that physical capacity was necessary to function, they put less emphasis on the detailed workings of the body than on environmental and mental matters. This is not to suggest that therapists did not consider how occupation could be used to achieve specific motor improvement. Rather, the therapists' fundamental vision was of occupation as the dynamic force that, by employing body and mind in interaction with the environment, maintained the ability to function. This focal viewpoint was both holistic and dynamic.

Values

Early occupational therapy inherited from moral treatment a belief in the essential worth

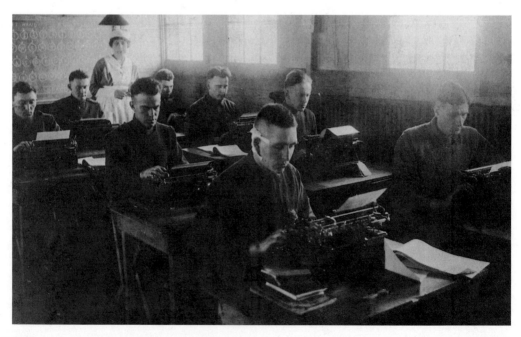

Soldiers injured in World War I learn new skills of shorthand and typing as part of a vocational rehabilitation program.

of individuals and in their right to humane care. Interwoven with this belief were the convictions that:

◆ The individual achieved dignity in the performance of everyday occupations.
◆ Meaning was realized in productive achievements and in creative and aesthetic pursuits.

Thus, occupation was valued for its role in human life. Early therapists saw the importance of culturally meaningful occupation as opposed to mere activity. Crafts, sports, recreation, and work were all valued because they embodied something important about the human spirit as reflected in the workmanship, sportsmanship, and craftsmanship. Because humans were by nature doers and creators, they were seen as having a right to engage in occupations. Finally, therapists valued holism, recognizing the connection between mind and body and seeing the person as connected to the environment through participation in occupations (Hall & Buck, 1915; Slagle & Robeson, 1941).

Summary

Occupational therapy's early paradigm focused on occupation, its role in human life and in health, and its potential as a therapeutic tool. The core constructs, focal viewpoint, and values of this paradigm (as shown in Table 3–1) shaped early occupational therapy practice. This practice approached people largely in terms of their motivation, emphasizing the importance of occupations as therapeutic media (e.g., crafts, dance, music, games, sports, and work activities). As a result of this early paradigm, occupational therapy identified itself as a field that appreciated the importance of occupation in human life, addressed problems of occupational disengagement, and used occupation as a therapeutic measure.

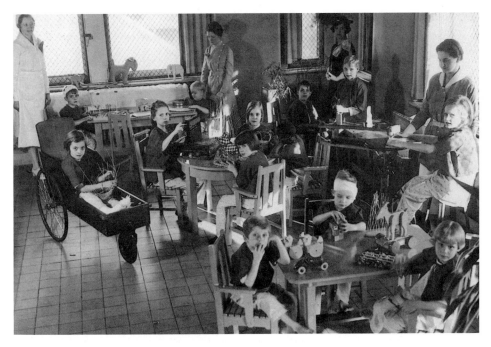

Play and crafts provide opportunities for children with physical impairments to develop a sense of enjoyment and mastery while developing their capacities.

TABLE 3-1. THE PARADIGM OF OCCUPATION	
Core Constructs	• Occupation plays an essential role in human life and influences each person's state of health.
	• Occupation consists of alternation between modes of existing, thinking, and acting and requires a balance of these in daily life.
	• Mind and body are inextricably linked.
	• Idleness (lack of occupation) can result in damage to body and mind.
	• Occupation can be used to regenerate lost function.
Focal Viewpoint	• Environment, mind, and body, with a focus on motivation and environmental factors in performance.
Integrated Values	• Human dignity as realized in performance.
	• Importance of occupation for health.
	• Holistic viewpoint.

Crisis in Occupational Therapy

In the late 1940s and the 1950s, occupational therapy came under pressure from medicine to establish a theoretical rationale and empirical evidence for practice. The following typifies the kind of criticism that physicians leveled at the field:

No one who has seen a good occupational therapy program in action can doubt that it seems to result in great help for some patients, and some help for many. There appears, however, to be no rigorous and comprehensive theory which will explain who is helped, how, by what, or why; and there is little objective evidence that occupational therapy is actually effective. (Meyerson, 1957, p. 131)

> **As a result of this early paradigm, occupational therapy identified itself as a field that appreciated the importance of occupation in human life, addressed problems of occupational disengagement, and used occupation as a therapeutic measure.**

Occupational therapists responded to medicine's criticisms by questioning their paradigm. Forging a closer alliance with medicine, the field began to explain its practice in terms of a biomedical perspective (Rerek, 1971). This move brought the occupational therapy's paradigm into a confrontation with reductionism.

Reductionism in Medicine

In the 20th century medicine increasingly embraced the highly successful reductionist scientific approach of the physical sciences (Riley, 1977). Reductionism assumes that the world is a vast mechanism in which laws of cause and effect govern the interrelationships of its parts (von Bertalanffy, 1968). Consequently, scientists seek explanation by reducing phenomena to measurable units whose relationship to other units can be specified (Weiss, 1969). Reductionism also assumes that any phenomenon can best be understood by dissecting and examining it in the same way that a machine can be understood through analysis of its parts and their cause-and-effect connections. Following this line of reasoning, scientists reduced living organisms to organs, organs to tissues, tissues to cells, and cells to the molecular structures of which they are composed.

Taken as a whole, reductionism in medicine sought to explain health and illness through careful identification and analysis of the building blocks of the human psyche and body. Medicine viewed health as analogous to a well-working machine and illness as the equivalent of damage to, or malalignment in, a machine's parts (von Bertalanffy, 1968; Buhler, 1962). Medical intervention in such a framework aimed at identifying and repairing broken or maladjusted parts through such means as surgery, chemotherapy, and psychotherapy.

When viewed from medicine's reductionistic perspective, occupational therapy's holistic view of body, mind, and environment and its focus on occupation as a means of therapy were misunderstood. For example, medicine focused on the medical practitioner as an external agent repairing the person. Hence, occupational therapy's viewpoint of self-repair through active agency of the person did not make sense.

As a consequence of the discrepancy between medicine's and occupational therapy's paradigms, the latter was dismissed as insufficiently grounded in theory and research. Many occupational therapists also came to see their paradigm as unsuitable to explain and justify the field's practice. Along with criticizing occupational therapy's knowledge base, physicians[1] and occupational therapy leaders recommended replacing it with

concepts derived from medicine. For example, it was proposed that psychodynamic concepts used by psychiatrists were more important to mental health practice than concepts of occupation:

> According to our point of view occupation is neither the aim nor the mechanism operating in this field that uses the media now in operation in an occupational therapy situation. Hence, occupational therapy taken as such is undefinable if the framework within which it seeks theoretical clarification is psychodynamics. (Azima & Azima, 1959, p. 216)

From the psychoanalytic perspective, the concept of occupation as an organizing force in therapy was too vague. Instead, it was proposed that the therapeutic impact of the client's engaging in occupation was that it served as a vehicle for expressing unconscious emotion. Similarly, critics writing from the physical disabilities perspective called for a refocusing to a neuromuscular perspective:

> A commonly accepted justification of the use of crafts and games as therapeutic media is the emotional value to the patient of an interesting and creative experience. The reasoning is accepted as a basic and important assumption empirically but not scientifically demonstrated. While the interest and pleasure of a creative activity are important, they do not provide the most fundamental and vital concept underlying occupational therapy of physical disabilities... Realization of the importance of neurophysiological mechanisms in the treatment of the motor system is increasing.

[1]To be fair, it must be recognized several of the early occupational therapy theorists were physicians (e.g., Adolf Meyer, William Rush Dunton, and Herbert Hall). These physicians clearly understood and helped articulate the first paradigm. It was the next generation of physicians who found fault with the field's paradigm. This may reflect the fact that medicine itself had undergone a profound change in its orientation; that is, it increasingly aligned itself with biochemistry and with laboratory research and the reductionist methods associated with them.

A study of them increases understanding of how the neuromuscular system operates in terms of purposeful function. (Ayres, 1958, p. 300)

Such criticisms of existing ideas and recommendations for rethinking what went on in practice fueled a crisis of confidence in the first paradigm.

In response, some leading occupational therapists called for a fundamental reorientation in the discipline's view of the therapeutic process. They proposed that occupational therapy needed to understand function and dysfunction in terms of underlying neurological, anatomical, and intrapsychic mechanisms. They also argued that the value of occupational therapy depended on its ability to influence these inner mechanisms.

Although the transition to a focus on inner mechanisms was gradual and subtle, by the end of the 1950s it had revolutionized occupational therapy. This revolution resulted in the emergence of a new paradigm, which in turn ushered in a new professional culture. One writer presaged the new paradigm in the following words:

As we talk of techniques let us think of underlying principles and build procedure on scientific fact. The clues lie in the basic concepts of psychology, physiology and anatomy. (McNary, 1958, p. 203)

 ## The Mechanistic Paradigm

The new paradigm promised to bring occupational therapy recognition as an efficacious medical service with an accepted rationale (Ayres, 1963; Fidler, 1958; Rood, 1958). In shifting to a new paradigm, the field sought to articulate discrete, tangible objectives for modifying dysfunctional parts of the client. Occupational therapy also

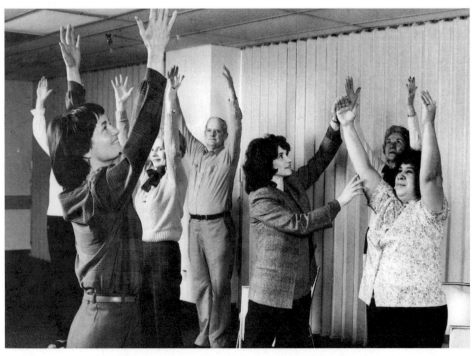

Clients engage in a range-of-motion dance exercise while the therapist helps them position their hands and arms properly to maximize the therapeutic value of the exercise.

aimed to gain a measure of scientific respectability in the medical community by adopting a perspective that paralleled that of biomedicine. In order to achieve these ends, occupational therapists reformulated their core constructs, focal viewpoint, and values.

Focal Viewpoint

The focal viewpoint of the new paradigm centered on the internal intrapsychic, neurological, and kinesiological mechanisms of which the client was composed. The new paradigm looked inward to these mechanisms and how they influenced function and dysfunction. The following quote by Ayres (1972) illustrates the new viewpoint:

Much of the time both the sensory and the psychotherapeutic situation are dealing with semi- or non-conscious experiences. The psychotherapist thinks in terms of subconscious psychological complexes and dynamics; the sensory integrative therapist includes many subcortical integrative mechanisms in his thinking and treatment planning. While one therapist is considering the Oedipus complex, the other is considering brain stem integrating processes. In both cases the underlying mechanisms are recognized, their effect on behavior analyzed, and methods of dealing with them contemplated. (p. 266)

Core Constructs

As the focal viewpoint refocused on inner mechanisms, the core constructs of the paradigm also shifted. The orientation provided

A. JEAN AYRES

A. Jean Ayres was born in 1920 and died in 1988 in California. She attended the University of Southern California, receiving bachelor and master's degrees in occupational therapy and a Ph.D. in educational psychology. She did postdoctoral training in child development and neuroscience.

As a therapist, Ayres worked with children. Her observations of learning-disabled children sparked an interest in exploring perceptual and motor contributions to learning. She devoted her career to developing a theory explaining relationships among neural functioning, sensorimotor behavior, and early academic learning. She identified specific subtypes or patterns of sensorimotor dysfunction and developed specific intervention strategies for them. She was the first to identify and describe sensory integration dysfunction, previously thought to be a broad spectrum of unrelated and unexplained cognitive and perceptual-motor problems. She developed standardized tests as nonstandardized observations to better understand children's problems. Ayres developed a rigorous research program to validate her tests and to test her theoretical arguments and clinical approaches.

In 1976, she founded the Ayres Clinic, which served as her private practice and as a training context for educating therapists in sensory integration principles and therapy. Her theory building and research always aimed to improve direct service. Ayres wrote numerous books and articles addressing her theory and techniques for clinical application. Her most definitive works on sensory integration theory include two books, titled *Sensory Integration and Learning Disorders* (1972) and *Sensory Integration and the Child* (1979).

In sum, Ayres devoted her career to the development of a specific applied theory. With her focus on the mechanisms underlying function and dysfunction, Ayres influenced development of the field's second paradigm. Her work exemplifies how knowledge should be generated for practice. She combined theory, research, and practice, developing tools to apply her theory in practice and conducting research to test the theory and its application. Her development of sensory integration was the first well-developed example of what is termed in this text a conceptual practice model.

by this new paradigm is characterized in the following constructs:

♦ All ability to perform is directly determined by the degree of integrity of the nervous, musculoskeletal, and intrapsychic systems.

♦ Dysfunction can be traced to damage or abnormal development in the nervous, musculoskeletal, or intrapsychic systems.

♦ Functional performance can be restored by using activity to improve the internal systems and/or by adapting equipment, tasks, or environments to compensate for permanent limitations in these systems.

The first construct directed attention to the neurological, musculoskeletal, and intrapsychic systems underlying function. For example, recognizing that function requires coordinated movement, the neurological and musculoskeletal principles underlying movement were applied to practice (Smith, 1978). The new paradigm, consequently, emphasized detailed analysis of the neuromuscular features of task performance. The following is an example of such analysis:

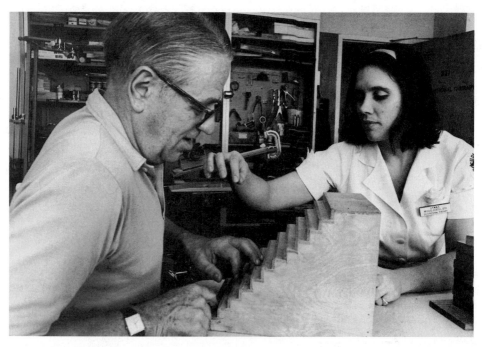

A client engages in a tabletop activity designed to provide appropriate exercise for his fingers.

Synergistic muscles may be used to prevent an unwanted movement, thus assisting in the performance of a task. Forcefully gripping a tool is used to illustrate this concept; the long finger flexors cross more than one joint and have the potential to act on each joint they cross. Forceful gripping of a tool would cause the wrist to flex if the wrist extensors did not contract synergistically to prevent this unwanted motion. (Smith, 1978, p. 86)

As the quote illustrates, occupational therapy focused on amassing information about what movement patterns were used in tasks.

The psychodynamic perspective stressed the relationship of unconscious processes to performance and the development of this relationship in the course of psychosexual maturation (Azima & Azima, 1959; Fidler & Fidler, 1958; Fidler & Fidler, 1963). From this perspective, therapists saw activities as opportunities for individuals to achieve emotional need satisfaction and as vehicles to express unconscious emotions.

Emphasis on understanding the underlying disordered mechanism led to increasing efforts to analyze and describe the disorder and its relationship to functional incapacitation. Precision in determining which neurological structures and processes were involved in a given problem was important so that the therapist could address the problem. Similarly, it was considered important to know how deficits in movement (e.g., limitations of range of motion, strength, and endurance) disallowed performance of daily activities. Therapists analyzed activities to

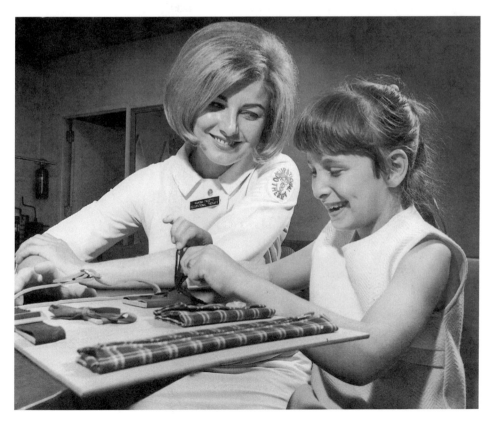

Practicing fine motor skills, a client manipulates zippers, buttons, and ties on a fastener board.

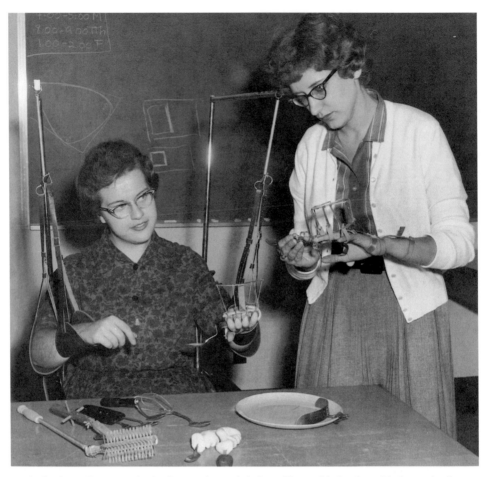

A client practices use of adaptive equipment designed to enable her to eat independently.

determine the particular movements they required so that they could identify and bridge any gaps between a person's capacity and those demands.

From the psychodynamic perspective, dysfunctional behavior was seen as a result of internal tension (i.e., anxiety) or of early blocked needs that prevented maturation of the ego (Azima & Azima, 1959; Fidler & Fidler, 1958; West, 1959). Therapists sought to determine the underlying conflicts or unfulfilled needs that interfered with functioning because these were the mechanisms to be altered in therapy. Often, the therapists used activities to diagnose the person's hidden feelings and unconscious motives by inter-

preting the unconscious meaning of colors, themes, and other characteristics of a person's creations (Llorens & Young, 1960; West, 1959).

The common focus in intervention was to identify the specific cause or problem underlying the inability to function and to change and/or compensate for it. In cases of neurological disorders, new treatment methods stressed identification of abnormal movement patterns and techniques to inhibit them and facilitate normal movement (Bobath & Bobath, 1964; Rood, 1958; Stockmeyer, 1972). Other approaches used activities and specialized equipment to stimulate the malfunctioning nervous system in order to elicit normal responses (Ayres, 1972, 1974). Therapists tried to provide a therapeutic rationale for every activity used in therapy, and the rationale had to be in terms of the impact on underlying mechanisms affecting movement. For example:

Sensory stimulus is developed through adapted cutaneous contact with tools, the beater of the loom, or the handle of a sander.... Gross motor reaching and throwing activities stimulate proprioception and kinesthetic awareness.... Use of a skateboard attached to the forearm for directed range of motion activities stimulates upper arm active movements. (Spencer, 1978, p. 355)

As illustrated in this quote, therapists sought, through understanding the nervous system and its various components, to influence the inner mechanisms that determined everyday functioning.

Under the new paradigm, therapists developed new treatment methods for musculoskeletal dysfunction, including splinting and positioning for optimal performance, passive and active range of motion, and exercises to develop muscle strength. Therapists analyzed activities to determine the movements needed in crafts and other activities. They made or prescribed adaptive devices to bridge the gap between persons' limited motion and the tasks they had to perform. Therapists also taught people compensatory techniques of self-care, dressing, and other functional performances.

Occupational therapy in psychiatry was predicated on the belief that if a person could learn to fulfill needs and could recapitulate

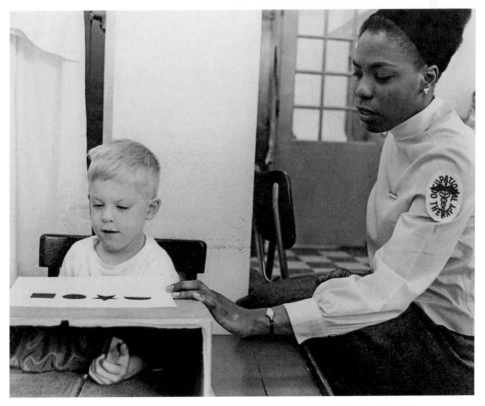

A client engages in an activity designed to develop perceptual motor skills

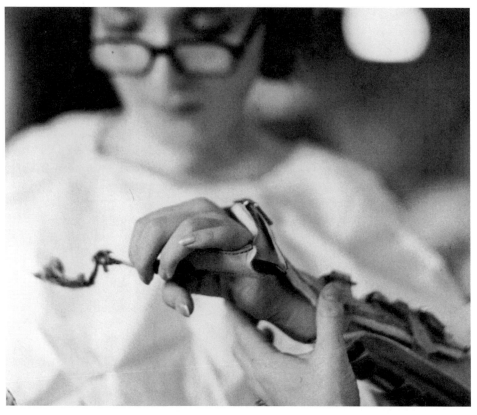

A client practices using an adaptive hand splint and an adapted utensil to eat independently.

and satisfy blocked childhood needs, the intrapsychic conflict could be removed, and the person would return to healthy functioning (Fidler, 1969; Llorens & Young, 1960; West, 1959). Another aim of psychiatric occupational therapy was to guide the person in regression to developmental stages that had not been completed. The following quote by Fidler (1958) exemplifies this approach:

> Occupational therapy can offer opportunities for the expression and satisfaction of unconscious oral and anal needs in an actual or symbolic way through activities which involve sucking, drinking, eating, chewing, blowing and those which use excretory substitutes such as smearing or building with clay, paints, or soil. (p. 10)

Overall, psychiatric occupational thera-

pists conceptualized treatment as a means to act out or sublimate feelings (Fidler & Fidler, 1963).

In a related approach, therapists used activities to establish a therapeutic relationship that would permit the person to develop healthy means of resolving intrapsychic conflict and fulfilling needs. As indicated in the following quote, activities themselves were less important than the therapist's therapeutic use of self:

> The effective therapeutic approach in occupational therapy today and in the future is one in which the therapist utilized the tools of his trade as an avenue of introduction. From then on his personality takes over. (Conte, 1960, p. 3)

Across the three mechanistic approaches

GAIL FIDLER

Born in 1916, Gail Fidler spent her early childhood in South Dakota. She later moved to Pennsylvania, where she attended Lebanon Valley College earning a bachelor's degree in education and psychology. Fidler worked briefly as a high school history teacher before securing a job as a hospital attendant at Wernersville State Hospital (Miller & Walker, 1993). There, Fidler encountered occupational therapy and was impressed with its impact on patients. She subsequently enrolled in the University of Pennsylvania and earned a certificate in occupational therapy. Later, Fidler once more returned to school, attending the William Alanson White Institute of Psychiatry and Psychology in New York. There, she studied and was influenced by interpersonal theory, particularly theories surrounding ego development, self-esteem, and competence (Miller & Walker, 1993).

In a career of more than 60 years, Fidler has served as an occupational therapy practitioner, administrator, educator, and theorist. She also served as associate executive director and briefly as Interim Executive Director of the American Occupational Therapy Association (Miller & Walker, 1993).

Although Fidler made important contributions throughout her career, her early work rooted in psychodynamic theory was the most influential on the field's paradigm development. Fidler's early writing envisioned the occupational therapist as an integral part of the psychodynamic process.

The 1963 text *Occupational Therapy: A Communication Process in Psychiatry*, coauthored with her psychiatrist husband Jay Fidler, discusses how activity can be used to express thoughts and feelings nonverbally (Fidler & Fidler, 1963). The Fidlers asserted that communication that emerges through activity is more likely to reveal unconscious emotions (Miller & Walker, 1993).

A consistent theme in Fidler's work is activity analysis. She proposes that, through the analysis of activity, the occupational therapist can glean information on the specific needs, interests, and abilities of the client and use this information to design action-oriented experiences to benefit the client. Fidler's early work on activity analysis focused on the psychodynamic elements of activities. Over the years she expanded this idea to include motor, sensory integrative, psychological, cognitive, sociocultural, and interpersonal skills (Miller & Walker, 1993). Fidler's view on the rehabilitative process includes the concept that activities should be used to explore and express unconscious emotions, to provide gratification of needs, to teach functional skills and adaptive ego defenses, to sustain intact functions, and to enhance works skills, habits, and independent functioning of activities of daily living.

In sum, Fidler's work for over 60 years as a clinician, educator, administrator, and advocate have made numerous contributions affecting mental health practice and the field as a whole. Her early theories based on the principles of psychodynamics contributed significantly to mental health practice and to the development of the field's second paradigm.

to treatment (intrapsychic, neurological, kinesiological), the common denominator was the attempt to isolate particular effects that the activity was meant to have on the neurological, musculoskeletal, or psychodynamic mechanisms. This aim for such approaches was to achieve more specificity in intended effects of therapy.

Values

The values of the new paradigm reflected its focus on scientific precision. Therapists came to emphasize the values of objectivity and exactness in problem identification and measurement. The value of scientific meticulousness was predicated on the belief that the therapist who specifically targeted the components of the disability was more effective. Consequently, therapists focused on how dysfunction of inner systems translated into limitations of capacity and how reduction of the dysfunction allowed persons to become more functional. Therapists also changed their value orientation toward therapeutic media. Therapists previously valued media's relationship to occupation in life and media's usefulness in motivating people to participate. Now, therapists began to appreciate the opportunities for muscle strengthening, expression of unconscious desires, and so on, that media could provide. Occupational therapy began to see the use of media as a therapeutic agent that targeted specific disordered mechanisms with precision.

Summary

By the 1960s occupational therapy's professional culture had changed in important ways. New patterns of thinking and practice constituted a new paradigm of inner

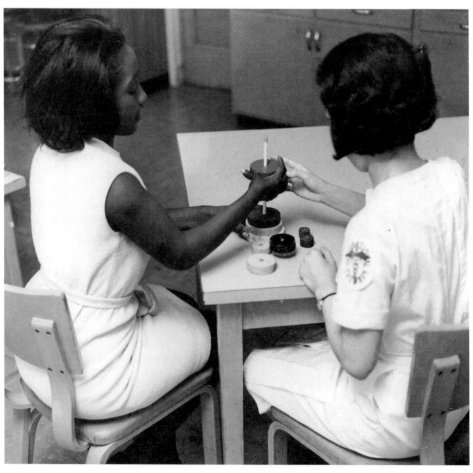

A client engages in grasp and release exercises after hand surgery.

TABLE 3-2. MECHANISTIC PARADIGM	
Core Constructs	• The ability to perform depends on the integrity of the nervous, musculoskeletal, and intrapsychic systems.
	• Damage or abnormal development in the inner systems can result in incapacity.
	• Functional performance can be restored by improving/compensating for limitations in inner systems.
Focal Viewpoint	• Internal mechanism, that is, internal intrapsychic, neurological, and kinesiological workings.
Integrated Values	• Precise knowledge and understanding of the inner workings.
	• Value of the inner workings to function.
	• Value of media as a means to reduce incapacity.

mechanisms, summarized in Table 3–2. This mechanistic paradigm resulted in some important advances in the field. Among the gains was a substantially increased technology for remediating specific problems. Occupational therapy's potential to modify persons' impairments was clarified. The paradigm also resulted in a deeper understanding of how bodily structures and processes facilitated or limited performance. The technology for adapting devices and environments to the needs of persons with motor impairment improved. The psychodynamic perspective increased understanding of how emotional problems might interfere with competent performance.

The changes in occupational therapy's professional culture transformed its practice. The transition from the paradigm of occupation to the mechanistic paradigm is manifest in important changes in thinking about and conducting occupational therapy practice. Such transformations of deep professional culture are never neat and precise. Rather, some ideas and practices from the first paradigm were still preserved in aspects of practice and occasionally expressed as part of the philosophy of the field. Nonetheless, a new culture of occupational therapy permeated the thoughts, attitudes, and practice of therapists.

🌿 The Second Crisis

Although the mechanistic paradigm achieved much of its promise, it also had some unforeseen and undesirable consequences for the field. Occupational therapy's fundamental perspective toward human beings had been altered radically. The early appreciation of the occupational nature of human beings, mind-body unity, self-maintenance through occupation, and the dynamic rhythm and balance of organized behavior were replaced with a new depth perspective.

Holistic thinking was replaced with a reductionist emphasis on the internal workings of the human psyche and body. In the same way, the therapeutic rationale changed drastically. The earlier rationale of therapy, which used such concepts as morale building, habit regeneration, and stimulation of interest, was replaced

> **Although the mechanistic paradigm achieved much of its promise, it also had some unforeseen and undesirable consequences for the field.**

with psychodynamic, neurophysiological, and kinesiological rationales that emphasized pathology reduction.

Practice also began to change. In some cases occupational therapists completely dropped participation in meaningful occupation from their therapeutic programs. This should not be surprising. As we saw earlier, the psychoanalytic approach included the argument that activity was merely a convenient method for therapeutic interaction. It was not difficult to conclude that activity is not really necessary at all, leading to occupational therapy approaches that resembled verbal psychotherapy. Similarly, in physical disabilities practice the primary focus of an activity was often to achieve greater strength. Consequently, therapists often abandoned activity altogether in favor of pure exercise.

In other cases the trappings of occupations were retained but without the underlying rationale provided by the first paradigm. Sometimes this change was taken to such an extreme that clients were placed in rather absurd circumstances. For example, some clinics maintained the use of such activities as sanding wood or working on a weaving loom, but these activities were disembodied. Clients sanded boards that were never used in woodworking projects (Spackman, 1968); they pushed the beaters of looms that were not strung for weaving. In parallel fashion, persons receiving therapy in mental health settings painted and did other creative activities, but their artwork was not recognized or appreciated as art. Rather, its value was as a medium for revealing unconscious feelings. In such cases the pale form of occupations was retained in practice, but they were only considered as mere vehicles for exercise or catharsis.

> **The mechanistic paradigm had diverted the field from its original mission and eclipsed the field's most seminal idea, the importance of occupation as a health-restoring measure.**

Therapists also came to have less appreciation of the person's experience of the process of engaging in occupations. As therapists focused on the impact of activity on underlying mechanisms, they tended to lose sight of the meaning of the activity to the person. The concept of purpose was substituted for the concept of meaning. Purpose referred to goal-directed activity, but it implied no obligation to consider either the personal or cultural relevance of the activity. The profession had strayed far from the original idea that meaning in occupations came from the fact that occupations were an essential part of the fabric of everyday life.

Therapists operating under the first paradigm considered the client's experience within the therapeutic occupation to be critical. Under the mechanistic paradigm, therapists lost concern for the client's experience.

As the field took on a new identity closely aligned with that of the medical model, there was an uncomfortable misfit between the activities used as therapy and the new concepts used to explain them. When the concern for occupations shrank to a more narrow concern for function, and when therapeutic occupations became media-directed toward reduction of pathological states, therapists were left with a shallow notion of their work and without a unique professional identity. The misuse of occupation (as illustrated above) and the growing embarrassment over the ordinariness of crafts, daily living tasks, and other therapeutic activities were symptomatic of the lack of a clear and compelling identity.

In addition to its own uneasiness with the new explanations for practice, occupational therapy was also influenced by new interdisciplinary thinking that challenged the reductionist view of the world. Biologists and behavioral scientists pointed out that reductionism was an inadequate scientific framework (von Bertalanffy, 1966). Many writers called for new, holistic scientific frameworks (Boulding, 1968; Koestler, 1969; Weiss, 1969). They criticized reductionism for creating a passive and mechanistic version of human behavior (von Bertalanffy, 1968). The call to move beyond reductionism created an intellectual climate in which occupational therapy's reductionistic paradigm of inner mechanisms was recognized as incomplete and as providing insufficient explanations for the effects of occupation on clients (Reilly, 1962, 1974).

The reductionist medical model especially failed to address the full range of problems of disabled persons. These problems extended beyond deficits of internal mechanisms and included the struggle to achieve meaningful lives and to thrive within society (Dubos, 1959; Safilios-Rothschild, 1970). In occupational therapy there was growing recognition of the limitations of practice based solely on mechanistic concepts (Reilly, 1962).

During the late 1960s and 1970s it became increasingly apparent that occupational therapy lacked a unifying identity (Gillette, 1967; Johnson, 1973; Mosey, 1971; West, 1968). Occupational therapy was becoming too diverse and fractionalized and lacked unity across specialty groups (Gillette & Kielhofner, 1979; King, 1978; Task Force on Target Populations, 1974). The alliance with medicine resulted in an orientation to specific disease categories without recognizing underlying occupational therapy principles (Mosey, 1971; Shannon, 1977). Moreover, the mechanistic paradigm had diverted the field from its original mission and eclipsed the field's most seminal idea, the importance of occupation as a health-restoring measure (Rerek, 1971; Shannon, 1977). Occupational therapy was jeopardizing its existence by abandoning the insights that engendered the profession (Shannon, 1977).

 # The Call for a New Paradigm

In the 1960s and 1970s Reilly and others developed a cluster of concepts aimed at recapturing elements of the field's first paradigm. This school of thought, called occupational behavior, embodied the following tenets:

♦ A return to the central focus on occupation (Michelman, 1971; Reilly, 1962; Robinson, 1977; Shannon, 1972; Task Force on Target Populations, 1974)
♦ Recognition of the human motivation for occupation (Burke, 1977; Florey, 1969)
♦ Study of the human sense of time, purpose, and personal responsibility for adaptation (Kielhofner, 1977; Watanabe, 1968; Woodside, 1976)
♦ Examination of the organizing influence of occupational roles on behavior (Heard, 1977; Matsutsuyu, 1971)
♦ The importance of the environment in supporting or impeding adaptation (Dunning, 1972; Gray, 1972; Reilly, 1966; Watanabe, 1968)
♦ The integration of interdisciplinary knowledge needed for this perspective under a holistic framework (Heard, 1977; Kielhofner, 1978; Matsutsuyu, 1971; Reilly, 1974; Robinson, 1977)

In time, the theme of resurrecting occupational therapy's original concepts and ideals began to be echoed by others (Task Force on Target Populations, 1974; West, 1984; Wiemer, 1979). By the beginning of the 21st century, occupational therapy had developed its third paradigm.

 # Conclusion

This chapter has described the genesis and transformation of occupational therapy's professional culture as represented in a series of paradigms (see Fig. 3–2). Occupational

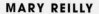

MARY REILLY

Born in Massachusetts, Mary Reilly graduated from the Boston School of Occupational Therapy. Early in her career she entered military service as Chief Therapist at the Lovell General and Convalescent Hospital at Fort Devens, Massachusetts. Her later work at Fourth Service Command included supervising occupational therapy programs in 11 general, 2 convalescent, and 6 regional and station hospitals. Reilly retired from the army in 1951 with the rank of captain. She earned a doctorate in education in 1959 and later became Chief of the Rehabilitation Department at the Neuropsychiatric Institute at UCLA. She served as a professor at the University of Southern California until retiring in 1977.

As early as 1958, Reilly began to advocate for a change in occupational therapy education and knowledge to incorporate a broader focus on the meaning of productivity and engagement in society and in individual lives. She argued that the human need for engagement in play and work was the foundation and *raison d'être* of the profession. In her 1962 Eleanor Clarke Slagle lecture, Reilly proclaimed occupational therapy to be "one of the greatest ideas of 20th century medicine." She stated that the field's bold hypothesis was that "man, through the use of hands as they are energized by mind and will, can influence the state of his own health" (Reilly, 1962, p. 2). In this paper, Reilly challenged the field to move beyond its mechanistic focus and recommit to the focus on occupation.

Although Reilly's writings are not extensive, her work was critical in shaping the movement from the paradigm of inner mechanisms to the contemporary paradigm. This was accomplished largely through her work in directing graduate students at the University of Southern California. She led them to develop a body of knowledge that she termed "occupational behavior" to emphasize that the field's knowledge should focus on occupation. She envisioned occupational behavior as the therapeutic framework for practice and education. Reilly contributed to this body of knowledge with her book *Play as Exploratory Learning* (Reilly, 1974). This text was the first serious treatment of the topic of play in the field.

In sum, Reilly was a pivotal figure in shaping the contemporary directions of the field. Her call for a refocus on the theme of occupation came at the time when the field was steeped in the mechanistic paradigm and went unheeded for a period of time. Through her own writings and those of her students, she was able to provide the field with a broad and scholarly understanding of the complex phenomena with which occupational therapists work. Her contribution in shaping the direction of the field places her as one of the most influential scholars in modern occupational therapy history.

therapy emerged at the beginning of the 20th century, drawing on principles and perspectives of 18th and 19th century moral treatment. The field originally embraced a paradigm of occupation, which incorporated a holistic outlook focused on mind-body and person-environment unity. This paradigm recognized that participation in everyday occupations influenced mental and physical well-being. It envisioned practice as participation in meaningful occupations that had broad therapeutic effects.

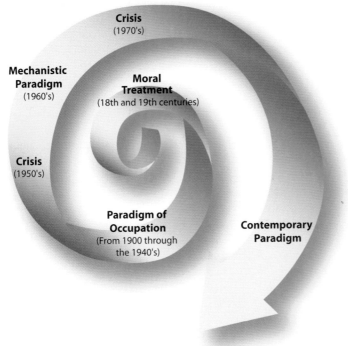

Figure 3-2. Paradigm changes in occupational therapy.

Beset by criticism from the medical profession, occupational therapy began to question its original orientation and identity. This crisis resulted in the field adopting the reductionist viewpoint of the medical model. The resulting paradigm stressed recognition of the inner mechanisms (musculoskeletal, neurological, and intrapsychic) underlying the capacity for performance. It envisioned practice as the application of activities to reduce pathological states in these inner mechanisms. Although this new professional vision resulted in advances in certain knowledge, it also created confusion about professional identity and a loss of respect for and confidence in the therapeutic impact of occupation.

Consequently, in constructing its third paradigm, occupational therapy has returned to a focus on occupation. This contemporary paradigm is the topic of the next chapter.

References

Ayres, AJ. (1958). Basic concepts of clinical practice in physical disabilities. American Journal of Occupational Therapy, 12, 300–302.

Ayres, AJ. (1963). The development of perceptual motor abilities: A theoretical basis for treatment of dysfunction. American Journal of Occupational Therapy, 17, 221.

Ayres, AJ. (1972). Sensory Integration and Learning Disorders. Los Angeles: Western Psychological Services.

Ayres, AJ. (1974). The Development of Sensory Integrative Theory and Practice. Dubuque, IA: Kendal & Hunt.

Ayres, AJ. (1979). Sensory Integration and the Child. Los Angeles: Western Psychological Services.

Azima, H & Azima, F. (1959). Outline of a dynamic theory of occupational therapy. American Journal of Occupational Therapy, 13, 215–221.

Barrows, M. (1917). Susan E. Tracy, R.N. Maryland Psychiatric Quarterly, 6, 53–62.

Barton, G. (1919). Teaching the Sick: A Manual of Occupational Therapy and Re-education. Philadelphia: WB Saunders.

von Bertalanffy, L. (1966). General systems theory and psychiatry. In Arieti, S. (ed.). American Handbook of Psychiatry, vol 3, pp 705–721. New York: Basic Books.

von Bertalanffy, L. (1968). General Systems Theory. New York: George Braziller.

Bing, R. (1981). Occupational therapy revisited: A paraphrastic journey. American Journal of Occupational Therapy, 35, 499–518.

Bing, RK. (1967). William Rush Dunton, Jr.: American psychiatrist and occupational therapist 1868–1966. American Journal of Occupational Therapy, 21, 172–175.

Bobath, K & Bobath, B. (1964). The facilitation of normal postural reactions and movements in the treatment of cerebral palsy. Physiotherapy, 50, 246–262.

Bockoven, JS. (1972). Moral Treatment in Community Mental Health. New York: Springer Publishing.

Boulding, K. (1968). General systems theory: The skeleton of science. In Buckeley, W. (ed.). Modem Systems Research for the Behavioral Scientist, pp 3–10. Chicago: Aldine.

Bryan, W. (1936). Administrative Psychiatry. New York: WW Norton.

Buhler, C. (1962). Values in Psychotherapy. New York: Free Press.

Burke, J. (1977). A clinical perspective on motivation: Pawn versus origin. American Journal of Occupational Therapy, 31, 254–258.

Cameron, RG. (1917). An interview with Miss Susan Tracy. Maryland Psychiatric Quarterly, 6, 65–66.

Conte, W. (1960). The occupational therapist as a therapist. American Journal of Occupational Therapy, 14, 1–3.

Creighton, C. (1993). Graded activity: Legacy of the sanatorium. American Journal of Occupational Therapy, 47, 745–748.

Dubos, R. (1959). Mirage of Health. New York: Harper & Row.

Dunning, H. (1972). Environmental occupational therapy. American Journal of Occupational Therapy, 26, 292–298.

Dunton, WR. (1915). Occupational Therapy: A Manual for Nurses. Philadelphia: WB Saunders.

Dunton, WR. (1919). Reconstruction Therapy. Philadelphia: WB Saunders.

Dunton, WR. (1922). The educational possibilities of occupational therapy in state hospitals. Archives of Occupational Therapy, 1, 403–409.

Dunton, WR & Licht, S. (eds.). (1950). Occupational Therapy; Principles and Practice. Springfield, IL: CC Thomas.

Fidler, G. (1958). Some unique contributions of occupational therapy in treatment of the schizophrenic. American Journal of Occupational Therapy, 12, 9–12.

Fidler, G. (1969). The task-oriented group as a context for treatment. American Journal of Occupational Therapy, 23, 43–48.

Fidler, G & Fidler, J. (1958). Introduction to Psychiatric Occupational Therapy. New York: Macmillan.

Fidler, G & Fidler, J. (1963). Occupational Therapy: A Communication Process in Psychiatry. New York: Macmillan.

Florey, L. (1969). Intrinsic motivation: The dynamics of occupational therapy theory. American Journal of Occupational Therapy, 23, 319–322.

Fuller, D. (1912). Introduction: The need of instruction for nurses in occupations for the sick. In Tracy, S. (ed.). Studies in Invalid Occupation. Boston: Whitcomb and Barrows.

Gilfoyle, EM. (1984). Transformation of a profession. American Journal of Occupational Therapy, 38, 575–584.

Gillette, N. (1967). Changing methods in the treatment of psychosocial dysfunction. American Journal of Occupational Therapy, 21, 230–233.

Gillette, N & Kielhofner, G. (1979). The impact of specialization on the professionalization and survival of occupational therapy. American Journal of Occupational Therapy, 33, 20–28.

Gray, M. (1972). Effects of hospitalization on work-play behavior. American Journal of Occupational Therapy, 26, 180–185.

Hall, HJ & Buck, MM. (1916). Handicrafts for the Handicapped. New York: Moffat, Yard & Company.

Hall, HJ & Buck, MMC. (1915). The work of our hands: A study of occupations for invalids. New York: Moffat, Yard & Company.

Hass, L. (1944). Practical Occupational Therapy. Milwaukee: Bruce Publishing.

Heard, C. (1977). Occupational role acquisition: A perspective on the chronically disabled. American Journal of Occupational Therapy, 31, 243–247.

Johnson, J. (1973). Occupational therapy: A model for the future. American Journal of Occupational Therapy, 27, 1–7.

Kidner, TB. (1922). Work for the tuberculous during and after the cure. Archives of Occupational Therapy, 1(5), 363–375.

Kidner, TB. (1924a). President's address. Archives of Occupational Therapy, 3(6), 423–431.

Kidner, TB. (1924b). Work for the tuberculous during and after the cure. Part II. Archives of Occupational Therapy, 3(3), 169–194.

Kidner, TB. (1925). Editorial. Archives of Occupational Therapy, 4(1), 73–75.

Kidner, TB. (1930). Occupational Therapy: The Science of Prescribed Work for Invalids. Stuttgart, Germany: W Kohlhammer.

Kielhofner, G. (1977). Temporal adaptation: A conceptual framework for occupational therapy. American Journal of Occupational Therapy, 31, 235–242.

Kielhofner, G. (1978). General systems theory: Implications for theory and action in occupational therapy. American Journal of Occupational Therapy, 32, 637–645.

Kielhofner, G. (1997). Conceptual Foundations of Occupational Therapy, 2nd ed. Philadelphia: FA Davis Company.

Kielhofner, G & Burke, JP. (1977). Occupational therapy after 60 years: An account of changing identity and knowledge. American Journal of Occupational Therapy, 31(10), 675–689.

King, LJ. (1978). Toward a science of adaptive responses. American Journal of Occupational Therapy, 32, 429–437.

Koestler, A. (1969). Beyond atomism and holism: The concept of the holon. In Koestler, A & Smythies, JR. (eds.). Beyond Reductionism, pp 192–232. Boston: Beacon Press.

Kuhn, T. (1970). The Structure of Scientific Revolutions, 2nd ed. Chicago: University of Chicago Press.

Licht, S. (1947). Modern trends in occupational therapy. Occupational Therapy and Rehabilitation, 26, 455–460.

Licht, S. (1948). Occupational Therapy Sourcebook. Baltimore: Williams & Wilkins.

Licht, D. (1967). The founding and founders of AOTA. American Journal of Occupational Therapy, 21(5), 269–277.

Lidz, T. (1985). Adolf Meyer and the development of American psychiatry. Occupational Therapy in Mental Health, 5(3), 33–53.

Llorens, LA & Young, GG. (1960). Fingerpainting for the hostile child. American Journal of Occupational Therapy, 14, 306–307.

Loomis, B. (1992). The Henry B. Favill School of Occupations and Eleanor Clarke Slagle. American Journal of Occupational Therapy, 46(1), 34–37.

Macintyre, A. (1980). Epistemological crises, dramatic narrative, and the philosophy of science. In Gutting, G. (ed.). Paradigms and Revolutions, pp 54–74. Notre Dame: University of Notre Dame Press.

Magaro, P, Gripp, R & McDowell, D. (1978). The Mental Health Industry: A Cultural Phenomenon. New York: John Wiley & Sons.

Marsh, C. (1932). Borzoi: Suggestions for a new rallying of occupational therapy. Archives of Occupational Therapy, 11, 169–183.

Matsutsuyu, J. (1971). Occupational behavior: A perspective on work and play. American Journal of Occupational Therapy, 25, 291–294.

McNary, H. (1958). A look at occupational therapy. American Journal of Occupational Therapy, 12, 203–204.

Meyer, A. (1922). The philosophy of occupational therapy. Archives of Occupational Therapy, 1, 1–10.

Meyer, A. (1931). Psychobiology: A Science of Man. Springfield, IL: Charles C Thomas.

Meyerson, L. (1957). Some observations on the psychological roles of the occupational therapist. American Journal of Occupational Therapy, 11, 131–134.

Michelman, S. (1971). The importance of creative play. American Journal of Occupational Therapy, 25, 285–290.

Miller, RJ & Walker, KF. (1993). Perspectives on Theory for the Practice of Occupational Therapy. Gaithersburg, MD: Aspen Publishers, Inc.

Mosey, A. (1971). Involvement in the rehabilitation movement: 1942–1960. American Journal of Occupational Therapy, 25, 234–236.

Obituary (1932). Occupational Therapy and Rehabilitation, 11(4), 321–323.

Parsons, SE. (1917). Miss Tracy's work in general hospitals. Maryland Psychiatric Quarterly, 6, 63–64.

Peloquin, SM. (1990). Occupational therapy service: Individual and collective understandings of the founders, Part 2. American Journal of Occupational Therapy, 45, 733–743.

Presidents of the American Occupational Therapy Association: 1917–1967. (1967). American Journal of Occupational Therapy, 21, 290–298.

Quen, JM & Carlson, ET. (1978). American psychoanalysis: Origins and development. New York: Brunner/Mazel Publishers.

Quiroga, VA. (1995). Occupational Therapy: The First 30 Years 1900–1930. Bethesda, MD: American Occupational Therapy Association.

Reilly, M. (1958). An occupational therapy curriculum for 1965. American Journal of Occupational Therapy, 12(6), 293–299.

Reilly, M. (1962). Occupational therapy can be one of the great ideas of 20th century medicine. American Journal of Occupational Therapy, 16, 1–9.

Reilly, M. (1966). A psychiatric occupational therapy program as a teaching model. American Journal of Occupational Therapy, 20, 61–67.

Reilly, M. (ed.). (1974). Play as Exploratory Learning. Beverly Hills: Sage.

Rerek, M. (1971). The depression years: 1929 to 1941. American Journal of Occupational Therapy, 25, 231–233.

Riley, JN. (1977). Western medicine's attempt to become more scientific: Examples from the United States and Thailand. Social Science and Medicine, 11, 549–560.

Robinson, A. (1977). Play: The arena for acquisition of rules for competent behavior. American Journal of Occupational Therapy, 31, 248–253.

Rood, M. (1958). Everyone counts. American Journal of Occupational Therapy, 12, 326–329.

Safilios-Rothschild, C. (1970). The Sociology and Social Psychology of Disability and Rehabilitation. New York: Random House.

Schultz, RL & Hast, A. (eds.). (2001). Women Building Chicago 1790–1990: A Biographical Dictionary. Bloomington, IN: Indiana University Press.

Shannon, P. (1972). Work-play theory and the occupational therapy process. American Journal of Occupational Therapy, 26, 169–172.

Shannon, P. (1977). The derailment of occupational therapy. American Journal of Occupational Therapy, 31, 229–234.

Slagle, EC. (1922). Training aides for mental patients. Archives of Occupational Therapy 1, 11–17.

Slagle, EC & Robeson, H. (1941). Syllabus for training of nurses in occupational therapy, 2nd ed. Utica, NY: State Hospitals Press.

Smith, HB. (1978). Scientific and medical bases. In Hopkins, HL. and Smith, ND. (eds.). Willard and Spackman's Occupational Therapy, 5th ed., pp. 82–99. Philadelphia: JB Lippincott.

Spackman, C. (1968). A history of the practice of occupational therapy for restoration of physical function: 1917–1967. American Journal of Occupational Therapy, 22, 67–71.

Spencer, EA. (1978). Functional restoration. In Hopkins, HL. and Smith, ND. (eds.). Willard and Spackman's Occupational Therapy, 5th ed. pp. 335–398. Philadelphia: JB Lippincott.

Stockmeyer, SA. (1972). A sensorimotor approach to treatment. In Pearson, P & Williams, C. (eds.). Physical Therapy Services in the Developmental Disabilities. Springfield, IL: Charles C Thomas.

Takata, N. (1969). The play history. American Journal of Occupational Therapy, 23, 314–318.

Task force on target populations. (1974). American Journal of Occupational Therapy, 28, pp. 158–163.

Tracy, S. (1912). Studies in invalid occupation. Boston: Whitcomb & Barrows.

Training of teachers for occupational therapy for the rehabilitation of disabled soldiers and sailors. (1918). Federal Board for Vocational Education, Washington, DC: Government Printing Office.

Watanabe, S. (1968). Four concepts basic to the occupational therapy process. American Journal of Occupational Therapy, 22, 439–450.

Weiss, P. (1969, November 29). Living nature and the knowledge gap. Saturday Review, 56, pp 19–22.

West, W. (ed). (1959). Psychiatric Occupational Therapy. New York: American Occupational Therapy Association.

West, W. (1968). Professional responsibility in times of change. American Journal of Occupational Therapy, 22, 9–15.

West, W. (1984). A reaffirmed philosophy and practice of occupational therapy. American Journal of Occupational Therapy, 38, 15–23.

Wiemer, R. (1979). Traditional and nontraditional practice arenas. In Occupational therapy: 2001, 42–53. [monograph]. Rockville, MD: American Occupational Therapy Association.

Winters, E. (ed.) (1952). The collected papers of Adolf Meyer: Volume IV: Mental hygiene. Baltimore: Johns Hopkins Press.

Winters, E. (ed.) (1951). The collected papers of Adolf Meyer: Volume II: Psychiatry. Baltimore: Johns Hopkins Press.

Woodside, H. (1976). Dimensions of the occupational behavior model. Canadian Journal of Occupational Therapy, 43, 11–14.

Chapter 4

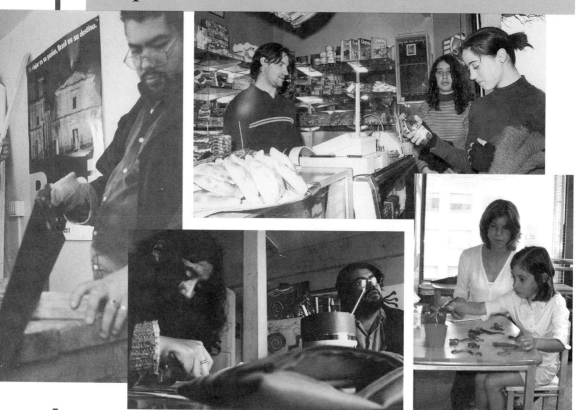

The Contemporary Paradigm: A Return to Occupation as the Professional Core

Contemporary occupational therapy has rediscovered the importance of engaging clients in everyday occupations. Whether it be learning to shop in a local store in order to be more independent, engaging in carpentry to develop work-related skills, exploring creative outlets for leisure, or engaging in play to develop perceptual motor abilities, contemporary practice is increasingly occupation-based. Such trends reflect the changing landscape of the field's paradigm in the last part of the 20th century.

By the late 1970s occupational therapy leaders began to call for a return to a focus on occupation. For instance, Wiemer (1979) argued:

> Ours is, and must be, the basic knowledge of occupation. It is that knowledge which permits the occupational therapist to look at an activity of daily living in a unique way, and so determine best how to facilitate the patient's or client's goal achievement. Our exclusive domain is occupation. We must refine, research, and systematize it so that it becomes evident, definable, defensible and salable. The "impact of occupation upon human beings" was spelled out as our sole claim to professionalism by our founders in 1917. It is our latent power if we will but keep it as our focus and direction. (p. 43)

Within two decades the field's paradigm had, once again, shifted so that occupational therapy became what Polatajko (1994) called "a discipline focused on occupation" (p. 591).

This contemporary paradigm was forged by integrating useful concepts gained through the mechanistic paradigm with the focus on occupation that characterized the field's original paradigm. Among other things, this synthesis has involved:

◆ Moving beyond the reductionist framework of the mechanistic paradigm toward more contemporary thinking.
◆ Incorporating what was learned about reducing impairments into a more holistic framework of enabling persons to adapt their occupational lives.
◆ Modernizing the understanding of occupation in light of contemporary knowledge from many disciplines.

This chapter examines these and other features of the contemporary paradigm.

Recall that a paradigm includes a focal viewpoint, core constructs, and values. The focal viewpoint provides a way of thinking about the phenomena addressed in theory and practice. The core constructs elucidate occupational therapy's view of humans, the problems that occupational therapists solve, and the global rationale underlying therapy. The values identify what is most important in practice. These three elements form the conceptual perspective and professional culture through which occupational therapists see their profession and its practice.

🌿 Focal Viewpoint

In the previous chapter, we saw that during the first occupational therapy paradigm, the focal viewpoint embraced a holistic picture of the interdependence of mind, body, and environment. We also saw how this focal viewpoint was replaced during the second paradigm with a reductionist focus on underlying mechanisms. Reductionism assumed that any phenomena could be explained by examining the components of which it was composed.

In occupational therapy practice, reductionism led to a focus on the underlying performance components, the kinds of problems that could occur in these components (e.g., impairments of motion, sensation, or cognition), and how therapy could remediate those specific problems. This mechanistic approach led to more precision and focus in therapy. However, it also failed to address the full range of problems of disabled persons and eroded appreciation of occupation as a therapeutic agent.

While occupational therapists were recognizing the limitations of reductionism in practice, interdisciplinary scholars were calling for a move beyond reductionism to a more holistic outlook provided by systems theory. Over the past two decades systems theory has been incorporated into occupational therapy in a variety of ways. Systems concepts have resulted in a shift in how occupational therapy thinks about the phenomena it addresses.

The Systems Approach to Understanding Occupation

A key theme in systems theory is that no system (e.g., cell, person, or organization) can be fully explained by examining the component parts of which it is made. Rather, there is an order in the whole that transcends the parts of which the system is composed. Whereas reductionism led to a focus on the musculoskeletal, neurological, and psychological systems underlying occupation, systems theory portrays the human being as an integrated, self-organizing system (Kelso, 1995; Vallacher & Nowak, 1994). This means that all behavior emerges out of the total dynamics created when the person's musculoskeletal, neurological, and psychological components are coupled with conditions in the environment, including the nature of the occupation the person is doing (Kelso, 1995; Thelen & Ulrich, 1991). Although these underlying musculoskeletal, neuromuscular, and psychological components are necessary to performance they are not sufficient for performance. What completes the picture is the context of the occupation that the person is doing and the features of the environment in which it is done (Law et al, 1996).

This way of thinking also reframes what happens in occupational therapy. The mechanistic paradigm envisioned therapy as achieving changes in underlying performance components (e.g., strengthening muscles or increasing confidence). The contemporary view is that occupational therapy provides individuals with opportunities to reshape their performance and their lives into new patterns that meet personal needs and desires. Therapy provides opportunities and environmental resources that support the emergence of new patterns of performance and participation in everyday life. Consequently, therapeutic change involves complex reorganization that includes the person's relationship to life occupations and to the environment. Performance components, the occupations being performed, and environmental conditions (Law, 1991) are parts of the multiple factors that become coordinated into a new order. This vision of therapy returns the field to a more holistic viewpoint in which the person, environment, and the occupations that make up that person's life are considered together.

> **Therapy provides opportunities and environmental resources that support the emergence of new patterns of performance and participation in everyday life.**

 ## Core Constructs

As noted earlier, the contemporary paradigm has returned to a focus on occupation. The core constructs include three broad themes that reflect this focus:

- Occupational nature of humans
- Occupational problems/challenges
- Occupation-based practice

The following sections discuss these themes.

The Occupational Nature of Humans

There has been a growing recognition that occupation represents an important part of what it means to be human. Humans' occupational nature is reflected in the fact that:

- All people have a basic motive or need for occupation.
- Occupation constitutes a specific domain of human behavior.
- Occupation is the primary source of meaning in life.

The need for occupation is reflected in the fact that humans have a strong drive to do things and flourish by engaging in practical, productive, and playful pursuits (Clark et al., 1991; Wilcock, 1993). The motive for occupation derives from the urges to do things, to discover, to exercise capacity, and to experience oneself as competent. This motive is the product of an evolutionary process in which the complex nervous system of humans gives them a pervasive need to act (Kielhofner, 2002; Wilcock, 1993).

The need for occupation leads people to a wide range of behaviors. Occupation, nevertheless, constitutes a coherent domain of behavior comprising play/leisure, activities of daily living, and work. Play refers to activities undertaken for their own sake; exploring, pretending, celebrating, engaging in games or sports, and pursuing hobbies (DiBona, 2000; Lobo, 1999; Parham & Fazio, 1997; Passmore, 1998). Activities of daily living are tasks that maintain one's self and lifestyle. They compose much of the routine of everyday life and include self-care, ordering one's life space (e.g., cleaning and paying bills), and getting to resources (e.g., travel and shopping) (Christiansen, 1994). Work includes productive activity (both paid and unpaid) that contributes some service or commodity to others as well as participating in education or training that improve one's abilities to be productive (Kielhofner, 2002).

Play, activities of daily living, and work interrelate in everyday life and across the life span. For example, play provides learning opportunities that are necessary for competence in adult work. Play in adult life renews the individual for work. Activities of daily living are necessary to prepare oneself (e.g., grooming and dressing) for work. Taken together, these occupations are the means by which individuals fill their time, create the circumstances of their everyday existence, and make their place in the world (Christiansen, 1996; Wood, 1995).

Participating in occupation creates and affirms meaning in life (Christiansen, 1999; Hasselkus, 2002). The meaning experienced in occupations emanates from a variety of sources, including the actual experience of performing the occupation, sociocultural norms and values, and the performer's personal history. The meaning persons take from their occupations depends on narratives that employ or impart a framework for making sense of and understanding life events (Clark, 1993; Hasselkus, 2002; Helfrich, Kielhofner, & Mattingly, 1994; Johnsson, Borell, & Kielhofner, 1997; Mallinson, Kielhofner, & Mattingly,1996; Mattingly, 1991). These occupational narratives link together past, present, and future, allowing individuals to experience the events and actions of occupational life as a meaningful whole (Jonsson, Josephsson, & Kielhofner, 2000; Jonsson, Josephsson, & Kielhofner, 2001). People engage in their occupations so as to locate themselves in an unfolding narrative and to achieve a particular direction or outcome in that story (Kielhofner et al., 2002).

Although only briefly characterized here, the ideas that humans have a basic need for and achieve meaning in their occupations and that occupation constitutes a coherent domain of human life are growing themes in the field. They have supported the field's appreciation of the centrality and importance of occupation to human life. Linked with this appreciation of humans' occupational nature is the recognition that occupational therapy addresses this aspect of human nature and, in particular, addresses problems in the domain of occupation.

Occupational Problems/ Challenges

The contemporary paradigm recognizes problems of participating in occupations as the focus for service (Rogers, 1982). Since occupation is a basic human need, persons who are denied access to or have restrictions in their occupations may suffer and experience a reduction in quality of life (Christiansen, 1994). A lack or disruption of participation in occupation may also restrict development, resulting in reductions of capacity and lead to maladaptive reactions. Because of the potential negative consequences of such occupational disruption or deprivation, it is the central problem to which the field addresses its efforts.

This focus on occupational problems has led the field to look beyond impairment to consider their impact on the person's occupational life. It has also led to the recognition that limitations of capacity alone are not sufficient to understand the nature of occupational problems. Rather, how impairments interact with conditions in the environment and with the life of the person who experiences those impairments must be considered (Trombly, 1993). In sum, there has been a broadening of perspective beyond the concerns for reduction of impairment to considerations of how occupational restrictions and barriers can be removed to allow persons to more fully participate in necessary and desired occupations.

Occupation and the Dynamics of Therapy

The third thematic area of the core constructs addresses the means and the goals of therapy. The field has returned to a recognition that engagement in occupation is the basic dynamic and core of therapy.

The mechanistic paradigm focused occupational therapy's attention downward to the underlying occupational performance components. It assumed that improvement in these components would yield corresponding improvement in occupational performance. The new view recognizes two important flaws in this approach (Trombly, 1993; Wood, 1995). First, when underlying performance components cannot be fully restored, the adaptation to permanent disability requires something different: a reorganization of the whole. As discussed earlier, this reorganization can be attended to only at the level of the occupations that make up the parts of the person's everyday life and the level of the whole occupational life and its meanings for the persons. Second, as noted earlier, the order we find in behavior depends not only on the status of performance components but also the task and environmental context (Kielhofner, 2002; Trombly, 1995).

Performance abilities in real-life occupations cannot be explained by the status of performance components (Trombly, 1993; Wood, 1995). Rather, performance reflects the alignment of these components within the occupational context. Consequently, occupations that are employed in therapy may be carefully selected to invite and direct the organization of performance.

In the contemporary perspective, the use of occupation to improve health status is once again recognized as the core of occupational therapy (Fisher, 1998; Reilly, 1962; Wood, 1998). As shown in Figure 4–1, therapists employ the therapeutic agency of occupation through four primary pathways:

◆ Providing opportunities for clients to engage directly in occupations.
◆ Enabling clients to engage in occupations by modifying the task or the environment in which the person performs, including removing architectural and social barriers (e.g., attitudes, discrimination, unfair policies) (Dunn, Brown, & McGuigan, 1994; Kielhofner, 2002).
◆ Providing training of clients in the use of various technical devices that extend limited capacity or compensate for lost capacity (Hammel, 1996).
◆ Providing counseling and problem-solving to facilitate the client's participation in occupation outside of therapy.

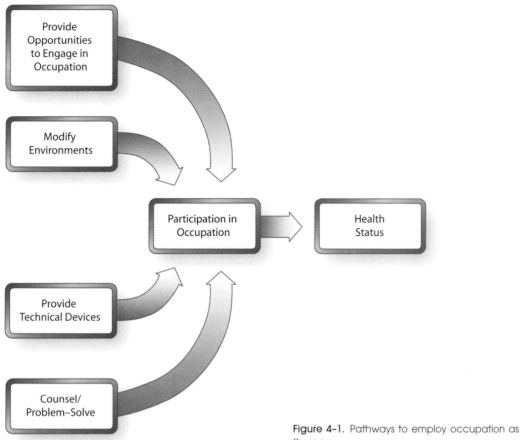

Figure 4-1. Pathways to employ occupation as therapy.

Underlying these efforts is the recognition that clients' engagement in occupations is the core of therapy that either achieves a needed change or maintains a desired situation.

Engagement in occupation involves not only what individuals do but also their subjective experience (Hasselkus, 2002; Yerxa, 1980). Therefore, the client must find meaning in the actions that constitute the therapy. This meaning ordinarily derives from the client's experiential background, the current impact of any impairments on the client's experience, and the significance of the therapeutic activity negotiated between the therapist and the client.

In the end, the meaning that is experienced in the therapeutic process determines the impact of the activity on the individual. Therapy is an event that enters into and becomes part of the occupational narrative of the client (Helfrich, Kielhofner, & Mattingly, 1994). The meaning that therapy has for the client is in relation to its relevance and impact upon this narrative. Moreover, in therapy the therapist helps clients to continue or reinvent their occupational narratives (Clark, 1993). Hence,

> **In the end, the meaning that is experienced in the therapeutic process determines the impact of the activity on the individual.**

new life meaning can be discovered and enacted in the course of therapy.

Values

By specifying what occupational therapy should be, the values of the paradigm shape the vision and decisionmaking of occupational therapists. Occupational therapy is guided by many values that are also shared with other professions. Two values that currently shape occupational therapy's unique orientation are respect for the value of occupation in human life and the concomitant importance of active engagement and empowerment of clients.

With the reorientation of the current paradigm, the centrality of occupation to well-being and quality of life has become a resonant theme in the field (American Occupational Therapy Association, 1993; Fondiller, Rosage, & Neuhas, 1990; Hasselkus, 2002). Related to this, it is recognized that the vision and mission of the field is to promote occupational well-being. Consequently, a core value defining the worth of occupational therapy is that it supports clients' desires to integrate themselves into the mainstream of life through participation in meaningful life occupations (Johnson, 1981; Yerxa, 1983).

It is also recognized that occupational therapy should always consist of the active and meaning-driven participation of the client, whose actions and investment determine effectiveness of the therapy (Wood, 1995). This value requires client-centered practice guided by a profound respect for and understanding of client's perspectives, desires, and needs as well as the client's right to make choices and exercise decision about the therapeutic process (Taylor, 2003; Townsend, 1993)

Conclusion

For a profession to be coherent, members must share a common culture and a vision of their work embodied in the field's paradigm.

This chapter aimed to provide an overview of the contemporary paradigm of occupational therapy. As with any shared perspective, this paradigm is a dynamic process in which members of the profession are constantly adding new depth and content. Any characterization of the paradigm can give only a broad-stroke interpretation of the ongoing discourse in the field, which shapes and reshapes its shared vision and culture. The true repository of the paradigm is, as noted earlier, in the ongoing dialogue of the field in its literature, practice, and shared oral traditions.

References

American Occupational Therapy Association (1993). Core values and attitudes of occupational therapy practice. American Journal of Occupational Therapy, 47, 1085–1086.

Christiansen, C. (1994). Ways of Living: Self Care Strategies for Special Needs. Rockville, MD: American Occupational Therapy Association.

Christiansen, C. (1996). Three perspectives on balance in occupation. In Clark, F & Zemke, R (eds.). Occupation Science, pp 431–451. Philadelphia: FA Davis.

Christiansen, C. (1999). Defining lives: Occupation as identity: An essay on competence, coherence, and the creation of meaning. American Journal of Occupational Therapy, 53, 547–558.

Clark, FA. (1993). Occupation embedded in a real life: Interweaving occupation science and occupational therapy. American Journal of Occupational Therapy, 47, 1067–1077.

Clark, FA, Parham, D, Carlson, ME, et al. (1991). Occupation science: Academic innovation in the service of occupational therapy's future. American Journal of Occupational Therapy, 45, 300–310.

DiBona, L. (2000). What are the benefits of leisure? An exploration using the leisure satisfaction scale. British Journal of Occupational Therapy, 63(2), 50–58.

Dunn, W, Brown, C & McGuigan, A. (1994). The ecology of human performance: A framework for considering the effect of context. American Journal of Occupational Therapy, 48, 595–607.

Fisher, AG. (1998). Uniting practice and theory in an occupational framework. American Journal of Occupational Therapy, 54(7), 509–521.

Fondiller, ED, Rosage, L & Neuhas, B. (1990). Values influencing clinical reasoning in occupational therapy: An exploratory study. Occupational Therapy Journal of Research, 10, 41–55.

Hammel, J. (ed.) (1996). Assistive Technology and Occupational Therapy: A Link to Function (Section 1). Bethesda, MD: American Occupational Therapy Association.

Hasselkus, BR. (2002). The Meaning of Everyday Occupation. Thorofare, NJ: Slack, Inc.

Helfrich, C, Kielhofner, G & Mattingly, C. (1994). Volition as narrative: Understanding motivation in chronic illness. American Journal of Occupational Therapy, 48, 311–317.

Johnson, J. (1981). Old value, new directions: Competence, adaptation, integration. American Journal of Occupational Therapy, 35, 589–598.

Johnsson, H, Borell, L & Kielhofner, G. (1997). Anticipating retirement: The formation of attitudes and expectations concerning an occupational transition. American Journal of Occupational Therapy, 51, 49–56.

Jonsson, H, Josephsson, S & Kielhofner, G. (2000). Evolving narratives in the course of retirement: A longitudinal study. American Journal of Occupational Therapy, 54, 463–470.

Jonsson, H., Josephsson, S & Kielhofner, G. (2001). Narratives and experience in an occupational transition: A longitudinal study of the retirement process. American Journal of Occupational Therapy, 55, 424–432.

Kelso, JAS. (1995). Dynamic Patterns: The Self Organization of Brain and Behavior. Cambridge, MA: MIT Press.

Kielhofner, G. (2002). A Model of Human Occupation: Theory and Application, 3rd ed. Baltimore, MD: Lippincott, Williams and Wilkins.

Kielhofner, G, Borell, L, Freidheim, L et al. (2002). Crafting occupational life. In Model of Human Occupation: Theory and Application, 3rd ed., pp. 124–144.

Law, M. (1991). The environment: A focus for occupational therapy. Canadian Journal of Occupational Therapy, 58, 171–179.

Law, M, Cooper, B, Strong, S, et al. (1996). Person–environment occupational model: A transactive approach to occupational performance. Canadian Journal of Occupational Therapy, 63, 9–23.

Lobo, F. (1999). The leisure and work occupations of young people: a review. Journal of Occupational Science (Australia), 6(1), 27–33.

Mallinson, T, Kielhofner, G & Mattingly C (1996). Metaphor and meaning in a clinical interview. American Journal of Occupational Therapy, 50, 338–346.

Mattingly, C. (1991). The narrative nature of clinical reasoning. American Journal of Occupational Therapy, 45, 998–1005.

Parham, LD, & Fazio, LS (eds.). (1997). Play in occupational therapy for children. St. Louis: Mosby.

Passmore, A. (1998). Does leisure support and underpin adolescents' developing worker role? Journal of Occupational Science (Australia), 5(3),161–165.

Polatajko, HJ. (1994). Dreams, dilemmas, and decisions for occupational therapy practice in a new millennium: A Canadian perspective. American Journal of Occupational Therapy, 48(7), 590–594.

Reilly, M. (1962). Occupational therapy can be one of the great ideas of 20th century medicine. American Journal of Occupational Therapy, 16, 1–9.

Rogers, J. (1982). Order and disorder in occupational therapy and in medicine. American Journal of Occupational Therapy, 36, 29–35.

Taylor, RR. (2003). Extending client-centered practice: The use of participatory methods to empower clients. Occupational Therapy in Mental Health, 19(2), 57–75.

Thelen, E & Ulrich, BD. (1991). Hidden skills: A dynamic systems analysis of treadmill stepping during the first year. Monographs of the Society for Research in Child Development, 565 (1, Serial No. 223).

Townsend, E. (1993). Occupational therapy's social vision. Canadian Journal of Occupational Therapy, 60, 174–184.

Trombly, C. (1993). The issue is anticipating the future: Assessment of occupational functioning. American Journal of Occupational Therapy , 47, 253–257.

Trombly, C. (1995). Occupation: Purposefulness and meaningfulness as therapeutic mechanisms. American Journal of Occupational Therapy, 49, 960–972.

Vallacher, RR & Nowak, A. (eds.). (1994). Dynamical Systems in Social Psychology. San Diego: Academic Press.

Wiemer, R. (1979). Traditional and nontraditional practice arenas. In Occupational therapy: 2001, 42–53 [monograph]. Rockville, MD: American Occupational Therapy Association.

Wilcock, AA. (1993). A theory of the human need for occupation. Journal of Occupational Science: Australia, 1(1), 17–24.

Wood, W. (1995). Weaving the warp and weft of occupational therapy: An art and science for all times. American Journal of Occupational Therapy, 49, 44–52.

Wood, W. (1998). It is jump time for occupational therapy. American Journal of Occupational Therapy, 52, 403–411.

Yerxa, EJ. (1983). Audacious values: The energy source of occupational therapy practice. In G. Kielhofner, G. (ed.) Health Through Occupation: Theory and Practice in Occupational Therapy, pp 149–162. Philadelphia: FA Davis.

Yerxa, EJ. (1980). Occupational therapy's role in creating a future climate of caring. American Journal of Occupational Therapy, 34, 529–534.

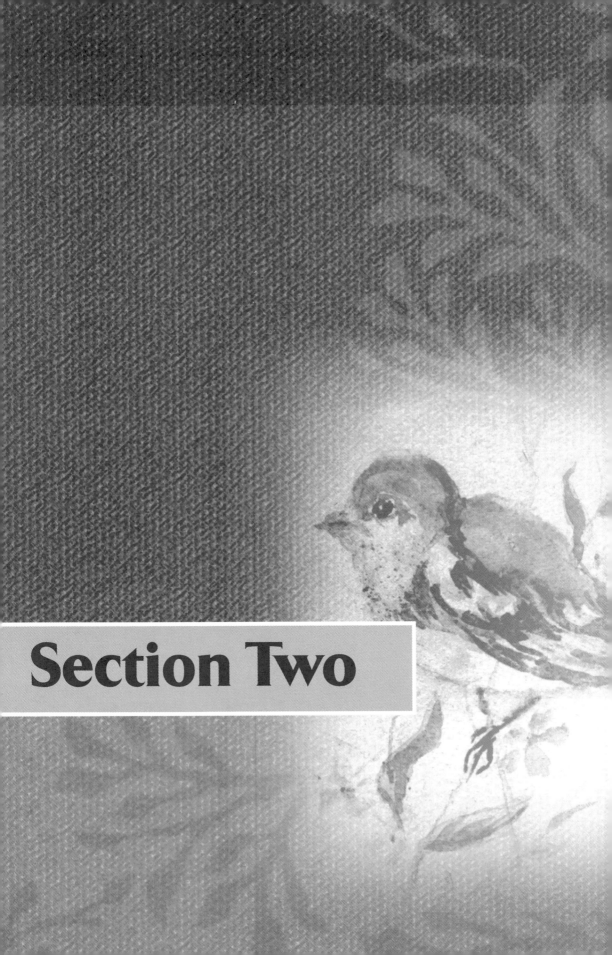

Section Two

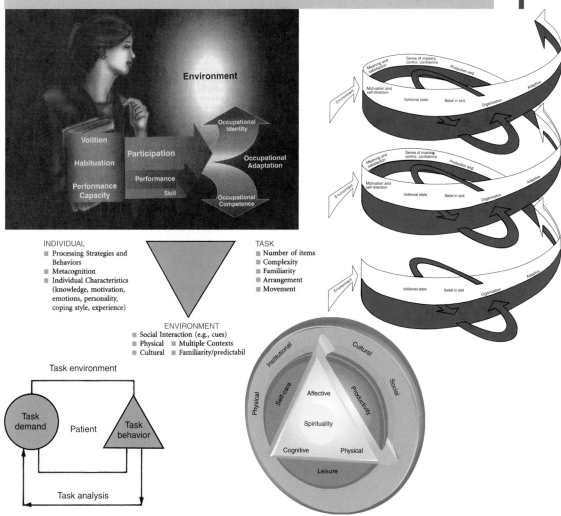

Chapter 5

Conceptual Practice Models

Conceptual practice models provide mental pictures that guide understanding of how people choose, experience, and do their occupations. They give insight into the occupational problems faced by clients, and they provide a rationale for practice. The various diagrams, verbal arguments, and research findings that characterize models are also linked to the concrete things that therapists do in everyday practice.

Occupational therapy practice creates a particular set of demands for knowledge. It challenges therapists with the following kinds of questions:

◆ How does one minimize the consequences of clients' physical or cognitive impairments in everyday occupation?
◆ How does one understand the sense of hopelessness in clients who have lost capacities necessary to their accustomed way of life? And, more, how does one help these clients retake control of their lives?

Such questions reflect the kinds of client problems that therapists are asked to solve. Occupational therapists have sought to create explanations for making sense of such problems and to develop therapeutic approaches. These efforts have resulted in conceptual practice models.

The Nature and Purpose of Conceptual Practice Models

A conceptual practice model involves, above all, a dynamic process of knowledge development. A model is never a finished product. Rather, a model is a way of thinking about and doing practice that is constantly refined and improved.

Conceptual practice models are developed to provide explanations of some phenomena of practical concern in the field and to provide a rationale and methods for therapy. Thus, a model has the dual purpose of explaining a group of phenomena and guiding practice related to those phenomena. It is the combined concern for

> **A model is a way of thinking about and doing practice that is constantly refined and improved.**

both theoretical explanation and practical action that make conceptual models of practice unique in their organization.

Components and Dynamic Processes of Models

A well-developed model has the following characteristics:

◆ It is built on an interdisciplinary base of knowledge.
◆ It articulates theory to explain particular phenomena.
◆ It yields a technology (e.g., procedures and materials) for therapeutic application.
◆ It is tested through research.

These characteristics of a model are developed as part of a dynamic flow of information, as illustrated in Figure 5–1. The interdisciplinary base provides information to support the theory. The theory provides the rationale for and guides the development of practical applications. Feedback from practice provides information for further theory development. Basic research tests the theoretical arguments. Applied research tests application of the theory in practice. Finally, models not only draw from but contribute theory and research to other disciplines and to other models in the field. This ongoing process of developing a model is influenced by and influences the field's paradigm. The following sections examine the characteristics of conceptual practice models in more detail.

Interdisciplinary Base

Models of practice in occupational therapy are influenced by and borrow from interdisci-

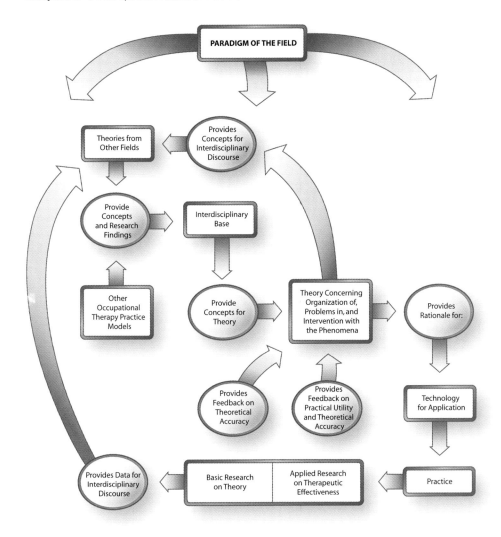

Figure 5-1. Components and proces of a conceptual model of practice.

plinary concepts. Those who develop models build theoretical concepts and propositions from both outside and inside the field that are relevant to the phenomena they are trying to explain. This use of concepts from other disciplines is not unique to occupational therapy. Because of the nature of knowledge development and the inevitable overlap among fields, the theoretical structures both in academic disciplines and applied fields are strongly influenced by developing knowledge in other disciplines. This is especially true today, since as disciplinary boundaries are not nearly as rigid as they once were.

Theory

Those individuals who develop conceptual practice models reinterpret, reorganize, and add to interdisciplinary concepts upon which they build are developing new theory. As they do this, they are influenced by the field's paradigm. The paradigm provides an intellectual

framework that influences both what interdisciplinary knowledge is selected and how it is
used in models. That is,
elements of the paradigm
are discussed in the literature, in conferences, and
other contexts. As those
who develop conceptual
practice models read, listen to presentations, and
enter into discussions, they
become part of that dis-
course and are influenced
by it in their own work.

> **In contrast to basic sciences such as biology or sociology in which theory is not designed for application, the applied theory of conceptual practice models focuses on problem identification and problem solution.**

cess is generally referred to as assessment.
Methods of assessment include formal, standardized procedures as
well as informal, naturalistic
methods. The theory of a
model should provide a
context within which the
therapists can make sense
of and draw conclusions
about the information gathered in assessment.

   Application of a model in
practice yields intervention
strategies. These may range
from methods for physically
handling clients to guidelines for interacting
with clients. Moreover, just as theory guides
the assessment process, it also allows therapists to make good decisions about selecting
and using intervention strategies in practice.

The theory in models
ordinarily addresses three practical concerns:

♦ How those aspects of occupation on
  which the model focuses (e.g., motivation,
  cognition, or movement) are ordinarily
  organized
♦ What happens when related problems
  arise
♦ How therapy can alleviate these problems

Because the theory in models is developed
in response to practical problems, it addresses
the resolution of those problems. In conceptual practice models, the theory is designed as an explanation-for-application. In
contrast to basic sciences such as biology or
sociology in which theory is not designed for
application, the applied theory of conceptual
practice models focuses on problem identification and problem solution.

Technology for Application

   Those who use models in practice require
supporting technology to apply the models.
The technology of models includes procedures, equipment, materials for assessment
and intervention, and examples that illustrate
application of the theory in practice.

   Application of a model in practice always
requires a way to gather and analyze data
about the phenomena addressed. This pro-

   Application of a model is often illustrated
through examples. The most common examples are case and program examples. Textbooks and articles that discuss application of
models typically include cases or programs to
show how the model's concepts are used in
practice. Cases illustrate the process of translating theoretical concepts to a particular
client. Programs illustrate how a model can be
used to identify and address the problems of a
client group.

Research

   Studies can test a model's theory and its
practical utility, encompassing the aims of
both basic and applied research. Basic
research aims to test the explanations offered
by a theory, whereas applied research examines the practical results of using a theory
to solve problems (Mosey, 1992a, 1992b).
Research that investigates conceptual practice models often integrates basic and applied research concerns. Moreover, when
studies are undertaken with primarily applied
or basic aims, their findings will tend to be
relevant for both applied and basic purposes.

WHAT IS THEORY?

Theory is an explanation of some phenomena that is composed of concepts and postulates (Mosey, 1992a). Concepts describe and define some entity, quality, or process. Concepts provide a specific way of seeing and thinking about the phenomena they refer to. Theories are often composed of both general concepts, which refer to larger chunks of reality, and specific concepts, which refer to the elements of which the general concepts are composed. Postulates are statements about relationships between concepts. They assert how the characteristics or processes to which concepts refer are organized.

When several concepts and postulates are linked together, they constitute a network of explanation. The key element of theory is explanation: giving a plausible account for how something works. Thus, theory does more than describe or state what is assumed or important. It provides insight into the nature and workings of specific phenomena.

As research evidence mounts, theoretical models can be altered to correct or elaborate existing concepts and propositions, strengthening the explanatory power of the theory. Empirical evidence that a model has practical utility is important for guiding evidence-based practice (Holm, 2000).

Development of Models of Practice

Each conceptual practice model has its own unique course of development. A model may begin as a collection of techniques or ideas in practice to which a comprehensive and coherent theory is added. Such an inductive approach begins with practical observations, borne out of clinical trial and error, which lead to articulation of the theory. The deductive approach begins with theory and goes on to address known problems in therapy. In this approach, clinical applications follow from the theory. Most models are developed by a combination of both approaches, although one or another approach may be dominant at different points in the model's development.

To gain acceptance and remain in use, a model of practice must have certain characteristics. First, the model has to be articulated formally. Model developers must publish articles and/or books on the model. Sometimes, however, model articulation begins with manuals, workshops, and other forms of organizing and sharing knowledge.

Models are made more credible when they have been subjected to research. Generally, research not only serves to test and refine the theory but also supports the development of the model's technology for application.

Finally, the model must be practical. A model should offer insights and tools that enhance practice and produce results desired by clients. This points to the importance of models being developed by collaborating teams of theoreticians, researchers, practitioners, and consumers.

Models, of course, vary in how well they are developed. Some models have well articulated theory but are weaker in application. Other models have appealing methods for

> **A model should offer insights and tools that enhance practice and produce results desired by clients.**

application, although their theory and research base are not as well developed. Although models may be adopted and survive for a while because of strength in one area, it is unlikely that a model can endure unless all elements are developed.

 Models in Perspective

Conceptual practice models are the major sources of theory building in occupational therapy. Moreover, they guide the research and clinical application efforts of the field. The quality of available conceptual practice models will determine to a large extent the competence of occupational therapists. Hence, these models are critically important to the profession.

 Current Models in Occupational Therapy

In practice, therapists encounter a wide range of occupational problems and related underlying impairments. Because of this diversity in what therapists must address in practice, occupational therapy requires a number of practice models. I emphasised in this chapter that models are dynamic and changing. This means not only that models will change over time but also that new models may emerge in the field and that some models may eventually fade from use.

One of the challenges in writing this book was to decide how to characterize the current conceptual practice models in occupational therapy. In deciding how to select from the literature those approaches that can be characterized as conceptual practice models, I asked whether they had articulated theory, a technology for application, and a research base. Based on these criteria, I identified the following seven conceptual practice models:

◆ The biomechanical model
◆ The Canadian model of occupational performance
◆ The cognitive disabilities model
◆ The cognitive-perceptual model
◆ The model of human occupation
◆ The motor control model
◆ The sensory integration model

They are the subjects of the chapters that follow.

References

Holm, M. (2000). Our mandate for the new millennium: Evidence-based practice: Eleanor Clarke Slagle Lecture. American Journal of Occupational Therapy, 54, 575–585.

Mosey, A. C. (1992a). Applied Scientific Inquiry in the Health Professions: An Epistemological Orientation. Rockville, MD: American Occupational Therapy Association.

Mosey, A. C. (1992b). Partition of Occupational Science and Occupational Therapy. American Journal of Occupational Therapy, 4, 851.

Chapter 6

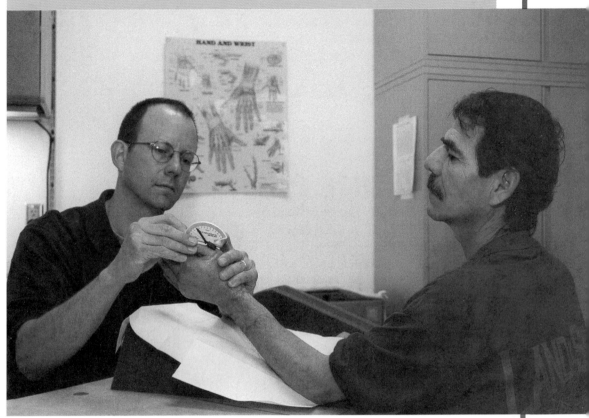

The Biomechanical Model

A therapist uses a goniometer (an instrument that measures the degrees of movement in a joint) to measure the finger range of motion of a client whose impairment includes restriction of hand motion. Based on this and other information about the client's movement capacity, the therapist will determine a treatment program aimed at increasing the client's functional use of the hand. This focus on precisely measuring and addressing limitations of functional movement is characteristic of the biomechanical model.

The biomechanical model has been present in some form throughout occupational therapy history. The basic concern of biomechanics is the musculoskeletal capacities that underlie **functional motion** in everyday occupational performance. The model's theory explains how the body is designed for and is used to accomplish motion. At one time this approach was called kinetic occupational therapy, a term that emphasized the goal of restoring abilities for motion (Ogden-Niemeyer & Land Jacobs, 1989).

Although much of the conceptual and empirical knowledge for this model comes from basic science, the practical applications have been accumulating throughout occupational therapy history. Many of the approaches and devices used today are based on decades of development.

The biomechanical model is applied to persons who experience limitations in moving freely, with adequate strength, and in a sustained fashion. These impairments result from disease or trauma in the musculoskeletal system, peripheral nervous system, integumentary system, or cardiopulmonary system. Problems of coordinated movement due to central nervous system impairment are more typically addressed through the motor control model or the sensory integrative model. Even in those cases, however, some biomechanical concerns, such as maintaining normal joint movement, are usually addressed.

Interdisciplinary Base

The biomechanical approach is based on principles of kinetics and **kinematics**, which concern the nature of movement and the forces acting on the human body as it moves.

Anatomy and physiology of the musculoskeletal system are also part of the interdisciplinary base of this model. This knowledge provides understanding of the architecture of bones, joints, and muscles that underlie motion as well as such processes as tissue healing, muscle strengthening, and the energy cost of activities that elaborate understanding of how humans produce and sustain movement. Finally, knowledge of how the cardiopulmonary system supports functioning of the musculoskeletal system is incorporated into this model.

Theory

Motion underlies occupational performance. Whether for manipulation of objects, gesturing in communication, or standing in a line while waiting a turn, all occupations involve persons stabilizing and moving their bodies. The theory of the biomechanical model concerns the ability to stabilize and move while performing occupations.

Organization

Theory in this model explains the biomechanical basis of the stability and movement required to perform occupations. Three broad concepts explain the capacity for motion. The first is the potential for motion at the joints, or **joint range of motion**. The second is **strength**, or the ability of muscles to produce tension for maintaining postural control and for moving body parts. The third is **endurance**, which is the ability to sustain effort (i.e., intensity or rate) over the time required to do a particular task.

Joint Range of Motion

Understanding the available motion at each joint comes from knowledge of the structure and function of the joint. "Each joint

> **Whether for manipulation of objects, gesturing in communication, or standing in a line while waiting a turn, all occupations involve persons stabilizing and moving their bodies.**

can move in certain directions and to certain limits of motion determined by its structure and the integrity of surrounding tissues" (Trombly & Radomski, 2002, p. 48). The connective tissue, muscle, and skin that surround joints have **elasticity,** which is the ability to stretch and to return to original shape and size after movement. The amount of elasticity of these tissues affects the extent of possible movement.

Range of Motion

Active range of motion refers to the range of movement that a person can produce using his or her own strength. **Passive range of motion** refers to the range of movement through which a joint can be externally manipulated.

Strength

Stability and motion are produced when skeletal muscles act on the joints of the body. Muscles cross one or more joints and exert force to control or produce movements allowed by the structure of the joints. Thus, tension produced in the muscles is necessary to stabilize or move joints.

The strength or ability of a muscle to produce tension is a function of the number and size of fibers in the muscle. The size, or diameter, of muscle fibers increases when the muscle is used to produce tension. Thus, the use to which a muscle is put in the course of everyday activities affects its strength.

In daily life, normal movement is not limited to the action of a single muscle across a single joint. Rather, performance depends on the simultaneous action of muscles across many joints. This produces the combination of stability and movement required for a task. Moreover, groups of muscles work together to produce each movement (Pedretti & Zoltan, 2001)

Endurance

The ability to sustain muscle activity (i.e., endurance) is a function of muscle physiol-

ogy. The variables involved are the work being done and the supply of oxygen and energy materials from the cardiopulmonary system. Thus, endurance is a somewhat more complex phenomenon than strength and motion since it depends on the musculoskeletal system, but also entails the functions of other body systems.

Dynamics of Movement Capacity

Several factors are considered in understanding movement. The potential for movement (joint range of motion) is a function of the anatomy of joints and soft tissues around joints. The production of movement is a function of muscle placement on the musculoskeletal system, of the coordinated work of muscles, and of the strength of individual muscles. Endurance is a function of muscle physiology and the ability of the body systems to transport needed material to and waste material out of muscle tissue.

Early understanding of how muscles produced movement was based primarily on the anatomical study of their position with respect to the skeletal system (i.e., where the muscles attached to bones and how they crossed joints). Such observations of anatomical organization led to the belief that specific movements and muscles would be used to perform a given task (Trombly, 1995).

As more sophisticated methods became available to study the process of movement, the understanding of how movement is used to accomplish occupations has changed. The actual movements produced during occupational performance can be described in terms of kinematics. For example, movement can be characterized by the actual movement path or displacement of a body part and the velocity (i.e., speed) and acceleration (i.e., rate of change in speed). Kinematics is an important part of the understanding of how the body actually accomplishes purposeful movements. For example, it is now understood that different persons use different combinations of movement to do the same purposeful task and that a person uses different combinations of movements to perform the same task at different times (Trombly, 1995).

Self-Maintenance of the Musculoskeletal System

One of the most important observations of this model is that the capacity for movement (i.e., strength, range of motion, and endurance) is correlated with occupational performance. That is, muscle strength increases and decreases according to how much muscles are stressed in the course of everyday occupations. Similarly, the structure of bones is also positively affected by how much weight-bearing they do, and joint mobility is affected by the nature of ongoing joint movement. Finally, the capacity for endurance waxes and wanes over time with changes in activity level.

> **Interventions based on the biomechanical model focus on the intersection of motion and occupational performance.**

Problems and Challenges

This model addresses problems and challenges related to producing the stability and movement for the performance of one's occupations. Such problems emanate from biomechanical impairments (i.e., restrictions of joint motion, strength, and/or endurance) (Trombly & Radomski, 2002). Thus, the central concern of the model is with problems that occur when persons cannot generate and/or sustain the stability or movement needed to perform their occupations. A variety of diseases or traumas may lead to such problems.

Joint range of motion may be limited because of joint damage, edema of tissues around the joint, pain, skin tightness, muscle spasticity (i.e., excess muscle tone producing tightness), or muscle and **tendon** shortening

as a consequence of prolonged immobilization. Examples of conditions that affect joint mobility are arthritis, trauma to the joint or to the surrounding connective tissue, and burns that limit the elasticity of skin over the joint.

Muscle weakness (i.e., reduced tension-producing capacity) can occur as a result of disuse or because of disease affecting muscle physiology. Loss of muscle strength may be due to diseases and trauma of the lower motor neurons (e.g., polio or amyotrophic lateral sclerosis), spinal cord, or peripheral nerves. which results in de-innervation of muscles. If muscles lose their innervation, they may completely atrophy and be incapable of producing tension. Muscle diseases, such as muscular dystrophy, directly affect muscle tissue. Finally, extended disuse or immobilization can result in weakness that impairs everyday performance (Pedretti & Zoltan, 2001; Trombly & Radomski, 2002).

Like strength, endurance can be reduced with any extended confinement or limitation of activity. Other factors, including pathology of the cardiovascular or respiratory systems and muscular diseases, can also reduce endurance.

Therapeutic Intervention

Interventions based on the biomechanical model focus on the intersection of motion and occupational performance. These interventions can be divided into three approaches:

- Preventing deformity and maintaining existing capacity for motion
- Restoration of capacity for motion
- Compensation for limited motion

In all three approaches, the overriding criterion for intervention is to minimize any gap between persons' existing limited capacity for movement and the movement requirements of their ordinary occupational tasks.

Maintenance and Prevention

As already noted, reasonable use is necessary to maintain function of the musculoskeletal system. The biomechanical model extends this principle to argue that muscles still able to produce contractions and move joints should be used to maintain the capacity for functional motion. When the person is not able to control stability or movement, joint range is maintained passively (i.e., by externally manipulating joints through their range of motion). Joint positioning, including the use of splints that maintain joints in proper positions, is also used to prevent joint deformity. The exception to this practice is when immobility of a joint is functionally advantageous for an individual.

Research has shown, and more and more people are aware, that many biomechanical problems are caused by how persons perform tasks in their daily occupations. Examples of this are back injury due to use of poor **body mechanics** while lifting and damage to soft tissues due to repetitive motions performed in work (Trombly & Radomski, 2002). This awareness has fueled interest in efforts to prevent occurrence or recurrence of such problems, especially in the workplace. Occupational therapists can teach proper body mechanics or recommend work-task or work-site modifications to avoid such problems.

Restoration

Restoration aims at increasing available motion, strength, and endurance. Principles of restoration are based on the understanding of normal biomechanical functioning. This model asserts that because movement in tasks maintains normal range, strength, and endurance, movement can also be used to restore or improve these.

Therapists provide clients opportunities to engage in occupations in which joint movements and muscle tension produced are gradually increased. These increases in demand result in increases in capacity until a desired level of functioning is reached. Goals for motion, strength, and endurance are determined according to the residual potential (i.e., how much improvement a person is likely to be able to achieve based on the nature of the disease or trauma underlying the impairment) and the movement demands of the occupations the person needs and/or wants to perform. For this approach to work, there must be the potential for the person to develop the motion, strength, and endurance necessary for the desired and/or necessary occupations.

For example, a client in occupational therapy who recently had hand surgery may be wearing a splint and doing things requiring finger movements in order to achieve the passive and active range of motion necessary for typing. Another client recovering from coronary bypass surgery may engage in graded occupations in order to increase endurance to a level required for self-care and leisure activities. Still another client after a work injury may be engaged in simulated work activities designed to increase lifting capacity to the level demanded on the job.

Compensation

Many people experience extended, permanent, or progressively greater limitations in their capacity for movement. **Compensatory treatment** aims to offset these limitations by bridging the gap between the person's capacity for stability or motion and what is required in everyday occupations (Trombly & Radomski, 2002). Compensation involves one or more of the following strategies:

◆ Using devices that are attached to the body or that mediate between the body and objects that need to be manipulated

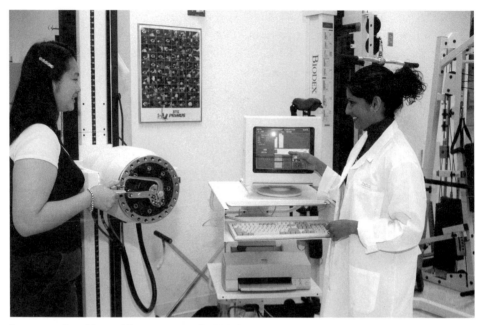

An occupational therapist measures a client's lateral pinch strength using a Baltimore Therapeutic Equipment Work Simulator.

◆ Modifying or replacing the physical environment and objects used to perform routine tasks

◆ Altering procedures for accomplishing tasks, including the use of other persons as assistants in accomplishing these tasks

✿ Technology for Application

An extensive technology has been developed to support the application of this model. Information about the technology exists in a wide variety of published sources, including those that focus on particular kinds of musculoskeletal impairments.

Assessment

Range of motion is usually measured with a goniometer calibrated to the degrees of movement about an axis. If the client is not capable of moving a joint voluntarily, the therapist passively moves it to evaluate available range. Range of motion is measured in degrees of movement about the axis of a joint.

Strength is normally tested as "maximum tension produced under voluntary effort" (Trombly & Radomski, 2002). The strength assessment used most often is **manual muscle testing,** in which the therapist (alone or using some instrument) tests the ability of the person to produce resistance and/or movement under standardized circumstances. In addition to examining strength of individual muscles and muscle groups, the evaluator may assess the pattern of muscle strength and weakness. Endurance is usually measured by determining duration or number of repetitions before fatigue occurs.

In addition to the more traditional and simple assessments of strength and endurance, several kinds of complex and computer-driven systems are available for muscle strength and endurance testing. These can produce very sophisticated analyses of a person's movement capacities.

Intervention

Methods of intervention are clearly delineated in this model. The method must match not only the targeted limitations of motion, strength, and endurance but also their underlying causes, because the latter may determine what is the most appropriate intervention. For example, if limited range of motion is due to tightness, stretching may be used to reduce tightness; if it is due to edema, compression may be used to reduce the edema. Active and passive range of motion and appropriate positioning may be used to prevent deformities. Special splints and other devices may also be used for these purposes.

Strength is developed by increasing the stress on a muscle through: (1) the amount of resistance offered to the movement; (2) the duration of resistance required; (3) the rate (speed of movement) of an exercise session; and (4) frequency of sessions. Different types of exercise regimens are available. Current approaches (such as work hardening) emphasize strengthening by performing the specific tasks required by the person's occupation (Ogden-Niemeyer & Land Jacobs, 1989). Therapists using this model may be involved in prescription, design, fabrication, checkout, and training in the use of orthoses (special devices attached to the body to substitute for lost stability or movement). Orthoses support, immobilize, or position a joint or joints and are used to correct for deformities and/or to increase function. An **orthosis** may be temporary or permanent. Orthotic splints either use existing movements to achieve functional motion or rely on sources of power external to the body. Occupational therapists are also involved in training clients to use prostheses (i.e., devices that replace amputated parts of the body).

Role of Occupation in Maintenance, Prevention, and Restoration

The traditional view in occupational therapy was that occupations provided natural and motivating circumstances for maintaining musculoskeletal functioning. This belief was based on the argument that involvement in

meaningful occupations employed attention, thereby encouraging greater effort, diminishing fatigue, and diverting attention from pain or fear of movement. Additionally, therapists argued that occupations provided a form of conditioning that more nearly replicated the normal demands for movement in everyday life. Reflecting this viewpoint, Trombly and Radomski (2002) suggest the following approach to selecting activities used as a therapeutic media:

> The best activity for remediation is one that intrinsically demands the exact response that has been determined to need improvement.... Contrived methods of doing an ordinary activity to make it therapeutic may diminish the value of the activity in the eyes of the patient. (p. 269)

As this quote implies, the therapist requires knowledge of the kind of functional movements that an activity will require from the participant. As noted earlier, it was assumed in the past that a therapist could determine what discrete movements would be required by doing a **biomechanical activity analysis**. Now it is recognized that while it may be possible to determine the overall type of movement required to complete a specific activity, it is not possible to predict the exact pattern of muscle action and joint motion with which a person will accomplish a given task. As Trombly (1995) notes:

> The next time the person does the same thing, his or her muscles may be more warmed up, or there may be a slight difference in placement of task object in relation to the active limb, so a new coordinative structure evolves. That is, different muscles may be recruited, or the same muscles used before may be more or less active in order to accomplish the movement goal in the most efficient way. The motor goal is constant

or invariant and requires a constant or invariant response, but this response can be fulfilled by a varying set of muscular contractions. (p. 965)

Perhaps for this reason, therapists have been shown in research to lack significant agreement about the biomechanical demands of activities (Trombly, 1995).

For this reason, biomechanical activity analysis is less concerned with specific motions and instead focuses on functional movements. That is, therapists pay more attention to the functional purpose of a task, because purpose does appear to exert an organizing influence on movement (Trombly, 1995). This means that when therapists analyze activities, they need to think about requisite movement in more functional terms such as grasping, lifting, climbing, carrying, and so on. These are the kinds of functional movements that may remain stable within occupations while the underlying combinations of muscle action and joint motion that accomplish the functional movements may vary considerably.

While the process of analyzing an activity is viewed differently than in the past, it is still an important element of this model since therapists need to modify occupational activities in order to achieve therapeutic goals. Activity may be modified so as to reduce or alter task demands and thereby prevent musculoskeletal problems.

Therapists may also adapt activity to better match permanently reduced musculoskeletal capacity. Finally, activity may be progressively modified to intensify task demands that will increase musculoskeletal capacity. Therapists have several ways to modify an activity including:

1. Positioning the task
2. Adding weights or other devices that provide assistance or resistance to movements performed in the activity
3. Modifying tools to reduce or increase demands
4. Changing materials or size of objects used
5. Changing the method of accomplishing the task

In doing activity adaptation, Trombly and Radomski (2002) caution that the therapist should not contrive the activity so much that it becomes meaningless. In all cases of using adapted activities, it is important that the client be involved in occupational performance that has some meaning and relevance.

Compensatory Technology*

Compensatory technology is used for clients who will live with a disability either temporarily or permanently. Underlying this technology is the principle that when persons do not have the biomechanical capacity to perform daily living, leisure, and work tasks in ordinary ways, special equipment and modified procedures can compensate. They are used to close the gap between the person's capacities and the task demands. As Trombly notes, the desired goal of the treatment is for the person to be able to use his or her remaining capacities (and by using, maintain them) while exercising the highest level of possible independence in occupational performance.

Evaluation includes assessment of actual performance in activities of daily living (e.g., toileting, bathing, feeding, grooming, dressing, mobility, and communication), leisure, work, and community living. When assessment is completed and the person's inability

---

*Trombly describes what she calls the rehabilitation approach as an alternative or complement to the biomechanical approach. However, purpose of this technology is to support compensation for biomechanical limitations. These rehabilitation techniques do not have an independent theory. Rather, the biomechanical model provides the rationale for the various rehabilitation strategies and equipment. Therefore, I am including what she calls rehabilitation techniques as a compensatory technology of the biomechanical model.

to perform necessary tasks is identified, the therapist determines the biomechanical limitations and assets. With this information, the therapist can recommend and train persons in the use of special equipment, modified procedures, or altered environments that make it possible for the person to perform the task. A wide range of adaptive equipment (commercially available or fabricated in therapy) is used to assist persons in performing every aspect of their daily occupations. The technology of adaptive equipment exists to interface between musculoskeletal capacities and environment and task demands. Some technology is quite simple, involving modification of ordinary tools and implements to make them easier to grasp and be manipulated. Some technology involves modification of the environment (i.e., adding ramps and grab bars) to make it easier for persons with limited biomechanical capacity to get around. There also exists more sophisticated technology for both restoration and compensation. This includes a wide range of equipment such as motorized wheelchairs, special communication devices, environmental controls, and modified workstations.

The occupational therapist identifies, in collaboration with the client, the most appropriate device and/or modified procedure to use in occupational tasks. The therapist also provides instruction and practice in how to make use of compensatory devices and procedures. This can include instructing persons in how to organize their tasks and time to make the best use of existing capacity to accomplish their occupational tasks.

The occupational therapy setting is often used for persons to try out adapted equipment and procedures. Also, as therapists increasingly provide services in homes, schools, and workplaces, they can work even more specifically in the natural setting in which the task is to be performed. Therapists may assist individuals in planning changes in their homes (if this is financially feasible) and in learning to access specialized transportation and community facilities.

Work Hardening

Work hardening is an individualized biomechanical approach to treatment aimed at returning an individual to work, usually to a specific job. One of the main methods used in work hardening is **physical reconditioning,** the use of simulated and real work activities along with exercise to improve the person's ability to perform specific work tasks.

Work hardening programs employ a range of equipment, including exercise and aerobic conditioning equipment, work capacity evaluation devices (that simulate the required movements of work tasks), work samples and workstations that simulate real jobs, and individualized simulations that reproduce a specific job requirement (Basmajian & Wolf, 1990; Riccio, Nelson, & Bush, 1990).

Research

Research related to the interdisciplinary theory of the biomechanical model is substantial and continues to grow. This research is producing new understanding of muscle physiology, the effects of exercise, and the dynamic role of muscles and muscle groups in movement (Basmajian & Wolf, 1990). As this body of knowledge develops, it influences the biomechanical model.

The proper area of occupational therapy research related to the biomechanical model will need further clarification, but some promising directions are emerging. One area of study is the relationship between musculoskeletal functioning and success in occupations. Such studies have examined the ability of measures of physical capacities to predict injured workers' return to work (Kircher, 1984), the potential for persons with muscular dystrophy to participate in specific occupational tasks (Schkade, Feilbelman, &

Cook, 1987), the relationship of wrist muscle tone to self-care abilities (Spaulding et al, 1989), and the relationship of grip strength to functional outcomes and work performance following hand trauma (Wahi Michener et al., 2001).

Other studies are beginning to examine the actual muscle action and kinematics patterns used in different task conditions (Follows, 1987; Mathiowetz, 1991; McGrain & Hague, 1987; Trombly & Cole, 1979; Trombly & Quintana, 1983; Wu, Trombly, & Lin, 1994). Such research helps to clarify how movement is produced and used in occupational performance.

In one promising area of inquiry, studies examine how the purpose or meaning of activities affects compliance, effort, fatigue, and improvement in movement capacity. One such study demonstrated the advantages of a dance program over normal range-of-motion exercises (Van Deusen & Marlowe, 1987a; Van Deusen & Marlowe, 1987b). A study of elderly women supported the conclusion that adding imagery to movement is more effective than rote exercise in eliciting frequency and duration of movement (Riccio, Nelson, & Bush, 1990). A study of women demonstrated that perceived exertion was less in a task with purpose than in a purposeless task in which the same effort was exerted (Kircher, 1984). A new dimension to the biomechanical model appears to be emerging from this line of research. This new dimension is the incorporation of the themes of experience and motivation into the understanding of human movement. Nelson and Peterson (1989), for example, differentiate between two motives that are intrinsic to movement: (1) pleasure in the sensory experience of moving and exerting effort and (2) the purpose added when

> **What makes the biomechanical model a unique model of practice in occupational therapy is the way biomechanical principles are applied to understanding occupational performance.**

movement is used to accomplish a goal. They argue that activities that add purpose to movement may enhance the quality of exercise both by increasing the goal orientation of the client and by providing environmental support that guides the client's attention and motor planning.

Finally, research has examined the outcomes of biomechanically based interventions. For example, one study examined the effects of body mechanics training on the performance of repetitive lifting (Lieber, Rudy, & Boston, 2000).

Trombly notes that much more investigation needs to be done to clarify relationships between musculoskeletal and occupational functioning and to document the effects of occupational therapy based on this model.

Discussion

The use of biomechanical knowledge is not unique to occupational therapy. For example, physical therapy also applies biomechanics. What makes the biomechanical model a unique model of practice in occupational therapy is the way biomechanical principles are applied to understanding occupational performance. Additionally, occupational therapy is unique in the use of occupations to influence changes in range, strength, and endurance. Increasingly, the health care system is demanding functional outcomes from intervention (e.g., whether the person will return to work or remain living at home). This trend encourages the use of occupations that present clients with real-life demands.

The use of physical agents (e.g., heat or electrical stimulation), passive manipulation (e.g., massage or joint mobilization), and pure exercise has been controversial in occupational therapy. Physical agents, passive manipulation, and pure exercise are used extensively in physical therapy and, in fact, characterize much of how that profession applies biomechanics. Nonetheless, occupational therapists also use these methods.

While the debates over occupational therapists' use of physical agents, exercise, and passive techniques have been heated, it seems that there are two legitimate sides to the argument. First, there is concern that occupational therapists who apply biome-

chanical knowledge can become overly reliant on, if not exclusively focused on, the non-occupational aspects of musculoskeletal function (West & Wiemer, 1991). Such practice brings into question whether occupational therapy is being practiced as it should be; that is, in accordance with how the field's paradigm identifies practice (Heater, 1992). Second, it is argued that there is a legitimate place for non-occupational techniques that may be used as an adjunct or prelude to occupational therapy's unique focus on occupational functioning (Ahl-

TERMS OF THE MODEL

Active range of motion	Degree of self-initiated movement possible at the joint.
Biomechanical activity analysis	Examination of the endurance, range of motion, and muscle strength needed for the completion of an activity.
Body mechanics	Position and movements of the body during the performance of occupations.
Compensatory treatment	Therapy involving adaptations to deal with existing limitations.
Elasticity	The capability of tissue to stretch and to return to its original shape and size.
Endurance	The ability to sustain effort over the time required to do a particular task.
Functional motion	Movement required for daily occupations.
Joint range of motion	The potential for motion at the joints.
Kinematics	The study of how the body moves in terms of movement path, velocity, and acceleration
Manual muscle testing	Examination of an individual's muscle strength by asking the client to produce movement against manual resistance.
Orthosis (pl, orthoses)	Device used to correct joint misalignment or to substitute for lost function.
Passive range of motion	Amount of movement at the joint when the joint is moved by means other than the individual.
Physical reconditioning	The process of returning the body to a state of fitness.
Strength	The ability of muscles to produce tension to maintain postural control and move body parts.
Tendon	Connective tissue that connects a muscle to the bone.
Work hardening	Program applying biomechanical principles by using simulations of the physical requirements of a work situation to recondition persons for work.

schwede, 1992). Current thinking suggests that use of these methods is "adjunctive" and has a legitimate purpose when they are necessary to develop or support the ability to engage in occupations (AOTA, 1992a; AOTA, 1992b). The focus on occupation is, thus, affirmed, and the use of adjunctive methods is recognized.

Given the centrality of movement problems in occupational therapy clients and the long history of this approach in occupational therapy practice, there is no doubt that the model will continue to be a vital part of occupational therapy science and practice. Further development is needed to increase its coherence and to articulate its position as a unique occupational therapy model of practice.

It is useful to consider that the biomechanical model was first developed as an occupational therapy approach under the previous paradigm and necessarily reflected the focus of that paradigm on inner mechanisms (i.e., musculoskeletal). As the field's paradigm has shifted to a focus on occupation, this model has had to be and is still being redefined.

🌿 Summary: The Biomechanical Model

Focus

- ◆ Musculoskeletal capacities that underlie functional motion in everyday occupational performance
- ◆ How the body is designed and used to accomplish motion for occupational performance
- ◆ Applied to persons who experience limitations in moving freely with adequate strength and/or in a sustained fashion

Interdisciplinary Base

- ◆ Kinetic and kinematic principles concerning nature of movement and forces acting on the human body as it moves

- ◆ Anatomy of musculoskeletal system
- ◆ Physiology of bone, connective tissue, and muscle and cardiopulmonary function

Theory
Organization

- ◆ Capacity for functional motion is based on:
  1. Potential for motion at the joints (joint range of motion)
  2. Muscle strength (ability of muscles to produce tension to maintain postural control and move body parts)
  3. Endurance (ability to sustain effort [i.e., intensity or rate] over time required to do a particular task)
- ◆ Joint range of motion depends on structure and function of joint and integrity of surrounding connective tissue, muscle, and skin
- ◆ Muscles cross one or more joints and exert force to control or produce movements allowed by structure of the joints
- ◆ Performance depends on simultaneous action of muscles across many joints producing stability and movement required for a task
- ◆ The ability to sustain muscle activity (i.e., endurance) is a function of muscle physiology in relationship to work being done and supply of oxygen and energy materials from cardiopulmonary system
- ◆ Movements produced during occupational performance are as much a function of dynamic circumstances of performance as they are of structure of the musculoskeletal system
- ◆ Capacity for movement (i.e., strength, range of motion, and endurance) affects and is affected by occupational performance

Problems and Challenges

- ◆ Problems exist when a restriction of joint motion, strength, and/or endurance interferes with everyday occupations
- ◆ Joint range of motion may be limited by joint damage, edema, pain, skin tightness,

muscle spasticity (excess muscle tone producing tightness), or muscle and tendon shortening (due to immobilization)

♦ Muscle weakness can occur as a result of:
1. Disuse
2. Disease affecting muscle physiology (e.g., muscular dystrophy)
3. Diseases and trauma of lower motor neurons (e.g., polio), spinal cord, or peripheral nerves, which result in de-innervation of muscles

♦ Endurance can be reduced by:
1. Extended confinement or limitation of activity
2. Pathology of cardiovascular or respiratory systems
3. Muscular diseases

Therapeutic Intervention

♦ Interventions focus on intersection of motion and occupational performance and can be divided into three approaches:
1. Prevention of contracture and maintenance of existing capacity for motion
2. Restoration by improving diminished capacity for motion
3. Compensation for limited motion

♦ Intervention aims to minimize any gap between existing capacity for movement and functional requirements of ordinary occupational tasks

Technology for Application

♦ Range of motion is usually measured with a goniometer calibrated to degrees of movement about an axis

♦ Strength is normally tested by manual muscle testing in which therapist (alone or using some instrument) tests the ability of a person to produce resistance and/or movement under standardized circumstances

♦ Endurance is usually measured by determining duration or number of repetitions before fatigue occurs

♦ Methods of intervention address not only targeted limitations of motion, strength,

and endurance but also their underlying causes because the latter may determine what is the most appropriate intervention

♦ Strength is developed by increasing stress on a muscle through:
1. Amount of resistance offered to the movement
2. Duration of resistance required
3. Rate (speed of movement) of an exercise session
4. Frequency of sessions

♦ Current approaches (such as work hardening) emphasize strengthening by having client perform tasks required by that person's occupation

♦ Prescription, design, fabrication, checkout, and training in use of orthoses to support, immobilize, or position a joint to prevent/correct contractures and/or enhance function

♦ Occupations:
1. Provide natural and motivating circumstances for maintaining musculoskeletal functioning
2. Employ attention, thereby encouraging greater effort, diminishing fatigue, and diverting attention from pain or fear of movement
3. Provide conditioning that more nearly replicates normal demands for movement in everyday life

♦ Attention to functional purpose of a task is important because purpose does appear to exert an organizing influence on movement

♦ Activity may be modified to:
1. Reduce or alter task demands and prevent musculoskeletal problems
2. Match permanently reduced musculoskeletal capacity
3. Intensify task demands that will increase musculoskeletal capacity

♦ Ways to modify an activity include:
1. Positioning the task
2. Adding weights or other devices that provide assistance or resistance to movements performed in the activity

3. Modifying tools to reduce or increase demands
4. Changing materials or size of objects used
5. Changing method(s) of accomplishing task

◆ When using adapted activities it is important that client be involved in occupational performance that has some meaning and relevance

◆ When persons do not have biomechanical capacity to perform daily living, leisure, and work tasks in ordinary ways, special equipment and modified procedures can compensate (i.e., close gap between a person's capacities and task demands)

Research

◆ Areas of study:
1. Relationship between musculoskeletal functioning and success in occupations
2. Muscle action and kinematic patterns used in different task conditions
3. How the purpose or meaning of activities affects compliance, effort, fatigue, and improvement in movement capacity

References

Ahlschwede, K. (1992). Views on physical agent modalities and specialization within occupational therapy: A rebuttal. American Journal of Occupational Therapy, 46, 650–652.

American Occupational Therapy Association. (1992a). Use of adjunctive modalities in occupational therapy. American Journal of Occupational Therapy, 46, 1075–1081.

American Occupational Therapy Association. (1992b). Position paper: Physical agent modalities. American Journal of Occupational Therapy, 46, 1090–1091.

Basmajian, JV & Wolf, SL (1990). Therapeutic exercise (5th ed.). Baltimore: Williams & Wilkins.

Follows, A. (1987). Electromyographical analysis of the extrinsic muscles of the long finger during pinch activities. Occupational Therapy Journal of Research, 7, 163–180.

Heater, SL. (1992). Specialization or uniformity within the profession? American Journal of Occupational Therapy, 46, 172–173.

Kircher, MA. (1984). Motivation as a factor of perceived exertion in purposeful versus non-purposeful activity. American Journal of Occupational Therapy, 38,165–170.

Lieber, S, Rudy, T & Boston, JR. (2000). Effects of body mechanics training on performance of repetitive lifting. American Journal of Occupational Therapy, 54, 166–175.

Mathiowetz, VG. (1991). Informational support and functional motor performance. Unpublished doctoral dissertation, University of Minnesota.

McGrain, P & Hague, MA. (1987). An electromyographic study of the middle deltoid and middle trapezius muscles during warping. Occupational Therapy Journal of Research, 7,225–233.

Nelson, DL & Peterson, CQ. (1989). Enhancing therapeutic exercise through purposeful activity: A theoretical analysis. Topics in Geriatric Rehabilitation, 4,12.

Ogden-Niemeyer, L & Land Jacobs, K. (1989). Work Hardening: State of the Art. Thorofare, NJ: Slack, Inc.

Pedretti, LW & Zoltan, B. (eds.). (2001). Occupational therapy practice skills for physical dysfunction (5th ed.). St Louis: CV Mosby.

Riccio, CM, Nelson, DL, & Bush, MA. (1990). Adding purpose to the repetitive exercise of elderly women. American Journal of Occupational Therapy, 44, 714–719.

Schkade, JK, Feilbelman, A, & Cook, JD. (1987). Occupational potential in a population with Duchenne muscular dystrophy. Occupational Therapy Journal of Research, 7, 289–300.

Spaulding, SJ, Strachota, E, McPherson, JJ, et al. (1989). Wrist muscle tone and self-care skill in persons with hemiparesis. American Journal of Occupational Therapy, 43,11–24.

Trombly, CA. (1995). Occupation: Purposefulness and meaningfulness as therapeutic mechanisms. American Journal of Occupational Therapy, 49, 960–972.

Trombly, CA & Cole, JM. (1979). Electromyographic study of four hand muscles during selected activities. American Journal of Occupational Therapy, 33, 440–449.

Trombly, CA & Quintana, LE. (1983). Activity analysis: Electromyographic and electrogoniometric verification. Occupational Therapy Journal of Research, 3, 104–120.

Trombly, CA & Radomski, M. (2002). Occupation Therapy for Physical Dysfunction (5th ed.). Philadelphia: Lippincott, Williams & Wilkins.

Van Deusen, J & Marlowe, D. (1987a). A comparison of the ROM dance, home exercise/rest program with traditional routines. Occupational Therapy Journal of Research, 7, 349–361.

Van Deusen, J & Marlowe, D. (1987b). The efficacy of the ROM dance program for adults with rheumatoid arthritis. American Journal of Occupational Therapy 41, 90–95.

Wahi Michener, SK, Olson, AL, Humphrey, BA, et al. (2001). Relationship among grip strength, functional outcomes, and work performance following hand trauma. Work, 16, 209–217.

West, WL & Wiemer, RB (1991). Should the representative assembly have voted as it did, when it did, on occupational therapists' use of physical modalities? American Journal of Occupational Therapy, 45, 1143–1147.

Wu, C-Y, Trombly, CA & Lin, K-C. (1994). The relationship between occupational form and occupational performance: A kinematic perspective. American Journal of Occupational Therapy, 48, 679–687.

Chapter 7

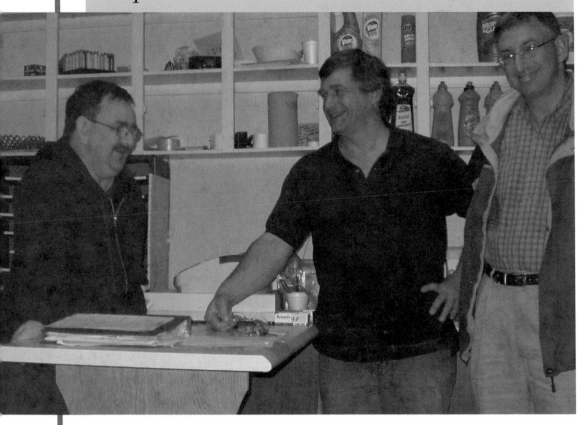

The Canadian Model of Occupational Performance

At Quick-Stuff, a consumer-run co-op, consumers own and operate the corner-store business. This business was developed in partnership with Connections Clubhouse, community support program for clients in Canada. Here, this client-centered approach reflective of the Canadian model of occupational performance is used by occupational therapists. Therapists support clients to engage in skill-building and empowering occupations designed to help them make a desired transition to full community living and participation.

The Canadian model of occupational performance grew out of efforts of a task force to develop national consensus guidelines for quality assurance in the practice of occupational therapy in Canada during the early 1980s. The *Guidelines for Client-Centered Practice of Occupational Therapy,* published in 1983 by the Department of National Health and Welfare and the Canadian Association of Occupational Therapists, included two key features: the client-centered perspective and a conceptualization called the occupational performance model. The principles of client-centered practice were elaborated in *Intervention Guidelines for the Client-Centered Practice of Occupational Therapy* (Department of National Health and Welfare & Canadian Association of Occupational Therapists, 1986) and *Toward Outcome Measures in Occupational Therapy* (Department of National Health and Welfare & Canadian Association of Occupational Therapists, 1987). From the outset this model was concerned with "the sequential interaction of events of the client with the occupational therapist" (Department of National Health and Welfare & Canadian Association of Occupational Therapists, 1983, p. 4).

With time, the ideas first proposed as guidelines for practice have evolved into three interrelated elements:

◆ Principles and other resources for client-centered practice
◆ A conceptualization of factors influencing occupational performance
◆ A process for implementing the conceptualization of occupational performance and client-centered principles in practice

In the literature, the second two elements are sometimes referred to as "models" (i.e.,

> **From the outset this model was concerned with "the sequential interaction of events of the client with the occupational therapist"**

the occupational performance model and the occupational performance processes model), but the usage of the term "model" in these instances is different than the term "conceptual practice model" in this book. To avoid confusion, the latter two components are not referred to as models in this chapter. Rather, the term model is reserved for collective approach represented in these three interrelated elements. Moreover, these three elements have been developed somewhat separately, with contributions by different combinations of leading authors. Thus, they are not as fully integrated as the elements of other conceptual practice models in this text. These three elements are treated here as components of a single conceptual practice model because they are used as such in practice, have been associated with each other in the literature, and have all been developed by Canadian authors.

The Canadian model of occupational performance is a generic model that is used with different types of clients and in any type of therapy setting. While it was originally developed to guide practice in Canada, its influence is now international. The literature on this model includes over 40 publications appearing the last 2 decades.

Interdisciplinary Base

This client-centered element of this model is based on the definition of client-centered practice proposed by the psychologist Carl Rogers (1951). Concepts of empowerment and justice from democratic principles have also been applied to the vision of client-centered practice (Townsend, 1993). Authors of this model have also used the occupational therapy perspective by Reed and Sanderson (1980) as the foundation for the original utilization of occupational performance. Other occupational therapy ideas concerning the nature and role of occupation in human life have also been incorporated into this model.

 Foci

This model has two primary foci. The first, **client-centered practice,** is concerned with the process of therapy and the relationship between client and therapy. The second focus of this model is on **occupational performance,** which is defined as "the ability to choose, organize, and satisfactorily perform meaningful occupations that are culturally defined and age-appropriate for looking after one's self, enjoying life, and contributing to the social and economic fabric of a community" (Law et al., 1997, p. 30).

Client-centered practice has been addressed over the course of development of this model through ongoing discussions of how to conduct such practice and by the development of a client-centered assessment. The conceptualization offered and the factors influencing performance are designed as a decision-making tool to orient the therapist to the client's needs and circumstances in the course of therapy. As noted earlier, the term Canadian model of occupational performance is used sometimes to refer specifically to the latter element. However, this conceptualization of occupational performance arose in conjunction with the concept of client-centered practice, and the two ideas are interrelated. Thus, as noted earlier, they are both presented here as elements of a single model.

 Theory

This model began with a process designed to identify guidelines for practice. The initial aim behind this model was not to create theory. However, as discussed by McColl and Pranger (1994), the guidelines, beginning with a definition of the field's domain of concern, were later elaborated into a conceptual model. This conceptual model has evolved as a variety of authors have contributed to it; many of the ideas of this model have evolved through consensus and through debate of issues among occupational therapists in Canada.

The most recent comprehensive discussion of the theory of this model was presented by Law et al. (1997) in a text published by the Canadian Association of Occupational Therapists entitled: *Enabling Occupation: An Occupational Therapy Perspective.*

Organization

The model includes a statement of values and beliefs, coupled with a conceptualization of occupational performance, and factors that impact occupational performance. The values and beliefs concern occupation, the person, the environment, health, and client-centered practice. For example, the values related to occupation are that it:

◆ Gives meaning to life
◆ Is important to health and well-being
◆ Organizes behavior
◆ Develops and changes over time
◆ Shapes and is shaped by the environment
◆ Has therapeutic effectiveness

These and the other values and beliefs are offered to "underpin a perspective on occupational performance and client-centered practice" (Law et al., 1997, p. 30).

The next component of this model is the conceptualization of occupational performance and its relationship to client-centered practice. It begins with the assertion that occupational performance is the "result of a dynamic relationship between persons, environment, and occupation over a person's life-span" (Law et al., 1997, p. 30). The major ideas in this model (see Fig. 7-1, p. 97) are as follows:

◆ The person is connected to the environment, and occupation occurs as an

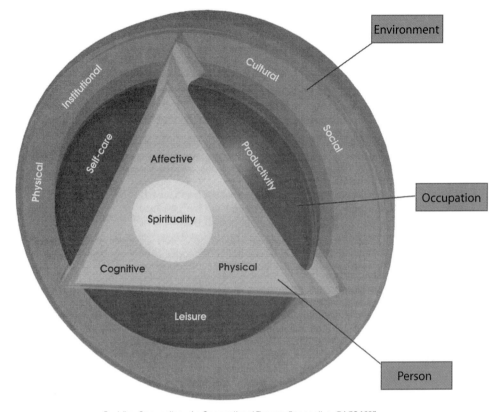

Enabling Occupation: An Occupational Therapy Perspective, CAOT 1997

Figure 7-1. Canadian Model of Occupational Performance (Reprinted from Enabling Occupation: An Occupational Therapy Perspective. Ottawa, Ontario: CAOT Publications ACE, 1997.)

interaction between persons and their environments

◆ Change in any part of the person-environment-occupation interaction affects the other parts and the consequent performance

◆ The person is illustrated at the center to highlight the client-centered perspective

◆ Spirituality is at the core of the person, shaped by the environment and giving meaning to occupations

The next component of the model includes definitions and elaborations of the key concepts. For example, occupation is conceptualized as including self-care, productivity, and leisure. It is elaborated as:

◆ A basic human need
◆ A health determinant

◆ A source of meaning and purpose, choice and control, and balance and satisfaction

◆ A means of organizing time, materials, and space and of generating income

◆ A descriptor of human behaviors that provides a unique perspective on human life

◆ A therapeutic medium

The person is seen as an integrated whole "who incorporates, spirituality, social and cultural experiences, and observable occupational performance components" (Law et al., 1997, p. 41).

Spirituality is presented as the central core of the person and is defined as "a pervasive life force, manifestation of a higher self, source of will and self-determination, and a sense of meaning, purpose and connectedness that people experience in the context of their environment" (Canadian Association of

Occupational Therapists, 1997, p. 182). This definition is one of many proposed views of spirituality in the model. For example, Urbanowski and Vargo (1994) propose a definition of spirituality as "the experience of meaning in everyday life activities" (p. 91). This definition is somewhat narrower than the following view of spirituality proposed by Egan and DeLaat (1994): "The individual's spirit is, in fact, the individual. At the core of each person is a being, a spirit, which is an integral part of the universe and exists and remains whole despite injury or illness" (p. 96). Consequently, the definition of spirituality continues to evolve in this model and depends on which author is writing about it.

Law et al. (1997) note that recognizing people as spiritual means:

◆ Recognizing their intrinsic value
◆ Respecting their beliefs, values, and goals

Social and cultural experiences, which are also proposed to be part of the person, are described as:

◆ Influencing people's view of themselves
◆ Shaping the meaning people experience in everyday life
◆ Connecting people to others

Performance components are the final components of the person. They are recognized as falling in three domains:

◆ Physical (sensory, motor, and sensorimotor functions)
◆ Affective (social and emotional functions)
◆ Cognitive (mental functions)

The **environment** is defined as "contexts and situations which occur outside individuals and elicit responses from them" (Law et al., 1997, p. 44). The environment includes institutional, physical, social, and cultural dimensions. The physical dimension includes the natural and built material environment. The social dimension includes social priorities about all elements of the environment, patterns of relationships of people living in an organized community, and social groupings based on common interests, values, attitudes, and beliefs. The cultural dimension includes the ethnic, racial, ceremonial, and routine practices based on customs and value systems of particular groups. The institutional dimension includes societal institutions and practices, including policies, decision-making processes, procedures, accessibility, and other organizational practices.

The final aspect of this model's theory is a developmental perspective. According to Law et al. (1997), this means that "the relationship between persons, the environment, and occupation changes over the lifespan in response to the opportunities and challenges that shape each person's occupational life course" (p. 47). It is recognized that the life course may include positive and negative transformations precipitated by personal, occupational, or environmental changes.

Problems and Challenges

The focus of problems in this model is occupational performance (i.e., difficulties engaging in productive, leisure, and self-care activities). Fearing, Law, and Clark (1997) list as examples of such problems a child's inability to participate in a previously valued activity such as a video game, an adult's inability to use public transportation, and an older person's inability to climb stairs and thereby gain access to the bathroom in the home.

It is recognized that problems of occupational performance may be precipitated by:

◆ Personal factors such as a developmental delay or acquired impairment
◆ Occupational factors such as an occupation becoming obsolete in the face of new technology

◆ Environmental factors such as limitations of access and inclusion in the community (Fearing, Law, & Clark, 1997; Law et al., 1997; Townsend, 1998)

While occupational performance problems may be precipitated by any of the above factors; the mismatch between person and environment or occupation is at their basis. Thus, occupational performance problems occur when:

◆ Changes in the person-environment-occupation balance can negatively influence occupational performance (i.e., the choice, organization, or ability to do occupations)
◆ Incompatibility of person-environment-occupation can negatively influence occupational performance (Fearing et al., 1997)

Therapeutic Intervention

As McColl and Pranger (1994) note, the model is not explicit in detailing a rationale or explanation of the therapeutic process. Consequently, the most important contribution of this model to explaining therapy has been discussion of the nature and process of client-centered practice.

While the model does not offer an explanation of the dynamics of such practice and how it achieves change, it provides a description of the process of such practice.

Law, Baptiste, and Mills (1995) note that client-centered practice is an approach that embraces a philosophy of respect and partnership with those receiving occupational therapy services. Fearing et al. (1997) define client-centered practice as "an alliance formed between client and therapist to use their combined skills and strengths to work

towards client goals related to occupational performance" (p. 8).

Law et al. (1997) note that client-centered practice refers to a collaborative approach that respects clients and involves them in decision-making. Recognizing the uniqueness of each client, client-centered practice is distinguished by the following elements that define the client-therapist relationship:

◆ The therapist maintains respect for the client's opinions regarding individual health care needs
◆ The responsibility for designing an individual's therapy program is shared by the client and therapist
◆ The therapist is responsible for providing information to facilitate the client's task of making decisions about his or her occupational needs. In addition, the therapist offers professional expertise that fosters a range of solutions to occupational performance issues

The client-centered approach recognizes the need to individualize the therapeutic assessment and intervention. This approach requires flexibility, places the emphasis on learning and problem solving, and maintains the focus on the client's goals. It is based on the beliefs that clients have unique knowledge of their own occupational lives and thus know their needs better than anyone else (Canadian Association of Occupational Therapists, 1997).

The basis for client-centered practice has been described as enablement (Polatajko, 1992). Enablement refers to a process in which things are done *with* clients instead of to or for them.

It is defined as "facilitating, guiding, coaching, educating, prompting, listening, reflecting, encouraging, or otherwise collaborating

> **The most important contribution of this model to explaining therapy has been discussion of the nature and process of client-centered practice.**

with people so that individuals, groups, agencies, or organizations have the means and opportunity to participate in shaping their own lives" (Law et al., 1997, p. 50). This process of enablement is guided by the following principles:

> **Enablement refers to a process in which things are done *with* clients instead of to or for them.**

◆ Basing practice on clients' values, meaning, and choice
◆ Listening to clients' visions
◆ Facilitating clients to envision possibilities
◆ Supporting clients' examination of risks and consequences
◆ Supporting clients to succeed
◆ Respecting clients' styles of coping or changing
◆ Guiding clients to identify needs from their perspective
◆ Facilitating clients to select meaningful outcomes (even if they differ from the therapist's perspective)
◆ Providing information to answer clients' questions
◆ Offering services without overwhelming bureaucracy
◆ Fostering open and clear communication
◆ Inviting clients to utilize their own strengths and community supports (Law et al., 1997).

Papers have also elaborated the idea that the client can be the family and other entities, including agencies and organizations (Darrah, Law, & Pollock, 2001; Law et al., 1997; Townsend, 1998). Moreover, it has also been emphasized that client-centered practice requires that therapists acknowledge economic, political, social, and other contextual factors that may influence a client's occupational performance and choices about how to cope (Canadian Association of Occupational Therapists, 1997; Townsend, 1993). It may also mean "working with organizations to reduce barriers and to create opportunities for safe and fair occupational conditions" (Townsend, 1998, p. 4).

Central to the client-centered process with this model is use of the Canadian Occupational Performance Measure (an assessment procedure discussed below) as part of a process of assessment and goal setting in therapy (Pollack, 1993). Clients are facilitated to identify and define their own problems and share responsibility with the therapist in deciding the goals and processes of therapy.

Technology for Application

The occupational performance process originally introduced by Fearing et al. (1997), elaborated by Stanton, Kramer & Thompson-Franson (1997) and more recently discussed by Fearing and Clark (2000), is proposed as an overall framework for implementing client-centered practice and for using the conceptualization of occupational performance. This process includes the following seven stages:

◆ Naming, validating and prioritizing the client's occupational performance issues (what the client considers to be important and requiring occupational therapy intervention)
◆ Selecting appropriate theoretical approaches to address the problems and guide the remaining steps of the process
◆ Identifying occupational performance components and environmental conditions contributing to the identified problems in occupational performance (this stage involves determining what to assess, selecting methods to gather information, and analyzing the findings)
◆ Identifying client strengths and resources

that can assist in resolving the occupational performance problems

◆ Negotiating targeted outcomes and developing action plans to achieve those outcomes

◆ Implementing the plans by reducing limitations in performance components and/or in the environment

◆ Evaluating the occupational performance outcomes

In addition to providing guidelines for achieving the aim of each stage, Stanton et al. (1997) offer a series of reflective questions that are designed to facilitate reasoning in each stage. The text, *Individuals in Context: A Practical Guide to Client-Centered Practice* (Fearing & Clark, 2000), provides a detailed discussion of the issues involved in each stage and offers principles, guidelines, and examples that illustrate how to undertake each stage.

While the occupational performance process is similar to occupational therapy processes described elsewhere (American Occupational Therapy Association, 2002), Stanton et al. (1997) emphasize that the performance process is specifically designed to illuminate the client-centered process. Discussion of the process does highlight how the process is undertaken as a partnership between the client and therapist.

 # The Canadian Occupational Performance Measure

The Canadian Occupational Performance Measure (COPM) was first published in 1990 (Law et al., 1990; Law et al., 1991). It has been revised to reflect research findings and insights from practice. The assessment is designed to assist the client and therapist in identifying problems in self-care, productiv-ity, and leisure (Carpenter, Baker, & Tydesley, 2001). It considers the client the expert on his/her own situation and aims to facilitate client's identification of priorities as guides for the therapy process. The COPM is intended to be used as an outcome measure and therefore is administered not only at the beginning of therapy but also at appropriate intervals or at discharge to capture change (Law et al., 1994). The COPM is supported by a user's manual and videotape.

The COPM includes a semi-structured interview designed to help the client identify and articulate occupational performance problems. The client first rates the importance of each of these issues and then selects the five that are most important or pressing. These five are then rated on two 10-point scales, one on which the client evaluates how well he/she performs and a second on which the client indicates satisfaction with performance. When the COPM is readministered to measure progress, the five identified areas are rated again by the client.

Identified strengths of this assessment are that it can be used with a wide range of clients (Pollack, 1993; Toomey, Nicholson, & Carswell, 1995) and actively engages clients in a collaborative process while encouraging responsibility for their own therapy (Carpenter et al., 2001; Mew & Fossey, 1996; Toomey, Nicholson, & Carswell, 1995).

There are a number of applications of the Canadian model of occupational performance described in the literature. For example, writers use the model to frame the challenges and needs of feeding infants with congenital heart disease (Imms, 2001), postmenopausal women with osteoporosis (Grant & Lundon, 1998), school-aged children with physical disabilities (Pollock & Stewart, 1998), and homeless persons in a shelter (Tryssenaar, Jones, & Lee, 1999). Waters (1995) provides a case example of using the COPM with a client recovering from a depressive episode.

Some papers describe programs based on this model. Healy and Rigby (1999) describe a program that promotes independent occupational performance in teenagers and young adults with physical disabilities, and Herzberg and Finlayson (2001) describe a program for persons in a homeless shelter. The texts *Client-Centered Occupational Therapy* (Law, 1998), *Enabling Occupation: An Occupational Therapy Perspective* (Canadian Association of Occupational Therapists, 1997), and *Individuals in Context: A Practical Guide to Client-Centered Practice* (Fearing & Clark, 2000) also provide a number of case and program examples.

Research

Over 20 studies have been published related to this model. Most of the research reported has focused on development and examination of the COPM. Some studies have also examined the influence of client-centered concepts on practice and its outcomes.

Studies Related to the COPM

Studies of the COPM have examined the reliability, validity, and clinical utility of the assessment. Overall, these studies provide evidence of the stability of the assessment, support its validity, and indicate that it can be a useful assessment. Some limitations identified in the literature are due to the lack of standardization of the assessment and its inappropriateness for clients who do not have insight into their own performance and goals. Below, some of the major studies examining the instrument are briefly reviewed.

Law et al. (1994) pilot-tested the COPM and found that it takes approximately 30 minutes to administer, effectively identifies a range of occupational performance issues, and is responsive to changes in clients' perception of change in occupational performance over time.

Sewell and Singh (2001) studied reliability and provided evidence that the COPM was stable across time in 15 clients with chronic obstruct pulmonary disease.

Chan and Lee (1997) examined the content and criterion validity of the COPM with clients with orthopedic and stroke-related impairments. Using a panel of experts, they concluded that the COPM's strength is in incorporating client perspectives and that its weakness is in measuring occupational performance and performance components of clients. They also found evidence of low concurrent validity (i.e., the COPM was not correlated as expected with other measures). They concluded that the instrument is less than desirable in providing "adequate information to directly enhance meaningful clinical reasoning of therapists" (Chan & Lee, 1997, p. 244), which they attribute to its nonstandardized testing processes.

Ripat et al. (2001) examined concurrent validity of the COPM with another self-report of performance. Although there was no correlation between the two measures, a secondary analysis that compared only areas of occupational performance rated by clients on the COPM produced an expected correlation.

McColl et al. (2000) examined the COPM with former consumers of occupational therapy. They found evidence of the construct validity of the COPM (i.e., COPM scores were correlated with measures of performance, life satisfaction, and community integration). They also reported that clients found the COPM understandable and useful in identifying and evaluating their problems.

Carpenter, Baker, and Tyldesley (2001) examined the COPM with clients in a pain management program and found mixed evidence concerning concurrent validity (i.e., the baseline COPM was not correlated with concurrent measures of psychological functioning; however, follow-up COPM was correlated with these measures). There were significant differences between baseline and outcome COPM measures, indicating the instrument was sensitive to capture change.

Chesworth et al. (2002) studied the COPM with clients who received mental health occupational therapy services. Their findings indicated that the COPM was appropriate for detecting significant changes in this group. Bodiam (1999) examined the COPM with 17 clients with neurological disorders and concluded that it was appropriate and sensitive to measure change in this group.

A study by Wressel, Marcusson, and Henriksson (2002) found that the COPM was helpful in goal setting and treatment planning, unless clients had poor insight or were seen in acute settings. Toomey, Nicholson & Carswell (1995) found that the COPM's usefulness depended on the extent to which therapists incorporated a client-centered approach to practice and could use it flexibly to fit the practice context. While the COPM has been designed to be an outcomes measure, the

results of the COPM can be misleading when used to capture change because of how the scores are calculated (Healy & Rigby, 1999).

Overall, the research on the COPM appears to have the following implications. The COPM works well as an overall process for enabling the client to identify personal concerns and priorities to be addressed in therapy. It provides a client-focused viewpoint on change in therapy, although care must be taken in interpreting the meaning of numerical scores obtained with the COPM. Mixed evidence concerning concurrent validity appears, in part, to be due to the selection of concurrent indicators. That is, the COPM tends to correlate well with other measures that capture the client's perception or experience but not so consistently with objective measures of performance. Such findings indicate that the COPM should not be confused with or considered a substitute for measures of actual performance. On the other hand, it is an appropriate place to begin when the goal is to obtain the client's view of his or her own situation. Finally, the COPM is most useful with clients who have the knowledge, insights, and attitudes consistent with what the instrument asks the client to do (i.e., to reflect on, evaluate, and prioritize areas of personal performance).

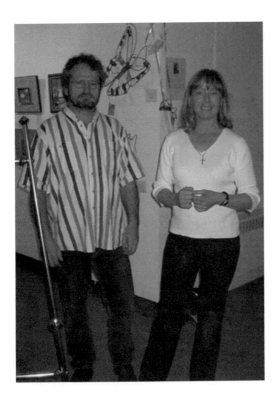

At an art exhibition and auction, Canadian occupational therapists provide opportunities, support, and social connections to empower mental health consumers to contribute to their communities and receive recognition for their talents.

Use and Outcomes of Client-Centered Principles in Practice

Blain and Townsend (1993) examined the impact of the guidelines produced in the 1980s on practice in Canada. This study found that the guidelines were most widely used in acute and rehabilitation services. It also pointed out that practitioners reacted with mixed interpretations of the model of occupational performance, especially the environmental and spiritual components.

Wilkins et al. (2001) examined barriers to implementing client-centered practice, identifying three types of barriers:

◆ Systems barriers related to the lack of an overall client-centered philosophy along with impeding policies and structures in the health services organization
◆ Therapists' understanding, acceptance, and skills for such practice
◆ Client factors, including the ability and willingness of clients to engage in a collaborative process

In a controlled study by Wressle et al. (2002), the researchers found that using the COPM improved client participation in the rehabilitation process.

Hammell (2001b) argues that the client-centered emphasis of this model requires qualitative research guided by client questions that illuminates the complexities of living with a disability and of clinical practice. While this kind of research has not been reported to date, it would appear that Hammell correctly identifies it as an appropriate direction for future inquiry.

🌿 Discussion

The Canadian model of occupational performance is widely used in Canada and has received attention in other parts of the world. In particular, the ideas of client-centered practice and the use of the COPM have been widely adopted. This model has two foci: (1) the concept of client-centered practice and (2) the conceptualization of occupational performance and the factors that influence it. The important contribution of this model has been to identify the importance of a client-centered collaborative approach to practice. It has helped the field to become more aware of the need to organize practice around client experience, knowledge, and desires. As stated in the original *Guidelines for Client-Centered Practice of* *Occupational Therapy* (Department of National Health and Welfare & Canadian Association of Occupational Therapists, 1983):

> The role of the occupational therapist is to facilitate the individual's engagement with his environment. An essential component of the therapeutic relationship is the therapist/client interaction and the exchange which occurs throughout the learning situation created by the occupational therapist. (p. 10)

This statement appeared to establish the therapist-client relationship as the central concern for this model. Given that the field's predominant view of the therapist-client relationship had previously been defined by psychodynamic concepts of the mechanistic paradigm, the prospect of a redefinition of this process from social science concepts that illuminated issues of power and decision-making in the therapeutic relationship was and remains important. It is interesting that this element of the model has received less attention then the conceptualization of occupational performance. Certainly, useful guidelines and procedures related to client-centered practice have been proposed, but the theoretical and empirical examination of the dynamics of the therapist-client relationship has not been a primary focus of this model, as might have been expected given its original vision.

The conceptualization of occupational performance offered by this model is still under development. McColl and Pranger (1994) offered a thoughtful critique of the COPM as it existed in the mid-1990s. They concluded that while the model is comprehensive it "leaves several important relationships unexplained (p. 258). To an extent, their criticism still holds, as the model is more descriptive than explanatory: it defines occupational performance and identifies personal and environmental factors that influence it. The model also states some assumptions and beliefs, and makes some statements concerning how factors influencing occupational performance are interrelated. However, inasmuch as no substantial explanatory theory is offered, this model serves as a broad framework for thinking about practice. The fact that one of the recommended steps in the occupational performance process is selection of appropriate theory (McColl, 2000) underscores the fact that this model's concepts do not directly address the dynamics by which intervention works.

Moreover, because the model offers limited theory to guide practice, it has to be used in conjunction with other practice models that are based on the specific needs of the client. This is recognized and recommended by the model's proponents (Canadian Association of Occupational Therapists, 1997; Fearing et al., 1997). Indeed, some consider it a strength that this model offers a unique perspective on client-centered practice, which can be combined with a range of other models that provide more specific details for intervention.

One of the more controversial aspects of this model's conceptualization of occupational performance is its inclusion of spirituality as a central component of the individual. Originally, spirituality was proposed as one component of the human being. However, following the recommendation of Egan and DeLaat (1994), spirituality was reconceptualized as the innermost core of the individual. Despite the centrality given to spirituality in the model, authors continue to debate the precise meaning of spirituality and its difference from both religiosity and from preexisting concepts in occupational therapy. Even proponents of spirituality have acknowledged that its imprecise definition and the semantic ambiguity of the term make it difficult to apply in practice (Urbanowski & Vargo, 1994). Smith (1997) objected to spirituality as the core and proposed instead that occupation should be the core of the model. Hammell (2001a) also criticized the centrality of spirituality, arguing that it leads to ambiguity and misunderstanding. She recommended replacing it with a concept of instrinsicality (a focus on personal values and priorities). Unruh, Versnel, and Kerr (2002) identify a number of concerns associated with the concept of spirituality, including practitioners' discomfort and the term's potential for harm. Identifying that the definition of spirituality does not coincide well with how it is defined in other fields, they recommend that the concept of occupational identity might be a more appropriate concept for the model. No matter what position is taken for or against the spirituality concept, authors appear to agree that

TERMS OF THE MODEL	
Occupational performance	The ability to choose, organize, and satisfactorily perform meaningful occupations
Client-centered practice	An alliance formed between client and therapist to use their combined skills and strengths to work toward client goals related to occupational performance
Spirituality	A pervasive life force; manifestation of a higher self; source of will and self-determination; and a sense of meaning, purpose, and connectedness that people experience in the context of their environment
Environment	Contexts and situations that occur outside individuals and elicit responses from them

its meaning and application in practice needs clarification.

While the concepts of client-centered practice and the COPM are primary strengths of this model, they can also be a limitation. Some clients are not able or ready to participate in the kind of collaboration envisioned in client-centered practice or required by the assessment (Law et al., 1990; Toomey, Nicholson, & Carswell, 1995; Trysenaar et al., 1999). Nonetheless, this model's attention to the dynamics of therapy and its espousal of a process that empowers and enables clients is an important contribution to the field.

Summary: The Canadian Model of Occupational Performance

◆ Began as guidelines for quality assurance in the practice of occupational therapy in Canada
Includes two key features:
   1. Client-centered perspective
   2. Occupational performance model
◆ A generic model used with different types of clients and in any type of therapy setting

Interdisciplinary Base

◆ Based on:
   1. Client-centered practice as proposed by Carl Rogers (1951)
   2. Concepts of empowerment and justice
   3. Occupational therapy perspective by Reed and Sanderson (1980)
   4. Occupational therapy ideas concerning nature and role of occupation in human life

Focus

◆ Process of therapy and relationship between client and therapist
◆ Occupational performance

Theory
Organization

◆ Includes a statement of a series of values and beliefs concerning occupation, person, environment, health, and client-centered practice
◆ Conceptualizes occupational performance as the result of a dynamic relationship among persons, environment, and occupation over the life span
◆ Person is seen as an integrated whole who incorporates spirituality, social and cultural experiences, and observable occupational performance components
◆ Environment is defined as contexts and situations that occur outside individuals and elicit responses from them; includes institutional, physical, social, and cultural dimensions
◆ Relationship among person, environment, and occupation changes over life span in response to opportunities and challenges that shape each person's occupational life course

Problems and Challenges

◆ The focus of problems in this model is occupational performance (i.e., difficulties engaging in productive, leisure, and self-care activities)
◆ These problems occur when:
   1. Changes in person-environment-occupation balance negatively influence occupational performance
   2. Incompatibility of person-environment-occupation negatively influences occupational performance

Therapeutic Intervention

◆ Focus on client-centered practice is distinguished by:
   1. Therapist's respect for client's opinions
   2. Responsibility shared by client and therapist
   3. Therapist providing information to

facilitate the client's task of making decision's about his/her occupational needs
◆ Basis for client-centered practice is enablement: facilitating, guiding, coaching, educating, prompting, listening to, reflecting on, encouraging, or otherwise collaborating with people to participate in shaping their lives
◆ Use of the Canadian Occupational Performance Measure is central

Technology for Application

◆ Occupational performance process includes seven stages:
  1. Naming, validating, and prioritizing client's occupational performance issues
  2. Selecting appropriate theoretical approaches to address problems
  3. Identifying occupational performance components and environmental conditions contributing to identified problems in occupational performance
  4. Identifying client strengths and resources
  5. Negotiating targeted outcomes and developing action plans
  6. Implementing plan
  7. Evaluating occupational performance outcomes
◆ Canadian Occupational Performance Measure:
  1. Designed to help client and therapist identify problems in self-care, productivity, and leisure
  2. Considers client as expert on his/her own situation and aims to facilitate client's identification of priorities for therapy
  3. Intended to be used as an outcome measure

Research

◆ Over 20 studies have been published
◆ Most focused on development and examination of the COPM

◆ Some examined influence of client-centered concepts on practice and its outcomes

Discussion

◆ Central contribution of this model has been to identify importance of a client-centered collaborative approach to practice
◆ Conceptualization of occupational performance offered by this model is still under development because it more descriptive than explanatory
◆ A controversial aspect of this model is inclusion of spirituality

References

American Occupational Therapy Association (2002). Occupational therapy practice framework: Domain and process. American Journal of Occupational Therapy, 56 (6), 609-639.

Blain, J & Townsend, E. (1993). Occupational therapy guidelines for client-centered practice: Impact study findings. Canadian Journal of Occupational Therapy, 60 (5), 271-285.

Bodiam, C. (1999). The use of the Canadian Occupational Performance Measure for the assessment of outcome on a neurorehabilitation unit. British Journal of Occupational Therapy, 62 (3), 123-126.

Canadian Association of Occupational Therapists (1997). Enabling Occupation: An Occupational Therapy Perspective. Ottawa, Ontario: CAOT Publications ACE.

Carpenter, L, Baker, GA, & Tyldesley, B. (2001). The use of the Canadian Occupational Performance Measure as an outcome of pain management program. Canadian Journal of Occupational Therapy, 68 (1), 16-22.

Chan, CCH & Lee, TMC. (1997). Validity of the Canadian Occupational Performance Measure. Occupational Therapy International, 4(3), 229-247.

Chesworth, C, Duffy, R, Hodnett, J, et al. (2002). Measuring clinical effectiveness in mental health: is the Canadian Occupational Performance an appropriate measure? British Journal of Occupational Therapy, 65(1), 30-34.

Darrah, J, Law, M & Pollock, N. (2001). Innovations in practice: Family-centered functional therapy—a choice for children with motor dysfunction. Infants & Young Children, 13(4), 79-87.

Department of National Health and Welfare and Canadian Association of Occupational Therapists (1983). Guidelines for the Client-Centered Practice of Occupational Therapy. Ottawa, Ontario: Minister of Supply and Services Canada, Cat. No. H39-33/1983E.

Department of National Health and Welfare and Canadian Association of Occupational Therapists (1986). Intervention Guidelines for the Client-Centered Practice of Occupational Therapy. Ottawa, Ontario: Minister of Supply and Services Canada, Cat. No.H39-100/1986E.

Department of National Health and Welfare and Canadian Association of Occupational Therapists (1987). Toward Outcome Measures in Occupational Therapy. Ottawa, Ontario: Minister of Supply and Services Canada.

Egan, M & DeLaat, MD. (1994). Considering spirituality in occupational therapy practice. Canadian Journal of Occupational Therapy, 60, 232-240.

Fearing, VG & Clark, J. (2000) Individuals in Context: A Practical Guide to Client-Centered Practice. Thorofare, NJ: Slack.

Fearing, VG, Law, M & Clark, J. (1997). An occupational performance process model: Fostering client and therapist alliances. Canadian Journal of Occupational Therapy, 64 (1), 7-15.

Grant, DD & Lundon, K. (1998). The Canadian Model of Occupational Performance applied to females with osteoporosis. Canadian Journal of Occupational Therapy, 66 (1), 3-13.

Hammell, KW. (2001a). Intrinsicality: Reconsidering spirituality, meaning(s) and mandates. Canadian Journal of Occupational Therapy, 68 (3), 186-194.

Hammell, KW. (2001b). Using qualitative research to inform the client-centered evidence-based practice of occupational therapy. British Journal of Occupational Therapy, 64(5), 228-234.

Healy, H & Rigby, P. (1999). Promoting independence for teens and young adults with physical disabilities. Canadian Journal of Occupational Therapy, 66(5), 240-249.

Herzberg, G & Finlayson, M. (2001). Development of occupational therapy in a homeless shelter. Occupational Therapy in Health Care, 13(4), 133-147.

Imms, C. (2001). Feeding the infant with congenital heart disease: An occupational performance challenge. American Journal of Occupational Therapy, 55(3), 277-284.

Law, M. (ed.). (1998). Client-Centered Occupational Therapy. Thorofare, NJ: Slack.

Law, M, Baptist, S, Carswell-Opzoomer, A, et al. (1991). Canadian Occupational Performance Measure. Toronto, CAOT Publications ACE.

Law, M, Baptist, S, McColl, MA, et al. (1990). The Canadian Occupational Performance Measure: An outcome measure for occupational therapy. Canadian Journal of Occupational Therapy, 57 (2), 82-87.

Law, M, Baptiste, S & Mills, J. (1995). Client-centered practice: What does it mean and does it make a difference? Canadian Journal of Occupational Therapy, 62 (5), 250-257.

Law, M, Polatajko, H, Baptiste, S, et al. (1997). Core concepts of occupational therapy. In Townsend, E. (ed.). Enabling Occupation: An Occupational Therapy Perspective. Ottawa, Ontario: CAOT Publications ACE.

Law, M., Polatajko, H, Pollack, N, et al. (1994). Pilot testing of the Canadian Occupational Performance measure: Clinical and measurement issues. Canadian Journal of Occupational Therapy, 61 (4), 191-197.

McColl, MA. (2000). Selecting a theoretical approach. In Fearing, VG & Clark, J (eds.). Individuals in Context: A Practical Guide to Client-Centered Practice. Thorofare, NJ: Slack.

McColl, MA, Paterson, M, Davies, D, et al. (2000). Validity and community utility of the Canadian Occupational Performance Measure. Canadian Journal of Occupationl Therapy, 67(1), 22-30.

McColl, MA & Pranger, T. (1994). Theory and practice in the occupational therapy guidelines for client-centered practice. Canadian Journal of Occupational Therapy, 61(5), 250-259.

Mew, MM & Fossey, E. (1996). Client-centered aspects of clinical reasoning during an initial assessment using the Canadian Occupational Performance Measure . Australian Occupational Therapy Journal, 43(3/4), 155-166.

Polatajko, HJ. (1992). Naming and framing occupational therapy: A lecture dedicated to the life of Nancy B. Canadian Journal of Occupational Therapy, 59(4), 189-200.

Pollack, N. (1993). Client-centered assessment. American Journal of Occupational Therapy, 47(4), 298-301.

Pollock, N & Stewart, D. (1998). Occupational needs of school-aged children with physical disabilities in the community. Physical and Occupational Therapy in Pediatrics, 18(1), 55-68.

Reed, K & Sanderson, SR. (1980). Concepts of occupational therapy. Baltimore: Williams & Wilkins.

Ripat, J, Etcheverry, E, Cooper, J, et al. (2001). A comparison of the Canadian Occupational Performance Measure and the Health Assessment Questionnaire. Canadian Journal of Occupational Therapy, 68(4), 247-253.

Rogers, CR. (1951). Client-Centered Therapy: Its Current Practice, Implications, and Theory. Boston: Houghton Mifflin.

Sewell, L & Singh, SJ. (2001). The Canadian Occupational Performance Measure: Is it a reliable measure in clients with chronic obstructive pulmonary disease? British Journal of Occupational Therapy, 64 (6), 305-310.

Smith, L. (1997). Spirituality questioned as profession's center. Canadian Journal of Occupational Therapy, 64, 271.

Stanton, S, Kramer, C & Thompson-Frason, T. (1997). Linking concepts to a process for organizing occupational therapy services. In Townsend, E. (ed.). Enabling Occupation: An Occupational Therapy Perspective. Ontario, Ontario: CAOT Publications ACE.

Toomey, M, Nicholson, D & Carswell, A. (1995). The clinical ability of the Canadian Occupational Performance Measure. Canadian Journal of Occupational Therapy, 62(5), 242-249.

Townsend, E. (1998). Using Canada's 1997 guidelines for enabling occupation. Australian Occupational Therapy Journal, 45, 1-6.

Townsend, EA. (1993). Occupational therapy's social vision. Canadian Journal of Occupational Therapy, 60, 174-184.

Tryssenaar, J, Jones, E & Lee, D. (1999). Occupational performance needs of a shelter population. Ergotherapie, 66(4), 174-184.

Unruh, AM, Versnel, J & Kerr, N. (2002). Spirituality unplugged: A review of commonalities and contentions and a resolution. Canadian Journal of Occupational Therapy 69(1), 5-19.

Urbanowski, R & Vargo, J. (1994). Spirituality, daily practice, and the occupational performance model. Canadian Journal of Occupational Therapy, 61(2), 88-94.

Waters, D. (1995). Recovering from a depressive episode using the Canadian Occupational Performance Measure. Canadian Journal of Occupational Therapy, 62(4), 84-92.

Wilkins, S, Pollack, N, Rochon, S, et al. (2001). Implementing client-centered practice: Why is it so difficult to do? Canadian Journal of Occupational Therapy, 68 (2), 70-79.

Wressle, E, Marcusson, J & Henriksson, C. (2002). Clinical utility of the Canadian Occupational Performance Measure—Swedish version. Canadian Journal of Occupational Therapy, 69(1), 40-48.

Wressle, E, Eeg-Olofsson, AM, Marcusson, J, et al. (2002). Improved client participation in the rehabilitation process using a client-centered goal formulation structure. Journal of Rehabilitation Medicine, 34, 5-11.

Chapter 8

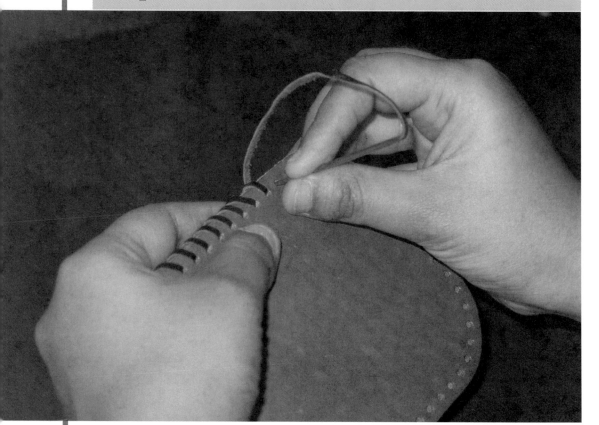

The Cognitive Disabilities Model

A client works with a small piece of leather with pre-punched holes. Following instructions given by the therapist, the client attempts to complete a leather lacing stitch. Based on the client's performance in this task, the therapist will draw conclusions about the client's extent of cognitive impairment. The leather lacing task used to assess the client's cognitive level reflects one of the key tenets of the cognitive disabilities model: that deficiencies in cognitive processing result in observable limitations in performance.

The cognitive disabilities model originated as an approach to persons with mental illness, and it is now applied to other groups of clients in whom **cognitive limitations** are observed (e.g., those with traumatic brain injury and dementia). This model began with an interest in describing the kinds of limitations persons exhibited in processing information during task performance. It continues to focus on impairments that result from medical or psychiatric conditions and emphasizes evaluation of clients' functional limitations (Allen & Earhart, 1992). There is also a strong emphasis on issuing warnings about clients' restricted capacity and on achieving necessary supervision, environmental modification, and/or legal restriction of patients to prevent hazardous situations (Allen & Earhart, 1992).

As the name of the model implies, the approach to functional limitations is based on concern for underlying **cognitive capacity.** According to this model, cognitive disability refers to an "incapacity to process information necessary to do ordinary activities safely" (Allen, 1992, p. 1) that results from medical conditions that restrict how the brain operates.

This model conceptualizes cognition as a single hierarchical continuum from more to less cognitive ability. The model describes the cognitive abilities and limitations in terms of cognitive levels graded hierarchically from the highest level of function to profoundly impaired function. Use of these cognitive levels to describe the extent of functional limitation and to guide the therapist's decision-making about client care is the core feature of how this model is applied. Consequently, the model seeks to achieve a description of clients' cognitive impairment (in terms of the level of cognitive functioning), from which therapists can determine appropriate intervention goals and advise others about the potential of clients to be safe and to learn.

Interdisciplinary Base

The cognitive disabilities model is derived from several sources. It began with attempts to classify the performance difficulties of clients by using concepts from Piaget's work on cognition, particularly his description of the sensorimotor period of development. The originator of this model, Claudia Allen, originally expected that cognitive capacities could be redeveloped in persons who had lost them, but she later abandoned this idea.

This model originally claimed to be based on the concepts of neuroscience. However, there is minimal reference to current neurological concepts. Moreover, the model draws different conclusions about the possibility of improving functioning than do other occupational therapy approaches based on neuroscience. These other models emphasize neuroplasticity and the potential for bringing about change through therapy. The cognitive disabilities model recommends against a focus on changing the individual through therapy. Allen (1987) points out that she avoided theories that assumed learning or normal memory because she presumes that these capacities are permanently impaired in persons with chronic psychiatric disease and brain damage.

The cognitive disabilities model was initially influenced by the medical view that functional limitations are directly mediated by neurological damage and change according to the natural history of the disease and/or with medical interventions that directly alter the brain. More recent work (Allen 1992; Allen & Earhart, 1992) seeks to establish a unique focus apart from the medical model. While the medical model stresses the disease process and its eradication and/or control, the cognitive disabilities model focuses on the consequences of the disease (i.e., cognitive limitations that result from diseases). This focus built upon the World Health Organization's previous system* for classifying impairment, disabilities, and handicaps (World Health Organization, 2001). This classification system focused on incapacitation resulting from diseases.

The model also stresses occupational therapy's concentration on adjustment to residual limitations as differentiating occupational therapy from medicine, which is concerned with producing biological change.† According to this model, occupational therapy should acknowledge and focus on the measurement and management of permanent residual limitations, not on altering them.

🌱 Theory

Although the model assumes that brain organization and impairment are the bases of cognitive processing difficulties, it does not seek to explain the brain-behavior relationship or how specific brain impairments affect the quality of cognition underlying action. Rather, the emphasis of the model is on how impairment of cognition affects performance of daily living tasks (Allen, 1992; Allen & Earhart, 1992).

Voluntary motor action was originally specified as the focus for this model. The model defined voluntary motor action as "a behavior response to a sensory cue guided by the mind" (Allen, 1985, p. 6). More recently, communication abilities also have been incorporated into the model. Com-

> **According to this model, occupational therapy should acknowledge and focus on the measurement and management of permanent residual limitations, not on altering them.**

munication abilities are viewed as being a function of cognitive level. Therefore, this model anticipates restrictions in communication when cognition is impaired.

Organization

According to the model, the brain determines cognition, and cognition, in turn, guides behavior (voluntary motor actions). As noted earlier, the explanatory focus is not on the brain-cognition relationship but on the role of cognition in determining task performance. The model has concentrated on two features of cognition:

◆ The cognitive dimensions of task performance
◆ The continuum of cognitive functioning (i.e., the levels of cognitive functioning)

Cognitive Dimensions of Task Performance

Although cognition is not defined in this model, it is noted that cognition involves responding to sensory cues by forming purposes and processing information to guide motor activity. This view of cognition is further explicated in the identification of the following dimensions of task performance: attention, behavior, purpose, experience, process, and time. **Attention** is selective responsiveness to sensory cues. **Behavior** refers to the motor actions exhibited in task performance. **Purpose** connotes the person's intended objective, which guides the

---

*The current WHO classification system uses concepts of activity and participation instead of impairment and disability to de-emphasize focus on limitations reflected in a range of health care approaches and in the earlier system (World Health Organization, 2001).

†Some take issue with the assertion that biological change is the exclusive domain of medicine. Certainly, many of the models discussed in this book assert that participation in occupation can influence biological changes (e.g., muscle fiber size and synaptic connections) that are also manifest as functional changes (e.g., strength, sensory and perceptual abilities).

motor response to a sensory cue. **Experience** is what a person goes through when he or she is involved in a task. **Process** refers to the course of action that is followed to achieve a purpose. **Time** refers to the duration over which a person sustains sensorimotor associations as manifest in ongoing voluntary motor responses to sensory cues. These dimensions were originally used as a basis for describing qualities of task performance across the cognitive levels.

Cognitive Levels

The model proposes a hierarchical continuum divided into six cognitive levels.* While detailed criteria for each level has been developed, the following is an overview of how the levels describe function and impairment (Allen, 1992):

◆ Level 0: Coma

Coma is a prolonged state of unconsciousness, with a lack of specific response to stimuli.

◆ Level 1: Automatic Actions

Automatic actions are a response to a stimulus initiated by someone else and are invariable reactions to the stimulus.

◆ Level 2: Postural Actions

Postural actions are self-initiated gross body movements that overcome the effects of gravity and move the whole body in space.

◆ Level 3: Manual Actions

Manual actions are use of the hands and occasionally other parts of the body to manipulate material objects.

◆ Level 4: Goal-Directed Actions

Goal-directed actions sequence the self through a series of steps to match a concrete sample or a known standard of how the finished product should appear.

◆ Level 5: Exploratory Actions

Exploratory actions are discoveries of how changes in neuromuscular control can produce different effects on material objects.

◆ Level 6: Planned Actions

Planned actions estimate the effect of actions on material objects, but the objects do not have to be present for the estimate to occur. The significance of the effects of a sequence of steps permits anticipation of secondary effects.

These levels have been a part of the cognitive disabilities model from its beginning, although some revision of the definitions of levels has occurred. More recently, intermediate levels have been identified. For example, Level 1 has been subdivided into 1.0 withdrawing, 1.2 responding, 1.4 locating stimuli, 1.6 rolling in bed, and 1.8 raising body part. The addition of these intermediate levels was intended to allow a finer discrimination of cognitive function/limitation (Allen, 1992).

Problems and Challenges

The cognitive disabilities model originally defined **cognitive disability** as "a restriction in voluntary motor action originating in the physical or chemical structures of the brain and producing observable limitations in routine task behavior" (Allen, 1985, p. 31). As the more recent definition given at the beginning of this chapter suggests, the current emphasis is on problems of information processing that compromise safe performance of ordinary activities.

The model still assumes that brain impairment underlies a deficit in mental processes

---

*Although technically there are seven levels when coma is included, the literature consistently refers to six levels; convention is followed here.

or cognition, which, in turn, restricts functional capacity. However, the model does not attempt to explain the nature or etiology of various brain impairments that lead to cognitive disabilities. Rather, the medical model is recommended as the source for explanations for diseases. Medical explanations of the underlying causes of the disability are recommended as important background information for occupational therapy (Allen & Earhart, 1992). The medical model also provides information about prognoses, such as the expected length of current symptoms and prospects for improvement of the condition.

> **The unique view of client problems in this model is its description of the restrictions in task performance that occur in association with disease.**

The unique view of client problems in this model is its description of the restrictions in task performance that occur in association with disease. This model offers the cognitive levels to delineate the extent of cognitive disability. In this regard, it is more descriptive than explanatory.

Therapeutic Intervention

This model makes two important assertions about change. The first is that occupational therapy does not change the cognitive level of clients who have cognitive limitations resulting from brain pathology. Changes in cognitive level are considered either part of the natural course of the disease process or due to the effects of medication. More recently, Allen has qualified that occupational therapy may be associated with changes in cognitive level, but she does not claim a causative link. She argues that other factors, such as natural healing and psychotropic drugs, have more effect than therapy on brain pathology and, therefore, on cognitive changes.

The second assertion is that brain impairments place restrictions on learning; persons at or below Level 4 are considered to have severe restrictions in learning new behaviors. Specifically, it is argued that clients at or below Level 4 do not generalize (Allen, 1992) and that "novelty is ignored at levels one through four, making it impossible to teach new skills" (Allen, 1982, p. 738).

Given these two assertions, the approach to intervention emphasizes monitoring changes in cognitive level and adapting intervention to fit the level at which the client is functioning. Once a client's cognitive level of function is determined to be stable or deteriorating (as in progressive dementias) intervention focuses on environmental modification, providing information and guidelines to caregivers, and other strategies designed to accommodate and manage the client's functional limitations/capacities.

The model offers the following guideline for intervention once a client's level of function is determined. Clients should be offered opportunity to process information at a higher level for a brief period but should not be forced to sustain function that produces discomfort, frustration, or confusion. Clients can struggle with higher function if they desire but should not be pushed. This guideline is based on the argument that it is not useful for persons to work toward function requiring a higher cognitive level than that for which they are judged capable (Allen & Earhart, 1992).

Phases of Treatment

This model divides treatment into four phases of illness (acute, post-acute, rehabilitation, and long-term), each having its own implications for treatment. During the acute phase, the therapist evaluates the client's cognitive level. In the post-acute phase, clients can engage in activities suited to their cognitive level; the therapist continues to monitor any changes in cognitive level and makes recommendations for how much assistance will be needed on discharge. Allen (1992) argues that when clients are in the rehabilitation phase, there is little or no change in cognitive level expected. Therefore, the emphasis is on improving client performance by providing adaptive equipment, modifying the environment, and teaching caregivers to provide assistance. At this stage, activity analysis allows therapists to provide activities of an appropriate level to the client. Moreover, activities beyond the client's level of ability can be avoided or done with appropriate modification/supervision. Long-term care refers to the provision of a community-based activity program for people who are functioning at cognitive Levels 3 and 4 (Allen, 1992).

Environmental Compensation

The main approach to treatment is **environmental compensation** for the client's limitations in functional capacity. This approach emphasizes making adjustments to the residual effects of disease rather than addressing the disease process itself (Allen & Earhart, 1992). Since this model does not expect occupational therapy services to affect the cognitive level of clients, cognitive improvement is not a goal of occupational therapy.* Rather, the occupational therapist documents the level of cognitive impairment and provides a task environment in which a client can function (Allen, 1992). According to this model, giving clients tasks that they can do, even with their cognitive limitations, enables them to be more functional.

A further goal of therapy is to enable clients to comprehend and accept their permanent concrete limitations. This is accomplished by providing concrete feedback to the client on task performance. Moreover, the client's cognitive level is used to indicate the type of environment in which the client can

function on discharge. The goal is to identify the least restrictive environment in which a person with cognitive disabilities can function safely (Allen, 1992; Allen & Earhart, 1992). The therapist's role also includes providing caregivers with realistic information about disabled persons' limits and about necessary supports to allow the disabled person to function.

 ## Technology for Application

The cognitive disabilities model provides detailed, specific procedures for client assessment, task analysis, and task selection in treatment.

Client Assessment

Detailed assessments of functional level have been developed for use with the cognitive disabilities model; they include the Routine Task Inventory, Allen Cognitive Level test, and Cognitive Performance Test.

The Routine Task Inventory (RTI) is administered by interviewing the client or by observing the client's performance. Since the reliability of this assessment for clients at Levels 1 to 4 is considered questionable, the RTI may be administered by interviewing a caregiver. When observation is used, it is recommended that more than a single activity be observed, as a single performance may give a biased reading of the client's level. The RTI consists of 32 routine activities such as grooming, dressing, bathing, shopping, and doing laundry as well as more general behavior items such as following instructions, cooperating, and supervising. Each task is described according to each of the six cognitive levels of performance. Matching the client's reported or observed performance to the descriptions under each task enables the therapist to determine the client's level of cognitive functioning.

---

* It is acknowledged that clients functioning at Levels 5 and 6 are capable of learning. However, this model does not provide guidelines for allowing these persons to capitalize on their learning capacity.

The Allen Cognitive Level (ACL) test uses performance in a single activity to provide a quick estimate of the client's cognitive level. Leather lacing is the activity; the cognitive level is determined by the complexity of leather lacing stitch that the client can imitate. Allen has standardized the method of presenting the task and scoring client performance. There are three versions of the ACL. The first version (ACL-O) is designed to measure persons whose level ranges from cognitive Levels 2 to 6. "Lack of sensitivity and other flaws" (Allen, Kehrberg, & Burns, 1992, p. 32) led to the development of the two other versions. The ACL-E has a more detailed score sheet and a modified administration procedure (i.e., the therapist twists the leather lacing to see if the client can correct it). The ACL-PS modifies the presentation of the leather lacing task to see if the client can do it by looking or requires verbal instructions or demonstration. Further revision of the ACL has resulted in yet another version, the ACL-90; this version is commercially available and is the version that is typically used.

The Cognitive Performance Test (CPT) is composed of six activities of daily living tasks: dress, shop, toast, telephone, wash and travel. Each task employs standardized equipment and administration. For example, the dress task consists of asking a client to choose the appropriate attire for the cold, rainy day. The client chooses between a man and woman's heavyweight raincoat, a man and woman's robe, a man's straw hat, a man's rain hat, a woman's plastic rain scarf, a woman's sheer scarf, and an umbrella. The client's choice and behavior in putting on appropriate clothes is used to determine the cognitive level at which the client is functioning.

In addition to these more structured assessments, therapists may observe the client's task performance to monitor his or her cognitive level. Guidelines are provided for identifying the client's cognitive level. Further, the use of tasks with known levels of complexity can be used to gauge the client's functional level. The therapist analyzes the task to determine its cognitive demands and then observes whether the person can perform it.

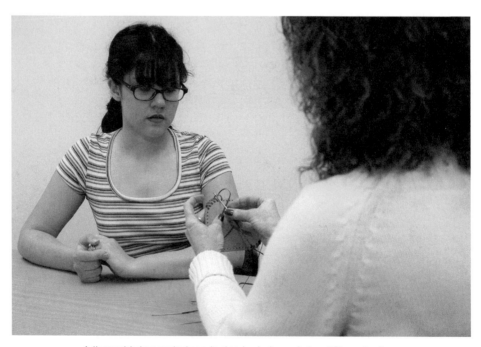

A therapist demonstrates a lacing technique during ACL evaluation.

Use of Assessment Data

Depending on the phase of the client's illness and/or treatment, assessment data may be used to evaluate the course of the disease or effects of medication or to determine the appropriateness of rehabilitation, discharge, supervision, and environmental accommodations. Evaluation is also used to make recommendations for appropriate placement of the client.

Allen and Earhardt (1992) emphasize that careful evaluation of a client's cognitive limitations has important implications for what a client can be considered capable and safe to do, what legal restrictions may be placed on a person, and the kinds of environmental safeguards and support are necessary to manage a person in the community. They link the idea of cognitive disability closely to the legal definitions of competence and the associated idea of ordinary care. **Ordinary care** is a legal term that refers to reasonable effort and judgment according to prevailing cultural norms. Allen and Earhardt indicate that cognitive Level 6 corresponds to what is legally defined as competence. Allen (1992) underscores the role of the occupational therapist in issuing warnings about client cognitive limitations. She indicates, "When necessary, therapists should take steps to initiate legal action (such as removing a driver's license or obtaining a legal guardian)" (p. 14).

Task Analysis

This model emphasizes the importance of **task analysis.** A text on this model includes a number of performance actions (e.g., sanding, gluing, cutting) and activities (e.g., grooming, dressing) that are analyzed according to the cognitive levels (Allen & Earhart, 1992). Analysis of task complexity underlies the entire assessment approach. Moreover, selection and adaptation of tasks for client performance is central to this model's treatment approach. Task analysis begins with determining the normal procedure for performing a task. Then the therapist identifies the relative complexity of steps in the task. It is argued that task analysis can be applied to any activity. Therefore, the client's cognitive

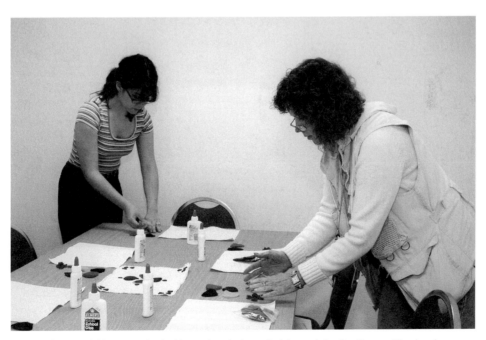

Craft activities are selected based on task analysis to match client's cognitive level.

level (functional ability) can be matched to any task, and it can be determined whether the client has the capacity to perform the task, given its complexity. Then, if necessary, the task can be adapted by changing or eliminating a troublesome step or adjusting the complexity of the task. For example, Allen (1982) notes the differences in complexity of pattern a client can create:

> At Level Three we see a disorganized use of one color; at Level Four the person can follow a checkerboard pattern; at Level Five the person follows a simple pattern and those people at Level Six create a unique pattern. (p. 734)

The final goal of all task analysis is to identify the steps in the process that the client cannot do. Tasks can then be adapted to avoid procedures that clients are unable to perform while allowing them to use remaining abilities. As Allen (1982) notes, the therapist uses "elements of the physical environment as substitutes for deficient patterns of thought that would normally be used to guide behavior" (p. 737). Figure 8-1, p. 119, illustrates the relationship of clients' task behavior, task analysis, and adjustment of task demands. According to this figure, task behavior is a function of the client (including the client's cognitive limitations) and the task demand. The model argues that, because the client's cognitive level cannot be changed, the therapist must analyze the task and adjust the task demand to accommodate the cognitive limitation of the client. This concept (whether applied in selecting tasks for use in therapy or in creating a functional environment for living) is central to how this model is applied.

A more recent feature of this model's approach to task analysis is the provision of guidelines for training in specific tasks, which take into consideration different levels of cognitive impairment. Guidelines are provided for determining what a person of a given cognitive level can do within given types of tasks along with information about how that person can be trained to do the task.

Treatment Applications

Application of the cognitive disabilities model is straightforward and requires very little adaptation for different settings. The model uses a very specific approach to identifying cognitive levels, to analyzing tasks of which persons are capable at those levels, and to providing such tasks as therapy. Descriptions in the literature of application of the model address a range of persons deemed to have cognitive limitations. These include, for example, papers illustrating its use with persons with dementia (Levy, 1988), persons with mental illness (Weissenberg & Giladi, 1989), and persons recovering from cerebrovascular accidents and traumatic brain injury (Allen, 1989).

Allen believes that purposeful activity is the treatment method of occupational therapy. She discusses the importance of focusing on routine tasks in the client's life. Allen (1987) writes that activity provides persons opportunity to use remaining capacities, thereby achieving meaningful involvement and a rightful place in community life. This treatment model strongly emphasizes the use of crafts during the acute phase of illness. According to the model, psychiatric clients prefer crafts because they are easily adapted to the client's functional level and provide tangible evidence of functional capacity (Allen, 1985; Allen, 1992).

> **The model uses a specific approach to identifying cognitive levels, to analyzing tasks of which persons are capable at those levels, and to providing such tasks as therapy.**

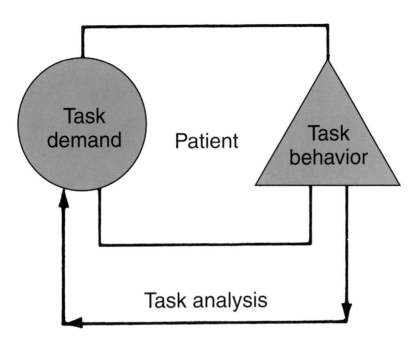

Figure 8-1. The therapist's awareness of the task environment.

🌿 Research

The cognitive disabilities model has generated 17 published studies. Almost all of this research is focused on examination of the psychometric properties of the assessments For example, studies have examined the reliability and concurrent validity of the ACL, RTI, and CPT (Bar-Yosef, Weinblatt, & Katz, 1999; Henry et al., 1998; Keller & Hays, 1998; Secrest, Wood, & Tapp, 2000). Other studies have examined the ability of cognitive level to predict community functioning. Results of these studies have provided mixed evidence concerning whether cognitive levels do predict community functioning (Roitman & Katz, 1996; Velligan et al., 1998). At best, there is sometimes a modest relationship between measures of cognitive level subsequent to community functioning. In some

studies, cognitive level was a poorer predictor of community adjustment than demographic variables such as age, sex, work history, record of hospitalization, and marital history. Such findings raise questions about how accurate and useful cognitive levels are for predicting community adjustment. This is an especially important question to answer as one of the primary uses of cognitive levels is to make decisions about the person's ability for and needs in community functioning (Earhart, 1999).

One pilot study (Raweh & Katz, 1999) examined outcomes of intervention with the cognitive disabilities model. They found that clients receiving services based on this model showed a slightly greater increase in functional performance over a control group as measured by the RTI but not in awareness of disability.

 # Discussion

The cognitive disabilities model seeks to objectively describe limitations in functional performance. The model's view of the nature of cognitive impairment is concise and provides specific methods of assessment and intervention. The model provides specific means for assessing client capacity and matching that capacity to task demands.

The cognitive disabilities model proposes a nontraditional view of the role of participation in activities and its relationship to functional capacity. The issue of whether clients improve and/or maintain capacity from participation in occupation is an important one that needs further scrutiny. Allen (1982) argues that occupational therapists have overstated the effect of activity in producing change as reflected in treatment goals of increasing or enhancing client capacity. She further argues that alternative explanations for improvement, such as the natural course of healing and the effects of other treatments such as medication, have not been sufficiently ruled out. Moreover, she asserts that occupational therapy has failed to recognize the permanent deficits of clients with cognitive disabilities, reasoning that "to deny mental deficits has led to false hope about our ability to resolve them" (p. 734).

Caution about possibly overstated claims for the impact of activity is useful. Furthermore, it is a useful argument that failure to recognize real limitations in persons' capacities may result in blaming them (i.e., attributing lack of performance on motivational factors) and in failing to provide them with necessary supports for functioning. On the other hand, denying that therapy can affect cognitive level and subsequent function is inconsistent with other views of the potential for changing or maintaining capacity in persons with brain injury or disease. While it is important to acknowledge any permanent limitations of capacity, the therapist must be careful not to limit unwittingly the client's opportunities to learn or to develop functional performance. Significant change in a person's functional capacity may take time and/or concentrated efforts. Therefore, it is possible to conclude that change cannot be affected by therapy when, instead, the current health care delivery system does not provide enough resources to bring about change. Moreover, the emphasis on clients' limitations could be used by those who control health policy to justify not expending time and resources to support clients to regain function.

The claim that learning does not occur within a wide range of functioning (Levels 1-4) is not yet substantiated. Because of the seriousness of this claim, it is critical to demonstrate through research whether permanent deficits exist in the learning capacities of persons with cognitive impairment. One pilot study suggested that, while learning differed in groups with different cognitive levels, all clients learned to master some new skills (Katz, Josman, & Steinmetz, 1988). This single study cannot rule out Allen's hypothesis that learning does not occur, but it indicates the importance of research to assess it. Moreover, it will be important to distinguish between those situations in which participation in occupation can produce an improvement and those in which significant improvement in discrete areas of function is not possible or likely.

Allen points out that disease can be a powerful explanation for much of the impairment therapists observe in clients with mental illness. Equally plausible is that the lack of opportunity to use or develop capacities is a source of functional limitation.

Since this model grew out of practice in psychiatric settings, it should also be noted that it represents a departure from traditional psychosocial models that emphasize motivational and emotional factors in functioning. This model has not been concerned directly with motivation, although Allen (1985) acknowledges humans have a need to engage in desirable activities. Moreover, she notes that persons suffer when left with nothing to do, and she argues that persons with disabilities should have access to activities that reflect their interests and desires (Allen, 1982). Her main concern is with the distress that occurs when persons do not have access to task performance. Despite this acknowledged concern, as Sweetingham (1996) points out, the "emphasis on observable behaviors may result in little attention being directed towards the individual's subjective experience" (p. 7).

In more recent work, Allen has recognized motivation as a possible factor influencing quality of performance (Allen & Earhart, 1992). This concern addresses the problem of how to achieve an accurate assessment of ability free of motivational factors. Allen's deemphasis of motivational factors is based on her view that differences in individual performance are more directly linked to actual functional limitations (i.e., the cognitive limitations) than to problems in motivation. No research, however, has demonstrated the relative importance of functional limitations and motivational factors.

Finally, the proposal that cognition can be reduced to a single hierarchical continuum differs from other occupational therapy approaches that argue that cognition is multidimensional. Such approaches suggest that an individualized picture of cognitive strengths and weaknesses is necessary and that a simple categorization of a person's cognitive capacity fails to recognize individual variability in cognitive styles and deficits.

Thus, while the cognitive disabilities model offers a concise formulation of cognitive factors that impact on occupational performance, this precision may be achieved at the expense of oversimplification. Finding the right balance between an adequate conceptualization of the phenomena of concern and having straightforward ideas for application is always difficult. No doubt, this issue will continue to challenge occupational therapists in the future both with regard to this and other conceptual practice models.

TERMS OF THE MODEL

Attention	Selected responsiveness to sensory cues
Behavior	Motor actions exhibited in task performance
Cognitive limitations	Deficits in mental processing that can be observed during task performance
Cognitive capacity	Potential for mental processing
Cognitive dimensions of task performance	Observable aspects of mental activity, including behavior, process, time, experience, and attention
Cognitive disability	Incapacity to process information necessary to do ordinary activities safely
Cognitive levels	System of classification based on complexity of sensorimotor associations demonstrated during performance of a task
Environmental compensation	Changing a task to accommodate for cognitive deficits
Experience	What one goes through when involved in a task

TERMS OF THE MODEL	
Ordinary care	Reasonable effort and judgment according to prevailing cultural norms; this concept is the point of reference for legally determining neglect
Process	Course of action that is followed to achieve a purpose
Purpose	The intended objective that guides the motor response to a sensory cue
Task analysis	Determination of the cognitive demands of an activity
Time	Duration over which a person sustains sensorimotor associations as shown by ongoing voluntary motor responses to sensory cues
Voluntary motor action	Behavioral response to a sensory cue that is guided by the mind

❧ Summary

Focus

◆ Originally an approach to persons with mental illness; now applied to other groups of clients in whom cognitive limitations are observed (e.g., those with traumatic brain injury and dementia)

◆ Focuses on residual limitations and emphasizes:
  1. Evaluation of patients' functional limitations
  2. Issuing cautions and warnings about clients' restricted capacity
  3. Achieving necessary supervision
  4. Environmental modification
  5. Legal restriction of patients to prevent hazards
  6. Cognitive levels (graded from highest function to profoundly impaired function) that are used to describe the extent of functional limitation

Interdisciplinary Base

◆ Piaget's work on cognition, particularly his description of the sensorimotor period of development

◆ Neuroscience (however, the model rejects neuroplasticity and the potential for bringing about change through therapy in persons with chronic psychiatric disease and brain damage)

◆ Emphasizes medical view that functional limitations result from neurological damage and change according to natural history of the disease and/or with medical interventions that directly alter brain

◆ World Health Organization classification of impairment, disabilities, and handicaps, which focuses on incapacitation resulting from diseases

Theory
Organization

◆ Function is based on the relationship of brain, cognition, and task behavior:
  1. Brain determines cognition
  2. Cognition guides behavior (voluntary motor actions)

◆ Concentrates on two features of cognition:
  1. The cognitive dimensions of task performance
  2. The continuum of cognitive functioning (i.e., levels of cognitive functioning)

◆ Cognitive dimensions of task performance (originally used as basis for describing performance across cognitive levels):
1. Attention (selective responsiveness to sensory cues)
2. Behavior (motor actions exhibited in task performance)
3. Purpose (person's intended objective)
4. Experience (what a person goes through when involved in a task)
5. Process (course of action followed to achieve a purpose)
6. Time (duration over which a person sustains sensorimotor associations)

◆ Hierarchical continuum is divided into six cognitive levels (not including coma):
1. Coma (prolonged state of unconsciousness without response to stimuli; not counted as a cognitive level because cognition is absent)
2. Automatic actions (response to stimulus initiated by someone else; invariable reactions to stimulus)
3. Postural actions (self-initiated gross body movements that move the whole body in space)
4. Manual actions (using hands and occasionally other body parts to manipulate objects)
5. Goal-directed actions (series of steps that match a sample or standard of a finished product)
6. Exploratory actions (discover how changes in neuromuscular control produce different effects on objects)
7. Planned actions (estimate effect of actions on objects that are present; anticipate secondary effects)

Problems and Challenges

◆ Brain impairment underlies a deficit in cognition, producing restrictions in task performance
◆ Cognitive levels describe extent of cognitive disability and extent of functional limitation

Therapeutic Intervention

◆ Assertions about change:
1. Occupational therapy does not change the cognitive level of clients who have cognitive limitations resulting from brain pathology (changes reflect the natural course of disease or effects of medication)
2. Brain impairments place restrictions on learning (persons at or below Level 4 have severe restrictions to learning new behaviors)

◆ Approach to intervention emphasizes:
1. Measuring and monitoring changes in cognitive level
2. Adapting intervention to fit level at which client is functioning
3. Maintaining that, although therapy can offer client an opportunity to process information at a higher level for a brief period, clients should not be pushed to struggle with higher function

◆ Treatment divided into four phases:
1. Acute (therapists evaluate client's cognitive level)
2. Post-acute (client can engage in activities; therapist monitors cognitive level and recommends how much assistance will be needed at discharge)
3. Rehabilitation (improving client performance by providing adaptive equipment, modifying the environment, and teaching caregivers to provide assistance; providing activities at an appropriate level to the client, avoiding supervising activities beyond the client's level of ability)
4. Long-term care (providing community-based activity program for people at cognitive Levels 3 and 4)

◆ Main approach to treatment is environmental compensation: making adjustments to the residual effects of disease rather than addressing the disease process itself
◆ Because occupational therapy services are presumed not to affect cognitive level of

clients, cognitive improvement is not a goal or outcome of therapy

◆ Goals are:
  1. Giving client tasks that can be accomplished
  2. Enabling client to comprehend and accept permanent limitations
  3. Identifying least restrictive environment in which person can function safely
  4. Providing caregivers with information about person's limits and necessary supports to function

Technology for Clinical Application

◆ Detailed, specific procedures are given for client assessment, task analysis, and therapeutic task selection

◆ Three formal assessments of functional level have been developed:
  1. Routine Task Inventory (administered by interviewing client or caregiver or by observing patient's performance; consists of 32 routine tasks, each described according to six cognitive levels)
  2. Allen Cognitive Level test (performance in leather lacing used to determine cognitive level)
  3. Cognitive Performance Test (composed of six daily living tasks and uses standardized equipment and administration)

◆ Informal observations of task performance and use of tasks with known levels of complexity gauge the client's functional level

◆ Evaluation of cognitive impairments is considered important to determine:
  1. What a client can be considered capable and safe to do
  2. What legal restrictions may be placed on a person

◆ Task analysis is central to treatment and includes:
  1. Determining normal procedure for performing a task.
  2. Identifying relative complexity of steps in a task

  3. Identifying steps in a process that client cannot do
  4. Adapting task to avoid procedures that clients are unable to perform

Research

◆ Studies focus on:
  1. Determining the reliability and validity of assessments
  2. Demonstrating associations between cognitive level and measures of mental status and psychiatric symptomatology

◆ Two studies raise questions about utility of cognitive level for predicting community adaptation

References

Allen, C. (1982). Independence through activity: The practice of occupational therapy (psychiatry). American Journal of Occupational Therapy, 36, 731–739.

Allen, C. (1985). Occupational Therapy for Psychiatric Diseases: Measurement and Management of Cognitive Disabilities. Boston: Little, Brown, & Co.

Allen, C. (1987). Cognitive disabilities: Measuring the social consequences of mental disorders. Journal of Clinical Psychiatry, 48, 185–191.

Allen, C. (1989). Treatment plans in cognitive rehabilitation. Occupational Therapy Practice, 1, 1–8.

Allen, C. (1992). Cognitive disabilities. In Katz, N. (ed.), Cognitive Rehabilitation: Models for Intervention in Occupational Therapy, pp 1–21. Boston: Andover Medical Publishers.

Allen, C & Earhart, C. (1992). Occupational therapy treatment goals for the physically and cognitively disabled. Rockville, MD: American Occupational Therapy Association.

Allen, C, Kehrberg, K & Burns, T. (1992). Evaluation instruments. In Allen, C, Earhart C & Blue, T. Occupational Therapy Treatment Goals for the Physically and Cognitively Disabled, pp 31–84. Rockville, MD: American Occupational Therapy Association.

Bar-Yoself, C, Weinblatt, N & Katz, N. (1999). Reliability and validity of the cognitive performance test (CPT) in an elderly population. Physical and Occupational Therapy in Geriatrics, 17(1), 65–79.

Earhart, C. (1999). Clinical interpretation of "Discharge planning in mental health: The relevance of cognition to community living." American Journal of Occupational Therapy, 53, 136–137.

Henry, AD, Moore, K, Quinlivan, M, et al. (1998). The relationship of the Allen Cognitive Level test to demographics, diagnosis, and disposition among psychiatric inpatients. American Journal of Occupational Therapy, 52, 638–643.

Katz, N, Josman, N & Steinmetz, N. (1988). Relationship between cognitive disability theory and the model of human occupation in the assessment of psychiatric and nonpsychiatric adolescents. Occupational Therapy in Mental Health, 8, 31–43.

Keller, S & Hayes, R. (1998). The relationship between the Allen Cognitive Level test and the life skills profile. American Journal of Occupational Therapy, 52, 851–856.

Levy, LL. (1988). Psychosocial intervention and dementia, Part II: The cognitive disability perspective. Occupational Therapy in Mental Health, 7, 13–36.

Raweh, DV & Katz, N. (1999). Treatment effectiveness of Allen's cognitive disabilities model with adult schizophrenic outpatients: A pilot study. Occupational Therapy in Mental Health, 14(4), 65–77.

Roitman, DM & Katz, N. (1996). Predictive validity of the Large Allen Cognitive Level test (LACL) using the Allen Diagnostic Module (ADM) in an aged, non-disabled population. Physical and Occupational Therapy in Geriatrics, 14(4), 43–57.

Secrest, L, Wood, AE & Tapp, A. (2000). A comparison of the Allen Cognitive Level test and the Wisconsin card sorting test in adults with schizophrenia. American Journal of Occupational Therapy, 54, 129–133.

Sweetingham, C. (1996). A critical appraisal of the cognitive disabilities model. New Zealand Journal of Occupational Therapy, 47, 5–9.

Velligan, DI, Bow-Thomas, CC, Mahurin, R, et al. (1998). Concurrent and predictive validity of the Allen cognitive levels assessment. Psychiatry Research, 80, 287–298.

Weissenberg, R & Giladi, N. (1989). Home economics day: A program for disturbed adolescents to promote acquisition of habits and skills. Occupational Therapy in Mental Health, 9, 89–103.

World Health Organization. (2001). International Classification of Functioning, Disability, and Health (ICF). Geneva: Author.

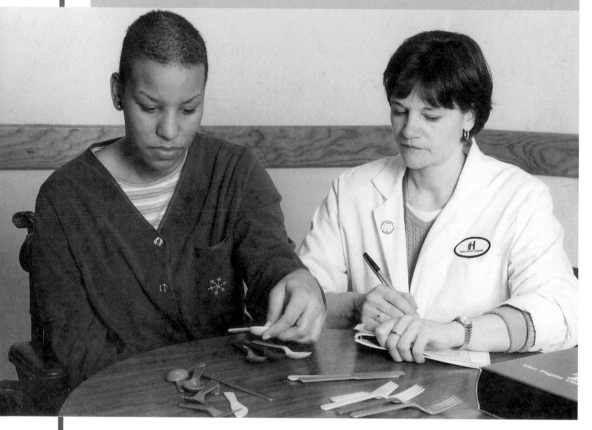

Chapter 9

The Cognitive-Perceptual Model

A client recovering from brain damage is seated with an occupational therapist. She is engaged in the task of sorting knives, forks, and spoons. By observing such things as how the client approaches the task, what mistakes she makes, and what aspects of the task are more challenging and why, the therapist will derive a picture of the client's cognitive-perceptual processes and problems. This approach to assessment, which examines the impact of cognitive and/or perpetual impairments in the context of task performance, is representative of current trends in the cognitive-perceptual model.

Persons with damage to the central nervous system (CNS) may experience a variety of perceptual and cognitive deficits. Approaches to addressing perceptual and cognitive problems* are widely represented in occupational therapy practice (Kunstaetter, 1988; Neistadt, 1986). Moreover, cognitive-perceptual literature and practice have grown dramatically in the last decade. Nonetheless, instead of a single, widely accepted formulation, there are a number of related conceptual schemes for understanding and addressing cognitive and perceptual problems.

These schemes overlap to an extent, and the trend in the literature appears to be toward an increasingly consistent view of cognitive-perceptual problems and their remediation. Recent efforts of a few authors to synthesize cognitive-perceptual themes and therapeutic approaches suggest that a cognitive-perceptual model of practice is being articulated and applied.

In this chapter I highlight the main concepts and applications that characterize this emerging conceptual practice model. My aim is to present convergent themes, concepts, and practices. Because the model is still being shaped, authors' use of terminology varies, including how the model or approach is labeled. In particular, it should be noted that the term *cognitive-perceptual* that I am using to label this model refers to what some have called cognitive-perceptual retraining or cognitive rehabilitation. This chapter integrates the work of several authors; I have used the terminology of particular authors when discussing their concepts.

The cognitive-perceptual model is built on an understanding of the brain's information-processing ability and its impairment in cases of injury. The model is concerned with how impaired cognitive and perceptual processes restrict occupational performance. One of the notable trends in the formulation of the model is toward an understanding of how cognitive and perceptual strategies and deficits are manifest in the midst of performing occupations.

Definitions of Perception and Cognition

Quintana (1995a) defines **perception** as the "integration of sensory impressions into psychologically meaningful information" (p. 201). Abreu and Toglia (1987) elaborate that perception is a dynamic process involving "sensory detection, sensory analysis, hypothesis formation, and a decision response" (p. 439). **Cognition** is defined by Quintana (1995) as the "ability of the brain to process, store, retrieve, and manipulate information" (p. 201). Abreu and Toglia (1987) note that cognition involves the abilities to "attend to, organize, and assimilate information" (p. 440). The three authors identify cognition as a process of using hindsight, foresight, and insight in determining a

> **Instead of a single, widely accepted formulation, there are a number of related conceptual schemes for understanding and addressing cognitive and perceptual problems.**

---

*The sensory integration and motor control treatment models have some overlapping concepts and methods with the cognitive-perceptual model (Neistadt, 1990). However, they differ in that both the sensory integration and the motor control models are primarily concerned with motor behavior, while the cognitive-perceptual model is more concerned with behavioral strategies. In addition, the sensory-integration model was developed to address problems of sensory processing unrelated to frank brain damage, whereas the cognitive-perceptual model is mainly applied to persons who have brain damage.

course of action. Thus, attention, memory, initiation, planning, reflection, and adaptive problem-solving are processes generally recognized as part of cognition. Noting that cognition is a global concept, Katz (1998) incorporates the following range of processes:

Metacognitive skills—knowledge and control—include awareness of abilities and disabilities and executive functions that consist of initiation, planning, problem solving, self-regulation, and self-correction. Cognitive skills comprise such areas as attention, orientation, perception, praxis, visual-motor organization, memory, and thinking operations. (p. x)

Perception and cognition cannot be entirely differentiated from each other; no borderline between the two has been clearly defined in the literature (Abreu & Toglia, 1987). Perception and cognition may be conceived as two ends of a continuum. On the perceptual end, action and awareness are more immediate and related to the concrete features of the environment and of experience. Perception involves immediate apprehension and appreciation of sensory data. Recognizing the smell of coffee, the taste of ice cream, and the sight of a flower are examples of perception. Yet perception is not merely a passive process of receiving sensory information. Rather, it is an active process of searching and judging the environment and recognizing its features (Abreu, 1981).

In contrast, cognitive action and awareness are more abstract and reflective, involving the formulation of intentions and action plans. Hence, processes normally termed "cognitive" involve more abstract and conscious reflection or anticipation not tied to immediate sensory data. Thus, cognition is involved in making coffee, in deciding between chocolate and strawberry ice cream, and in arranging flowers in a bouquet.

Abreu and Toglia (1987) make another important distinction. Some perceptual abilities are related to a particular sensory system, but cognition interfaces with all forms of sensory information. Perception can guide a range of action (e.g., driving and walking) at the same time that cognitive processes are actively involved in such unrelated acts as talking or planning ahead. Moreover, perception may guide actions (e.g., typing) that are in the service of higher cognitive processes (e.g., writing this book).

Thus, the continuum from perception to cognition is characterized by few to many sensory modalities and by spontaneous to reflective processes. The relationship between perception and cognition may also be considered in the following way: perceptual processes represent lower-level operations that are part of a broader set of processes referred to as cognition. The tendency for literature to refer to cognitive processes and cognitive rehabilitation as incorporating elements of perception (as does, for example, Katz's quotation above) suggests that perception may be increasingly seen as a component of cognition.

Interdisciplinary Base

The perceptual and cognitive concepts and related interventions used in occupational therapy are based on the work of neuroscience and neuropsychology (Abreu, 1981). One important influence has come from the work of scientists who have studied the effects of traumatic brain lesions on cognition and perception. Another influence has been research in the field of ecological perception. The researchers who created measures of specific perceptual and cognitive performances have also influenced occupational therapists' views of these phenomena. Theories from psychology, in particular learning theory that stresses information processing, have also been incorporated into this model. A more recent influence is dynamical systems theory, which is resulting in a move toward more process-oriented and occupationally contexted views of perception and cognition.

🌿 Theory

Because this model is in an early stage of development, no comprehensive, widely accepted theoretical explanation of the cognitive-perceptive processes in occupational performance has been articulated. However, definite themes are emerging so that it is possible to identify preliminary theory concerning organization, problems and challenges, and therapeutic intervention.

Organization

Underlying this model is the assumption that performance in occupations is based on the ability of persons to perceive and evaluate sensory information and the ability to conceive of, plan, and execute purposeful action. These cognitive-perceptual abilities are the basis for interaction with the environment in work, play, and daily living tasks.

The earlier efforts to explain cognition and perception and their role in everyday performance focused on specifying taxonomies of perceptual and cognitive abilities. While such taxonomies are still a component of this model, more recent literature emphasizes explaining the cognitive and perceptual processes manifest in occupational performance.

Taxonomies of Cognitive and Perceptual Abilities

Understanding of cognitive and perceptual abilities used in occupational performance first emerged from clinical observations of specific performance problems and from development of standardized tests designed to capture some component(s) of perception and/or cognition. For example, Quintana

(1995) offers the following list of cognitive-perceptual functions:

- ◆ Recognition of body scheme (i.e., spatial arrangement of one's body parts)
- ◆ Discrimination of right from left
- ◆ Identification of one's body parts
- ◆ Ability to name which finger is being touched (finger gnosia)
- ◆ Recognition of both sides of the body (the corresponding deficit is ignorance of one side of the body)
- ◆ Recognition of one's deficits
- ◆ Realization of the position of one's body in space
- ◆ Recognition of the relation of self to other objects
- ◆ Awareness of spatial relations
- ◆ Ability to find one's way from one place to another (topographical orientation)
- ◆ Distinguishing foreground from background (figure-ground)
- ◆ Carrying out purposeful movement (praxis)
- ◆ Carrying out drawing and constructional tasks (constructional praxis)
- ◆ Ability to get dressed (dressing praxis)
- ◆ Attention
- ◆ Orientation to person, place, and time
- ◆ Memory
- ◆ Problem-solving

Zoltan, Seiv, and Freishtat (1986) offer a similar collection of cognitive-perceptual areas of performance. Their taxonomy also includes such abilities as:

- ◆ Visual attention and visual scanning of the field of vision
- ◆ Ability to recognize faces
- ◆ Ability to initiate, plan, and organize performance
- ◆ Mental flexibility
- ◆ Abstraction

More recently, Unsworth (1999) offered a classification that includes:

◆ Cognitive processes (concentration, memory, and learning)
◆ Metacognitive processes (executive functions of insight and self-awareness)
◆ Perceptual processes (praxis and perceptual processing)

As these three examples show, there is no universally accepted taxonomy of perceptual and cognitive abilities. Moreover, there are a number of important limitations to these categories. They are not mutually exclusive, nor do they reflect a consistent approach to classification.

Because there is a great deal of overlap between these areas of cognitive-perceptual function, some authors have questioned just how useful they are (Toglia, 1992). In fact, Toglia suggests focusing instead on the underlying processing strategies and conditions that influence performance (Toglia & Finkelstein, 1991). It appears that the trend in this model is to de-emphasize the more specific taxonomies of cognitive-perceptual abilities and focus on explanations of the processes involved across cognitive and perceptual domains.

Explaining the Cognitive-Perceptual Process

Just as with the taxonomic approach, there is no single formulation of the processes involved in perception and cognition. Four themes seem to be important in modeling cognitive and perceptual processes:

1. Steps or stages in the organization of information
2. Cognitive strategies
3. Process of learning
4. Dynamic interaction among person, task, and environment

Cognitive-Perceptual Stages Abreu and Toglia (1987) offered one of the earliest conceptual schemes for explaining both perceptual and cognitive processes. Their schema, later elaborated by Abreu and Hinajosa (1992), identified three stages of information processing:

1. Detecting relevant stimuli
2. Discriminating and analyzing stimuli
3. Formulating responses based on hypotheses derived from comparing current sensory stimuli with past experiences

The importance of identifying stages of information processing is that it allows therapists to identify where along the process individuals may be having difficulty and need remediation and/or support.

Cognitive Strategies Abreu and Toglia (1987) point out that **cognitive strategies** affect how efficiently a person can process information. Cognitive strategies are the tactics that a person employs in occupational performance. Such strategies include planning ahead, choosing where to begin, varying one's speed, systematically searching for information, and generating alternatives. While the stages of cognitive-perceptual processing are universal and closely linked to organization of the human brain, cognitive strategies are learned methods of acquiring and dealing with information. Since these strategies affect how efficiently a person processes information, they have the ability to either limit or enhance cognitive-perceptual functioning.

Learning An important concept in this model is learning. **Learning** refers to a change in behavior (Neistadt, 1994) or in the capacity to respond to the environment that results from practice or experience. All learn-

> **Underlying this model is the assumption that performance in occupations is based on the ability of persons to perceive and evaluate sensory information and the ability to conceive of, plan, and execute purposeful action.**

ing reflects changes in the brain that result from interactions with the environment (Abreu & Toglia, 1987; Neistadt, 1994).

Closely related to the concept of learning is the idea of generalization or **transfer of learning.** The extent to which persons are able to transfer a cognitive-perceptual strategy from the activity in which it was learned to another activity or situation depends on the level of learning of which they are capable. Authors speak of the degree of learning transfer of which a person is capable. Neistadt (1994) incorporates the idea of transfer of learning into a conceptualization of the levels of information processing and learning of which persons are capable. She discusses three levels of learning:

1. **Association learning,** in which a person learns a connection between two events
2. **Representational learning,** which involves forming internal representations or images of events and their spatial-temporal organization
3. **Abstract learning,** which involves acquiring rules, knowledge, and facts that are not context-dependent

Persons capable of abstract learning will be able to generalize learning of conceptual and perceptual strategies to tasks and situations that are significantly different from those of the learning context, whereas persons restricted to association learning will not be able to generalize widely. Hence, persons in the latter group need to learn each task required for their occupational life individually, whereas those in the former group will learn strategies and apply them to a range of occupations.

Dynamic Interactional View　Toglia (1998) offers a dynamic interactional view that builds on information processing ideas and that incorporates a dynamical systems perspective (Fig. 9-1). According to her approach, cognition should be seen as the ongoing product of a dynamic process of interaction between an individual, the task being performed, and the environment. Within the individual she includes:

1. Processing strategies and behaviors, which are the approaches, routines, and tactics that the person uses to select and guide information processing (including prioritizing versus clustering information, discriminating between important versus unimportant information).
2. **Metacognition,** which refers to awareness and control of one's cognitive processes and capacities.

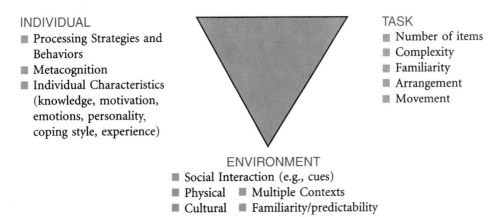

INDIVIDUAL
■ Processing Strategies and Behaviors
■ Metacognition
■ Individual Characteristics (knowledge, motivation, emotions, personality, coping style, experience)

TASK
■ Number of items
■ Complexity
■ Familiarity
■ Arrangement
■ Movement

ENVIRONMENT
■ Social Interaction (e.g., cues)
■ Physical　■ Multiple Contexts
■ Cultural　■ Familiarity/predictability

Figure 9-1. Dynamic interactional model of cognition. (From: Toglia, JP (1998). A dynamical interactional approach to cognitive rehabilitation. In Katz, N (ed.), Cognition and occupation in rehabilitation: Cognitive models for intervention in occupational therapy, p. 8. Bethesda, MD: American Occupational Therapy Association. Copyright 2004 by the American Occupational Therapy Association, Inc. Reprinted with permission.)

3. Individual characteristics, which include knowledge based on experience, motivation, and emotions.

The environment includes social, physical, and cultural elements that may influence the person's ability to process information within multiple contexts.

The task refers to the occupation the person is performing; it can be characterized by two parameters: surface characteristics and conceptual characteristics (Toglia, 1998; Toglia & Finkelstein, 1991). **Surface characteristics** refer to such things as the number, qualities, and arrangement of objects, types of stimuli, task directions, and movement demands. Surface characteristics are, therefore, readily observable features of a task. **Conceptual characteristics** are not directly observable; they include the kinds of skills and strategies the task demands based on its complexity and familiarity as well as the meaning it evokes.

According to Toglia (1998), cognition involves dynamic interaction of all these elements:

> The environment can mediate processing between the task and the individual. In some situations the task parameters may be the primary influence on information processing; in other situations the environment or the individual characteristics may be the most influential. (p. 15)

Understanding cognition requires attention to the interaction among the three elements. Cognition involves receiving, elaborating, and monitoring incoming information and using this information flexibly across tasks. Cognition also involves using efficient information-processing strategies, evoking previous knowledge, and using metacognition.

Cognitive processing, cognitive strategies,

and metacognition are all emergent phenomena that are influenced by environmental and task parameters. When those parameters change, cognitive processes and strategies may shift into different modes of operating. For example, a person may use one cognitive strategy until a task reaches a certain level of complexity and then shift to another strategy.

Toglia's dynamical systems-based framework appears to be the most comprehensive formulation of cognitive processes, and it shares features with other important occupational therapy conceptualizations. In addition, it is the approach that most clearly embraces contemporary systems concepts. As such, it appears to be the kind of articulation of cognitive-perceptual processes that will emerge in this model.

Problems and Challenges

Perceptual and cognitive impairments result from brain damage and disorganization. One of the major diagnoses that involves cognitive-perceptual problems is cerebrovascular accident (CVA). CVA is also one of the most frequently represented diagnoses in occupational therapy practice. This model is also applied to persons with traumatic brain injury, persons with CNS impairments (e.g., cerebral palsy), and persons who have developmental and learning disabilities. Individuals with brain damage present with reduced information-processing capacity:

> This reduction in information processing capacity can result in global or specific deficits depending on the nature of the brain damage.... The brain-damaged person has difficulty structuring and organizing information.... Clinically, the client may not automatically attend to the relevant feature of a task, group similar items together, formulate a plan, or break the task down into steps (Abreu & Toglia, 1987, p. 441)

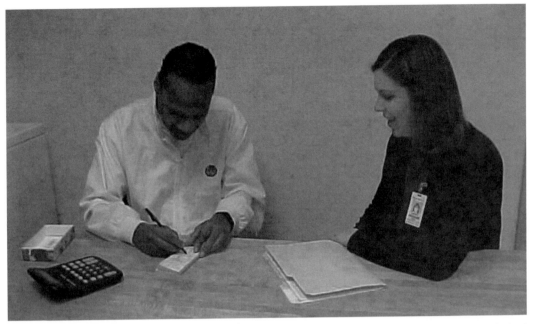

A client experiencing processing difficulties associated with Parkinson's disease works on the cognitive task of balancing his checkbook with support from the therapist.

Toglia also observes that cognitive impairments represent a decrease in efficient use of processing strategies to select, discriminate, organize, and structure incoming information (Toglia & Finkelstein, 1991). Neistadt (1994b) points out that brain damage can variously impact the ability for learning. Metacognition can also be impaired, as when persons are unaware of their cognitive-perceptual problems.

The basic view of this model is that when persons have CNS damage, a combination of information-processing abilities, learning abilities, and metacognition can be impaired (Neistadt, 1994b; Toglia, 1998). Hence, client problems are conceptualized in terms of the specific kinds of information processing difficulties they present, the amount of limitation in learning they experience, and their metacognitive status.

The cognitive-perceptual problems that persons demonstrate depend on the nature of insult to the CNS. These problems are also being recognized as dependent on task and environmental context (Neistadt, 1994b; Toglia, 1998). For example, persons with cognitive-perceptual problems may not have difficulty processing information in simple tasks but may show problems when task parameters change. The kinds of cognitive-perceptual problems a person demonstrates may be global, or they may be manifest in specific areas of cognitive-perceptual functioning, such as visual processing. For this reason, attention is still paid to specific areas of cognitive-perceptual impairment.

Classifying Specific Areas of Impairment

A number of specific areas of impairment are defined in this model. Some of these impairments are based on readily observable deficits, such as memory loss. Others are identified with specific assessments, which identify a type of impairment.

Some examples of common cognitive-perceptual impairment are disruption of body scheme, lack of left/right discrimination, difficulty with body-part identification, unilateral neglect (i.e., neglect of one side of the body), dyspraxia, attention deficits, problems with visual scanning, disorientation, and memory loss.

Disruption of Occupational Performance

Because the impaired brain is less capable of processing sensory information and is consequently unable to interpret and translate it into appropriate plans of action, the individual's occupational performance is impaired. Hence, difficulties in work, play or leisure, and self-care result from significant impairment of perceptual and cognitive capacities. In some cases, specific kinds of occupational performance difficulties have been shown to be associated with a given perceptual impairment. For example, persons with unilateral neglect have difficulty dressing because they do not recognize the affected side of the body. In other cases, the impairment is defined by its functional implication (e.g., dressing apraxia). A more global perceptual or cognitive impairment may have effects on all areas of performance. For example, memory loss or poor problem-solving may impair function through a whole range of occupational tasks. As will be noted later, there is a growing research literature that seeks to demonstrate the relationship between perceptual and cognitive deficits and functional performance problems.

Therapeutic Intervention

Authors discussing cognitive and perceptual approaches (Katz, 1998; Unsworth, 1999) to intervention note that although these approaches can vary in their techniques and emphases, they share overlapping principles and strategies. In the end, all interventions for cognitive-perceptual problems can be classified into remedial approaches, which seek to restore specific cognitive-perceptual abilities, and adaptive approaches, which emphasize enabling clients to use remaining abilities and compensate for deficits (Quintana, 1995). Treatment aimed at remediating perceptual and cognitive problems uses tasks that require the brain to process information in ways that target impaired information-processing capacities (Neistadt, 1990). The remedial approach is based on the idea that the brain has capacity to reorganize and, therefore, reclaim its informational processing capacity to an extent. Adaptive approaches help persons learn to capitalize on their existing potentials and to use strategies to substitute or compensate for limitations. The adaptive approach also stresses making individuals aware of their perceptual and cognitive limitations in order to compensate for their problems. Finally, this approach recognizes that performance will be enhanced if the environment or the task is modified to accommodate the particular limitations of the individual.

As Neistadt (1994b) argued, both remedial and compensatory cognitive-perceptual interventions involve learning, which depends on plasticity of the brain. This means that appropriate treatment approaches depend on the potential for recovery of information processing capacities and the potential for learning by persons with a brain injury. This potential for learning and recovery are influenced by "the person's general mental and physical health, the severity of the injury, and the amount and quality of environmental stimuli in that person's life" (Neistadt, 1994b, pp. 426-427). Occupational therapy enables learning and recovery by manipulating the environmental stimuli in the form of presenting occupational tasks and modifying the social context. How this is best done and what it can achieve depends on the other factors noted above.

Neistadt (1994b) suggests that therapy should be undertaken according to the level of information processing and kind of learning that persons are capable of (association, representational, and abstract learning). Depending on the kind of learning of which a person is capable, different treatment approaches will work best. For example, a person who relies on associative learning will have difficulty transferring learning to tasks that differ much from the learned task or to new contexts. Representational learners more readily transfer learning (i.e., they would be able to perform learned tasks under different conditions), but they have difficulty in transferring learning to new tasks or totally new situations. According to Neistadt (1994b) clients with the most ability to transfer learning would benefit from a remedial approach, which assumes transfer of learning, whereas those with less ability to transfer learning would benefit from an adaptive approach, which emphasizes learning specific functional tasks.

Toglia (1991) argues that transfer of learning exists on a continuum from near to far. Transfer is considered to be near when only one or two surface characteristics (e.g., physical features or arrangement of objects used, context, rules or directions) of the task are altered. Transfer is considered far when most or all surface characteristics are different. Like Neistadt, she argues that treatment should be graded to how much transfer of learning a client is capable of. As a client improves, tasks can be varied to further enhance transfer of learning (Toglia, 1991).

Metacognition also determines the client's ability to transfer learning and benefit from remedial and compensatory approaches. Metacognition includes knowledge of one's cognitive capacities, the ability to assess task difficulty, selection of appropriate cognitive strategies, and monitoring of one's performance (Toglia, 1998). When metacognition is impaired, the ability to transfer learning will also be impaired, and both remedial and compensatory strategies have more limited success (Toglia, 1991).

Traditional cognitive-perceptual treatment approaches tended to be deficit-specific; that is, aimed at remediating or compensating for specific areas of deficits identified in testing. Such a targeted approach assumed that cognitive-perceptual deficits could be differentiated into discretely meaningful categories and that these deficits could be specifically addressed. Moreover, it was often assumed that cognitive-perceptual skills were hierarchically organized so that the simpler ones should be retrained first, proceeding to more complex ones. Finally, it was assumed that once a particular area was improved, the client would show improvement in all tasks and situations requiring that ability (referred to as generalization or transfer of training).

Recent approaches have adopted a more holistic, process-oriented, and/or dynamical systems approach. Holistic approaches emphasize a top-down strategy that focuses on the highest level of cognitive-perceptual functioning and its role in integrating lower level or component functions (Warren, 1993). The process view emphasizes that activities should be selected to:

> involve specific processing at particular levels of the central nervous system. If the client attends to the stimulus events of the activities, then registering the stimulus event is feasible. If the client detects the information, then the ability to analyze information for use is feasible. If the client is able to analyze the information, then the client can compare the stimulus events with long-term memories and related the stimulus to the overall purpose and goal of the activities (Abreu & Hinajosa, 1992, p. 175).

Hence, activities should be chosen to elicit and challenge these information-processing capacities.

The dynamical approach emphasizes understanding how cognitive-perceptual behavior emerges under different task and contextual conditions (Toglia, 1998). This approach examines how and under what conditions a client shows a problem. For example, a client may have no difficulty in a cognitive-perceptual area until a task exceeds a certain threshold of complexity (number of component parts or steps) or until the environment is changed. Hence, the therapist simultaneously examines how the client processes information and how such strategies succeed and fail under different task and environmental conditions. In this way, the therapist can identify task and environmental dimensions that create difficulty for the client as well as client information-processing difficulties that create problems across different kinds of tasks. Next, individualized treatment, which takes this information into consideration, is developed.

Basic to individualized treatment is the estimation of the client's potential for change. Clients who are aware of errors, and who respond to cues and to modifications in tasks, will benefit from a multicontext approach in which their ability to process information across different situations is enhanced (Toglia, 1998). Clients without such awareness and responsiveness will most likely receive a functional approach that does not assume improvement of underlying abilities and transfer of training.

 # Technology for Application

Assessment

To determine whether perceptual or cognitive deficits exist, the therapist must rule out

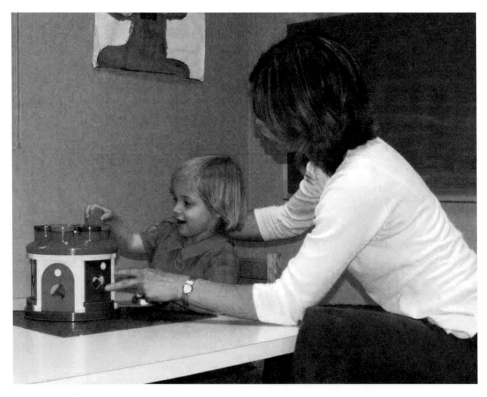

A pediatric client plays with keys to open doors to find hidden shapes. Finding and identifying these shapes develops shape recognition and perceptual-motor coordination.

other, more basic problems. For example, apraxia is defined as the inability to carry out purposeful movement when sensation is intact and the person has capacity for coordinated voluntary movement. Only when assessment determines that those sensory and coordination abilities are intact can the impairment be considered to be due to the inability to organize sensory information and plan and execute coordinated movement in order to accomplish tasks.

There are a wide range of standardized tests and informal procedures for evaluating cognitive and perceptual deficits (Brockmann Rubino & Van Deusen, 1995; Katz, 1998; Unsworth, 1999). Many of the standardized tests in use by occupational therapists have been developed by neuropsychologists, but several have been developed by occupational therapists. For example, The A-One is an assessment that links functional performance in occupations to neurobehavioral deficits (Arnadottir, 1990). It identifies both the level of independence in five activities of daily living (ADL) and the presence and severity of specific neurobehavioral impairments through analysis of how the impairments affect ADL tasks.

Another example is the Loewenstein Occupational Therapy Cognitive Assessment (LOTCA) (Cermak et al., 1995; Izkovich et al., 1990). Originally developed in Israel, it is now used widely. It consists of four major areas (orientation, perception, visuomotor organization, and thinking operations) represented by a total of 20 subtests. The LOTCA is designed to capture client abilities and limitations and to determine the capacity to cope with routine occupational tasks.

Therapists usually employ a battery of standardized tests in association with this model (Abreu & Toglia, 1987; Zoltan, Seiv, & Freishtat, 1986). Nonetheless, other methods of assessment are also considered important. Abreu and Toglia (1987) note that the standardized tests may provide only limited infor-

mation about the client's functioning because there is not a perfect relationship between perceptual and cognitive deficits and occupational performance. Consequently, Abreu and Toglia and Neistadt (1990) note the importance of going beyond standardized tests to gather qualitative information and to observe how the deficits affect persons' performance in their occupational tasks. As Abreu and Toglia (1987) point out, the occupational therapist's role is to evaluate function and impairment, and therefore cognitive-perceptual data must be viewed in terms of their occupational-performance implications.

A new approach to assessment based on dynamical principles emphasizes simultaneously examining the cognitive and perceptual processing of a person along with noting the impact of variation of task parameters and environmental conditions (Toglia & Finkelstein, 1991). For example, Toglia and Finkelstein developed the Dynamic Visual Processing Assessment, which examines scanning, object perception, unilateral inattention, and keeping track of visual information. This assessment determines how such parameters as number of items and their arrangement affects performance in these areas. It also examines the impact of environmental cuing and self-awareness of errors.

Treatment

As the earlier discussion of theory about intervention pointed out, there are essentially two different approaches to remediating cognitive and perceptual problems. That is, intervention aims either at improving or compensating for limitations of cognitive-perceptual abilities. These two approaches to treatment of cognitive-perceptual deficits are referred to as remedial and functional training (sometimes called adaptive training) (Abreu & Toglia, 1987; Neistadt, 1990; Zoltan, Seiv, & Freishtat, 1986).

According to Neistadt (1990), remedial training "seeks to promote the recovery or reorganization of impaired central nervous system functions" (p. 299). Remedial training is based on the premise that task training results not only in learning the specific task but also in increasing the cognitive or perceptual skill used in the task (Zoltan, Seiv, & Freishtat, 1986). Thus, training is expected to transfer to other situations and tasks in which the perceptual or cognitive skills are required. As noted earlier, use of this approach should depend on determination that the client is capable of learning in such a way as to effectively transfer training.

Functional (or adaptive) training does not rely on changing cognitive-perceptual capabilities but seeks to enable individuals to perform optimally despite such limitations. Neistadt (1990) refers to this approach as adaptive, pointing out that therapy provides "training not in the perceptual skills of functional behavior but in the activity of daily living behaviors themselves" (p. 299). Consequently, this approach emphasizes finding and using means for the person to accomplish necessary tasks and routines despite the presence of cognitive-perceptual deficits.

The functional approach has two categories:

1. Compensation, in which the client is made aware of the problems and taught to make allowances for them
2. Adaptation, or changing the environment to make up for the person's deficits

An example of the compensation approach is training to overcome visual scanning deficits. Usually, visual scanning occurs automatically in response to novel stimuli (i.e., something new or a change in the stimulus field) and when persons consciously search for information in the visual field. When deficits in visual scanning occur, clients can learn to override them. Once they are shown how visual scanning normally func-

tions and how their own is not functioning, they can be taught new, conscious visual behaviors that compensate for the lack of automatic visual scanning in situations such as reading and driving (Warren, 1993).

Environmental adaptation often involves establishing a particular set of circumstances in which the person performs tasks (e.g., an invariant routine, the use of sensory and cognitive cues to support the task process, or changing the materials needed to complete a task). Some environmental adaptations require a family member or caretaker to supervise and provide cues and other necessary support (Abreu, 1981).

In the past, it was believed that the sequence of treatment should recapitulate (repeat the stages of) developmental states (Kaplan & Hier, 1982). It was argued that, following brain injury and the disorganization of perceptual and cognitive abilities, persons best relearn and reorganize if they follow the developmental sequence with which the skills were first learned. Abreu and Toglia (1987) disagree. They argue that because of the store of knowledge in the adult brain, the circumstances for relearning perceptual and cognitive tasks after brain damage are very different from the conditions of initial developmental learning. Most approaches currently described in the literature do not recommend a developmentally sequenced approach. Rather, they argue for an approach tailored to the remaining capacities, nature of processing impairments, and learning potential of the client.

Finally, because metacognition affects clients' abilities to transfer learning and make use of adaptive strategies to compensate for problems, therapists seek to improve metacognition. This can include helping the client gain insight into problems, evaluate task demands, and assess outcomes of performance (Toglia, 1992).

Modalities Used in Therapy

The range of activities used in the remedial approach is wide. In many cases, therapists use testing materials to train cognitive-perceptual skills. That is, the tasks used to test perceptual and cognitive abilities are used as drills to exercise and develop these skills (Neistadt, 1990; Zoltan, Seiv, & Freishtat, 1986). For example, a client may practice connecting a series of dots or copying a simple design in order to overcome visual scanning deficits. Zoltan, Seiv, and Freishtat note that clients sometimes object to cognitive training as childish, degrading, and irrelevant. For this reason, training tasks based on normal occupation performance may be preferable. One challenge with using occupational tasks is the need to first analyze an activity to determine which perceptual and cognitive skills the activity calls for (Cermak, 1985). Development of protocols for training persons in the contexts of occupations is one way to standardize how clients are presented with perceptual and cognitive demands. An example of such an approach is a meal preparation treatment protocol developed by Neistadt (1994). With the increase of dynamical systems concepts, which stress the importance of task parameters in determining performance, and with improved methods of identifying task parameters, the use of occupational tasks for remediation will likely increase while training drills will decrease.

The use of computers for retraining many perceptual skills is increasing because of computers' greater acceptability to many clients and because of the wide range of available, relevant software. When computers were first introduced, enthusiasm for

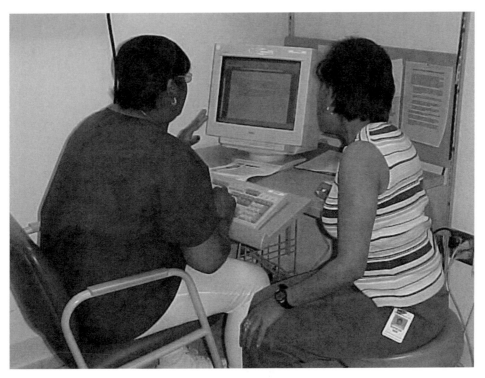

A client with perceptual difficulties works on computer skills such as attention, scanning, and discrimination in order to return to work.

computer retraining was great, but clinical observation suggests that this type of training does not generalize well into other areas of activity. Such computer exercises appear to be most useful in the early stages of recovery, when the most basic capacities are returning. Later, activities more nearly matched to desired life tasks appear more useful.

As this model is further developed, the modalities will be further refined and tested for their relevance and efficacy. It does appear, however, that occupational tasks that demand cognitive-perceptual abilities and that reveal deficits may be the most useful context for both remedial and adaptive intervention strategies.

🌿 Research

Research related to this model is varied. One active area of research is the development and testing of assessment tools (Baum & Edwards, 1993; Boys et al., 1988; Cermak, 1985; Van Deusen, Fox, & Harlowe, 1984; Van Deusen & Harlowe, 1987). Other studies have evaluated the incidence of cognitive-perceptual deficits in persons with various kinds of neurological impairments. One such project was a study of the patterns of impairment in motor planning, language, and memory in persons with Alzheimer's disease (Baum et al., 1988). Another study demonstrated that children with cerebral palsy lagged behind normal children in the development of visual-perceptual skills (Menken, Cermak, & Fisher, 1987). Other examples of this type of research are a study that investigated relationships between visual-perceptual motor abilities and clumsiness in non-

disabled and learning-disabled children (O'Brien, Cermak, & Murray, 1988) and studies of visual spatial, visual perception, and praxis deficits in persons who have experienced a stroke (Brockmann Rubino & Van Deusen, 1995; Kaplan & Hier, 1982; York & Cermak, 1995).

Other studies have sought to demonstrate the impact of cognitive-perceptual deficits on occupational performance. One study of persons 4 to 6 years after their strokes documented that perceptual deficits not only endured but also had as much impact on self-care performance as motor impairments did (Abreu & Hinajosa, 1992). Two studies (Kaplan & Hier, 1982; Nelle et al., 1991) found that deficits in perception were correlated with self-care problems. Two studies of stroke clients found that cognitive skills correlated with self-care skills and that cognitive improvement correlated with improvement in self-care skills (Carter et al., 1988). However, findings of these and other studies suggest that the relationship of perception and cognition to functional performance is not strong.

If measures of perceptual and cognitive ability that factor in occupational task and context are developed and used in such research, it is likely that stronger relationships will be demonstrated. Future research should certainly include efforts to more clearly show how perceptual and cognitive deficits relate to performance problems in daily occupations. Also needed are studies to evaluate the outcomes of different treatment approaches (Neistadt, 1990; Van Deusen, 1988; Van Deusen & Harlowe, 1987). Neistadt (1990) identified a number of research questions that could be posed to investigate the assumptions underlying treatment aimed at improving perceptual

> **This model is important to the field, given the pervasiveness of cognitive and perceptual impairments in occupational therapy's clients and the wide range of techniques occupational therapists employ to remediate such impairments.**

and cognitive deficits. One vital question is whether occupational therapy aimed at cognitive and perceptual skills enhances functional performance.

 # Discussion

Although the cognitive-perceptual model has been developing for some time, it still represents a multifaceted and loosely connected collection of concepts and approaches rather than a single well-integrated model. Nonetheless, this model is important to the field, given the pervasiveness of cognitive and perceptual impairments in occupational therapy's clients and the wide range of techniques occupational therapists employ to remediate such impairments.

One interesting aspect of this model is that research, as much as clinical application, has advanced interest in the whole area. The research literature is beginning to document both the extent of cognitive-perceptual deficits in persons with brain damage and the impact of these deficits on occupational performance. As this model is more clearly articulated, research is likely to lead to a cumulative and authoritative body of knowledge. This model appears to be moving in the direction of combining approaches that examine the nature of perceptual and cognitive impairments alongside their functional impact in the context of occupational performance. In this way it provides a multidimensional understanding and approach to cognitive and perceptual impairments and their impact in occupational life.

TERMS OF THE MODEL	
Abstract learning	Acquiring rules, knowledge, and facts that are not context-dependent
Association learning	Learning a connection between two events
Cognition	Ability to attend to, process, store, retrieve, manipulate, and assimilate information
Cognitive strategies	Tactics for processing information, including planning, choosing where to begin, varying one's speed, systematically searching for information, and generating alternatives
Conceptual characteristics	Kinds of skill and strategies a task demands and the meaning it evokes
Learning	Change in behavior or in capacity to respond to environment, which results from practice or experience
Metacognition	Awareness of one's own cognitive processes
Perception	Integration of sensory impressions into psychologically meaningful information
Representational learning	Forming internal representations or images of events and their spatio-temporal organization
Surface characteristics	Readily observable features of a task, including number, qualities, and arrangement of objects; types of stimuli; task directions; and movement demands
Transfer of learning	Ability to apply strategies learned in a task and situation to other tasks and situations

Summary: The Cognitive-Perceptual Model

Focus

- Addressed to persons with damage to the CNS
- Instead of a single, widely accepted formulation, there are many related conceptual schemes for understanding and remediating cognitive and perceptual problems
- Built on an understanding of the brain's information-processing ability and its impairment in cases of injury, the model is concerned with how impaired cognitive and perceptual processes restrict occupational performance

Definitions of Perception and Cognition

- Perception is:
  1. The integration of sensory impressions into meaningful information
  2. A dynamic process involving detection and analysis, hypothesis formation, and response to sensation
- Cognition is:
  1. Ability to attend to, process, organize, store, retrieve, and manipulate information
  2. A process of using hindsight, foresight, and insight to select action
  3. A composite of attention, memory, initiation, planning, reflection, and adaptive problem-solving
- Perception and cognition can be conceived as two ends on a continuum:
  1. Perception involves immediate action and awareness related to the concrete features of the environment
  2. Cognition involves abstract and reflective action and awareness

- Perception is increasingly seen as a component of cognition

Interdisciplinary Base

- Neuroscience, neuropsychology, ecological perception, learning theory are traditional influences
- A more recent influence is dynamic systems theory

Theory

- No comprehensive theoretical explanation of the cognitive-perceptive processes in occupational performance has been articulated, but definite themes are emerging

Organization

- Performance in occupations is based on the ability of persons to perceive and evaluate sensory information and the ability to conceive, plan, and execute purposeful action
- Early efforts explain cognition and perception and their role in performance-specified taxonomies, whereas more recent literature emphasizes explaining cognitive and perceptual processes
- There is no universally accepted taxonomy of perceptual and cognitive abilities
- Existing taxonomies do not reflect a consistent approach to classification
- Some authors have questioned utility of the taxonomies
- Four themes appear important in model of cognitive and perceptual processes:
  1. Steps or stages in the organization of information
  2. Cognitive strategies
  3. Process of learning
  4. Dynamic interaction between person, task, and environment

◆ Three stages of information processing:
1. Detecting relevant stimuli
2. Discriminating and analyzing stimuli
3. Formulating responses based on comparing current sensory stimuli and past experiences

◆ Cognitive strategies:
1. Affect efficiency of information processing
2. Include tactics of planning, choosing where to begin, varying speed, searching for information, and generating alternatives

◆ Learning refers to a change in behavior or in capacity to respond to environment, resulting from practice or experience, reflecting changes in the brain

◆ Three levels of learning:
1. Association learning (learning a connection between events)
2. Representational learning (forming internal representations or images of events)
3. Abstract learning (acquiring rules, knowledge, and facts that are not context-dependent)

◆ Dynamic interactional view sees cognition as the ongoing product of individual, task, and environment interaction

Problems and Challenges

◆ Perceptual and cognitive impairments result from brain damage and disorganization

◆ Individuals with brain damage present with reduced information-processing capacity that can affect all three stages of sensory information processing

◆ Cognitive impairment reflects decreased efficiency for selecting, discriminating, organizing, and structuring information

◆ Client problems are conceptualized in terms of specific kinds of information processing difficulties, amount of limitation in learning, and metacognitive status

◆ The cognitive-perceptual problems that persons demonstrate depend on:
1. Nature of insult to the CNS
2. Task and environmental context

◆ Reduction of brain capacity for processing, interpreting, and translating sensory information into appropriate plans of action impairs occupational performance

Therapeutic Intervention

◆ Remedial approaches seek to restore specific cognitive-perceptual abilities

◆ Adaptive approaches emphasize enabling clients to use remaining abilities and compensate for deficits

◆ Therapy enables learning and recovery by presenting occupational tasks and modifying physical and social context according to information processing and learning of which persons are capable

◆ Traditional cognitive-perceptual treatment approaches are aimed at remediating or compensating for specific areas of deficits, but recent approaches adopt a more holistic, process-oriented and/or dynamic systems approach

◆ Holistic approaches focus on the highest level of cognitive-perceptual functioning and its role in integrating lower level or component functions

◆ Process view emphasizes selecting activities to involve specific processing at particular levels of the CNS

◆ Dynamic approach emphasizes understanding how cognitive-perceptual behavior emerges under different task and contextual conditions

Technology for Application

◆ A wide range of standardized tests and informal procedures exists for evaluating cognitive and perceptual deficits. Tests developed by occupational therapists include:

1. A-One (assessment that links functional performance in occupations to neurobehavioral deficits)
2. Loewenstein Occupational Therapy Cognitive Assessment (consisting of orientation, perception, visuomotor organization, and thinking operations) designed to capture abilities and limitations and determine capacity to cope with routine occupational tasks

◆ Standardized tests may provide only limited information about functioning because there is no perfect relationship between perceptual and cognitive deficits and occupational performance

◆ Qualitative information and observation of how deficits affect occupational performance are important

◆ Assessment based on dynamic principles emphasizes examining cognitive and perceptual processing along with the impact of variation of task parameters and environment

Treatment

◆ Remedial training promotes recovery or reorganization of impaired CNS functions and is expected to transfer to other situations and tasks in which perceptual or cognitive skills are required

◆ Functional (adaptive) training enables individuals to perform optimally despite limitations and includes:

1. Compensation, in which the person is made aware of problems and taught to make allowances
2. Adaptation, or changing environment to make up for deficits

◆ Current approaches do not recommend a developmental sequence but rather one tailored to remaining capacities, nature of processing impairments, and learning potential of client

Research

◆ Research areas:

1. Development and testing of assessment
2. Evaluating incidence of cognitive-perceptual deficits
3. Demonstrating impact of cognitive-perceptual deficits on occupational performance

References

Abreu, BC. (1981). Physical Disabilities Manual. New York: Raven Press.

Abreu, BC & Hinajosa, J. (1992). The process approach for cognitive-perceptual and postural control dysfunction for adults with brain injuries. In Katz, N (ed.), Cognitive Rehabilitation: Models for Intervention in Occupational Therapy, pp 167–194. Boston: Andover Medical Publishers.

Abreu, BC & Toglia, JP. (1987). Cognitive rehabilitation: A model for occupational therapy. American Journal of Occupational Therapy, 41, 439–448.

Arnadottir, G. (1990). The Brain and Behavior: Assessing Cortical Dysfunction Through Activities of Daily Living. St. Louis: CV Mosby Co.

Baum, C & Edwards, DF. (1993). Cognitive performance in senile dementia of the Alzheimer's type: The Kitchen Task Assessment. American Journal of Occupational Therapy, 47, 431–436.

Baum, CM, Edwards, DF, Leavitt, K, et al (1988). Performance components in senile dementia of the Alzheimer type: Motor planning, language, and memory. Occupational Therapy Journal of Research, 8, 356–368.

Boys, M, Fisher, P, Holzberg, C & Reid, DW. (1988). The OSOT perceptual evaluation: A research perspective. American Journal of Occupational Therapy, 42, 92–98.

Brockmann Rubino, K & Van Deusen, J. (1995). Relation of perceptual and body image dysfunction to activities of daily living of persons after stroke. American Journal of Occupational Therapy, 49, 551–559.

Carter, LT, Oliverira, DO, Duponte, J, et al. (1988). The relationship of cognitive skills performance to activities of daily living in stroke patients. American Journal of Occupational Therapy, 42, 449–455.

Cermak, SA. (1985). Developmental dyspraxia. In Roy, EA (ed.), Advances in Psychology: Vol 23: Neuropsychological Studies of Apraxia and Related Disorder, pp 225–248. North Holland, New York: Elsevier Science.

Cermak, SA, Katz, N, McGuire, E, et al. (1995). Performance of Americans and Israelis with cerebrovascular accident on the Loewenstein Occupational Therapy Assessment (LOTCA). American Journal of Occupational Therapy, 49, 500–506.

Izkovich, M, Elazar, B, Averbuch, S, et al. (1990). LOTCA: Loewenstein Occupational Therapy Cognitive Assessment Manual. Pequannock, NJ: Maddak.

Kaplan, J & Hier, DE. (1982). Visuo-spatial deficits after right hemisphere stroke. American Journal of Occupational Therapy, 36, 314–321.

Katz, N. (1998). Preface. In Katz, N. (ed.), Cognition and Ocupation in Rehabilitation: Cognitive Models for Intervention in Occupational Therapy, pp ix-xiii. Bethesda, MD: American Occupational Therapy Association.

Kunstaetter, D. (1988). Occupational therapy treatment in home health care. American Journal of Occupational Therapy, 42, 513–519.

Menken, C, Cermak, SA & Fisher, A. (1987). Evaluating the visual-perceptual skills of children with cerebral palsy. American Journal of Occupational Therapy, 41, 646–651.

Neistadt, ME. (1986). Occupational therapy treatment goals for adults with developmental disabilities. American Journal of Occupational Therapy, 40, 672–678.

Neistadt, ME. (1990). A critical analysis of occupational therapy approaches for perceptual deficits in adults with brain injury. American Journal of Occupational Therapy, 44, 299–304.

Neistadt, ME. (1994a). A meal preparation treatment protocol for adults with brain injury. American Journal of Occupational Therapy. 48, 431–438.

Neistadt, ME. (1994b). The neurobiology of learning: Implications for treatment of adults with brain injury. American Journal of Occupational Therapy, 48, 421–430.

Nelle, D, Titus, M, Gall, NG, et al. (1991). Correlation of perceptual performance and activities of daily living in stroke patients. American Journal of Occupational Therapy, 45, 410–417.

O'Brien, V, Cermak, SA & Murray, E. (1988). The relationship between visual-perceptual motor abilities and clumsiness in children with and without learning disabilities. American Journal of Occupational Therapy, 42, 359–363.

Quintana, LA. (1995a). Evaluation of perception and cognition. In Trombly, C (ed.), Occupational Therapy for Physical Dysfunction, 4th ed, pp 201–223. Baltimore: Williams & Wilkins.

Quintana, LA. (1995b). Remediating cognitive impairments. In Trombly, C (ed.), Occupational Therapy for Physical Dysfunction, 4th ed, pp 539–548. Baltimore: Williams and Wilkins.

Toglia, JP. (1991). Generalization of treatment: A multicontext approach to cognitive perceptual impairment in adults with brain injury. American Journal of Occupational Therapy, 45, 505–516.

Toglia, JP. (1992). A dynamic interactional approach to cognitive rehabilitation. In Katz, N. (ed.), Cognitive Rehabilitation: Models for Intervention in Occupational Therapy, pp 104–143. Boston: Andover Medical Publishers.

Toglia, JP. (1998). A dynamical interactional model to cognitive rehabilitation. In Katz, N. (ed.), Cognitive Rehabilitation: Models for Intervention in Occupational Therapy, pp 4–50. Bethesda, MD: American Association of Occupational Therapy, Inc.

Toglia, JP & Finkelstein, N. (1991). Test protocol: The dynamic visual processing assessment. New York: New York Hospital–Cornell Medical Center.

Unsworth, C. (ed.) (1999). Cognitive and Perceptual Dysfunction: A Clinical Reasoning Approach to Evaluating and Intervention. Philadelphia: FA Davis.

Van Deusen, J. (1988). Unilateral neglect: Suggestions for research by occupational therapists. American Journal of Occupational Therapy, 42, 441–448.

Van Deusen, J, Fox, J & Harlowe, D. (1984). Construct validation of occupational therapy measures used in CVA evaluation: A beginning. American Journal of Occupational Therapy, 38, 101–106.

Van Deusen, J & Harlowe, D. (1987). Continued construct validation of the St. Mary's CVA evaluation: Bilateral awareness scale. American Journal of Occupational Therapy, 41, 242–245.

Warren, M. (1993). A hierarchical model for evaluation and treatment of visual perceptual dysfunction in adult-acquired brain injury, Part 1. American Journal of Occupational Therapy, 47, 42–54.

York, CD & Cermak, SA. (1995). Visual perception and praxis in adults after stroke. American Journal of Occupational Therapy, 49, 543–550.

Zoltan, B, Seiv, E & Freishtat, B. (1986). Perceptual and Cognitive Dysfunction in the Adult Stroke Patient. Thorofare, NJ: Slack.

Chapter 10

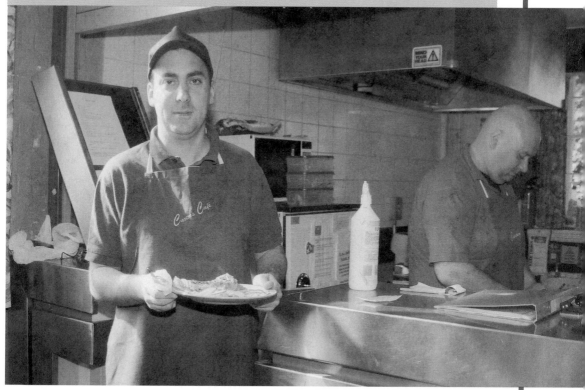

The Model of Human Occupation

A client works in a café that is operated to provide work training and experience for persons with mental health problems. With the support and guidance of an occupational therapist, the client has opportunities to develop a sense of competence and satisfaction in working. He will also develop the habits and skills necessary to success in the workplace. Importantly, the program also allows the client to take on the role of worker in a real-life context where the ordinary demands and expectations, as well as the social identity of the role, are present. Like other programs based on the model of human occupation, this one emphasizes engagement in meaningful occupations to address multiple personal and environmental factors that influence occupational adaptation.

The model of human occupation was introduced in the 1980s (Kielhofner, 1980a, b; Kielhofner & Burke, 1980; Kielhofner, Burke, & Heard-Igi, 1980) and has been more fully articulated in three editions of *A Model of Human Occupation: Theory and Application* (Kielhofner, 2002). This model is concerned with:

♦ The motivation for occupation
♦ Pattern for occupation
♦ Subjective dimension of performance
♦ Influence of environment on occupation

Unlike most models that are designed for specific types of impairment, this model is intended for use with any person experiencing problems in occupational life. It is also designed to be applicable across the life span.

 ## Interdisciplinary Base

This model draws on concepts from psychology and anthropology concerning human needs and motives. Concepts from sociology and social psychology and from early occupational therapy literature have been incorporated to understand how occupation is organized into everyday patterns. The view of performance capacity offered by this model is largely based on concepts of phenomenology from philosophy. The view of the environment in this model is influenced by literature from environmental psychology, sociology, and anthropology. Finally, this model uses systems theory to frame how these factors are organized together in human action and experience.

 ## Theory

The model conceptualizes humans as composed of three elements:

♦ Volition
♦ Habituation
♦ Performance capacity

Volition refers to the process by which persons are motivated toward and choose what they do. **Habituation** refers to a process whereby doing is organized into patterns and routines. **Performance capacity** refers both to the underlying objective mental and physical abilities and the lived experience that shapes performance.

Volition

According to this model, volition includes a deep human drive for action, combined with thoughts and feelings about doing things, shaped by previous experience and linked to the future. Volitional thoughts and feelings pertain to:

♦ How effective one is in acting on the world
♦ What one holds as important and meaningful to do
♦ What one finds enjoyable and satisfying to do

These three sets of thoughts and feelings are referred to as personal causation, values, and interests.

Personal Causation

Personal causation is reflected in awareness of one's abilities and the sense of how effective one is in achieving what one wants. It is influenced by one's sociocultural context and the extent to which it emphasizes and requires different capabilities (e.g., physical, interpersonal, or mental capacity). It is also influenced by the changing demands for capacity that occur across the developmental continuum. Consequently, **personal causation** is a dynamic unfolding set of thoughts and feelings about one's capacities and efficacy influenced by the ongoing awareness of personal performance and its consequences.

Values

Values are grounded in the commonsense understanding of the world provided by the sociocultural context. They define what is worth doing, how one ought to perform, and what goals or aspirations deserve commitment. Values are associated with strong emotions (e.g., feelings of security, worthiness, belonging, or accomplishment). Persons express their values when they see a course of action as how one ought to act and another as an improper or inferior way of doing things. Values determine one's view of the worth of different occupations. Therefore, they influence the sense of self-worth that one derives from succeeding at occupations. In short, **values** are what one finds important and meaningful to do.

Interests

Interests are what one finds enjoyable or satisfying to do. They begin with natural dispositions to enjoy different types of doing and develop through the experience of pleasure and satisfaction in engaging in occupations. Being interested in an occupation means that one feels an attraction based on anticipation of a positive experience. This attraction may come from positive feelings associated with the exercise of capacity, intellectual or physical challenge, fellowship with others, aesthetic stimulation, or other factors. Other pleasures associated with occupations may emanate from sensory experiences that arise during performance, aesthetic arousal, or intellectual intrigue. Since many occupations produce outcomes or products, satisfaction may also emanate from what is created or produced. Attraction to any particular occupation typically represents the convergence of more than one of these factors.

The Volitional Process

Volitional thoughts and feelings are embedded in a cycle of anticipation, choice, experience while doing, and subsequent interpretation (Kielhofner, 2002). The attraction to occupations, beliefs about capacity, and convictions about performance influence how people attend to the world and anticipate opportunities and requirements to do things. Volition also shapes the choices people make to engage in occupation and the way they experience and interpret what they have done. For example, a student who is committed to attending a competitive college may anticipate with anxiety, put forth substantial effort studying for, and react negatively to getting an average grade on an examination. Another student who plans to enter a skilled trade may be much less concerned with preparing for the examination and quite pleased with receiving an average grade. The way persons anticipate, choose, experience, and make sense of what they do is always based on their own unique volition.

Habituation

Habituation organizes one's doing into the recurrent patterns that make up much of daily routines. These patterns integrate people into the rhythms and customs of the physical, social, and temporal worlds.

Habituation connects people to and makes them functional within their familiar social, physical, and temporal context. Habituation also depends on and uses the regularity in these environments to guide action (e.g., the rhythms of day and week, the patterned actions of others, and the stable physical environment). It involves the ability to appraise the action-significance of various features of the environment. For example, the appearance of an acquaintance is recognized as occasion for a greeting, the buzzing of the alarm clock as time to rise, or the approaching landmark as the place to turn the car on the way to work. Such appreciations enable people, without deliberation or attention, to do what has become habituated in the right way, place, and time.

Habituated patterns of action are governed by habits and roles. Together, habits and roles weave the patterns with which people traverse their temporal, physical, and social contexts. Habits and roles give regularity, character, and order to what people do and how they do it.

Habits

Through repeated experience, individuals acquire ways of appreciating and behaving in familiar environments. These habits are learned ways of doing occupations that unfold automatically. Habits regulate behavior by providing a manner of dealing with environmental contingencies. They locate people in unfolding events, allowing them to steer their behavior toward familiar and expected circumstances. **Habits**, then, are acquired tendencies to automatically respond and perform in certain, consistent ways in familiar environments or situations.

Roles Through interaction with others, people also internalize attitudes and ways of behaving that belong to a given role. Once internalized, a **role** serves as a framework for looking out on the world and for acting. Enacting a role may be reflected in one's dress, demeanor, and the content of one's actions. Roles not only shape one's attitude and actions but also profoundly influence the sense of who one is. For example, people see themselves as students, workers, parents, friends, and so on.

The Influence of Habituation in Everyday Life Habituation regulates the patterned, familiar, and routine allowing people to automatically recognize and respond to features and situations in the environment. Importantly, habituation thus steers people through a host of routine circumstances that are managed without having to attend to them reflectively. By doing so, habituation

frees one up to engage consciously in other thoughts or actions while doing routine things. For example, while driving to work, we can plan aspects of the day, listen to the radio, or carry on a conversation. Such layering of activity characterizes much of each person's daily routine.

Performance Capacity

Performance capacity is the ability for doing things provided by the status of underlying objective physical and mental components and corresponding subjective experience. A number of practice models address capacities and impairments related to movement, perception, and cognition; therefore, the model of human occupation has not been directly concerned with performance capacity. However, new theory within the model (Kielhofner et al., 2002) offers a different but complementary way of understanding performance capacity that focuses on subjective or lived experience and its role in how people perform. This perspective asserts that experience, instead of being simply an artifact or consequence of doing something, is central to how people perform. The fundamental argument is that to learn any performance, one must discover how it feels (i.e., locate the experience within the lived body). The **lived body**, then, is the experience of being and knowing the world through a particular body. Performance is guided, then, by how it feels to engage in occupation.

The Environment

This model conceptualizes the environment as providing opportunities, resources, demands, and constraints (Kielhofner, 2002). How the environment affects each person depends on that person's values, interests, personal causation, roles, habits, and performance capacities. This unique influence of the environment in each individual is referred to as **environmental impact.**

Physical and Social Environment

Both the physical and social environment impact motivation for, patterning, and performance of occupation. The **physical environment** consists of the natural and human-made spaces (e.g., forest, pond, classroom, theatre) and the objects within them (e.g., trees, rocks, books, cars, and computers). The **social environment** consists of groups of persons and the occupational forms that individuals belonging to those groups perform. Groups provide and assign roles to their members, and groups constitute social space in which those roles are acted out according to group ambience, norms, and climate. **Occupational forms** are rule-bound sequences of action that are oriented to a purpose, sustained in collective knowledge, culturally recognizable, and named. Said simply, occupational forms are the things that are available to do in any social context. The **occupational settings** in which people perform (e.g., home, neighborhood, school, workplace) are made up of unique configurations of spaces, objects, occupational forms, and/or social groups that cohere and constitute a meaningful context for performance. So, for example, a person whose neighborhood is a small town in the countryside will have quite different opportunities and resources, demands, and constraints than someone whose neighborhood is the area surrounding public housing in an inner city.

> **Volition, habituation, performance capacity, and environmental conditions always resonate together, creating conditions out of which our thoughts, feelings, and behavior emerge.**

Organization of Occupation

The model of human occupation uses systems theory to frame how volition, habituation, performance capacity, and environment are interrelated and organized over time (Kielhofner, 2002). Two main points are emphasized:

◆ Occupation is dynamic and context-dependent.
◆ People shape who they are by what they do.

The first point underscores that a person's inner characteristics constantly interact with the environment to influence how one is motivated, what one does, and how one performs. What a person does is the result of a confluence of personal and environmental circumstances. Thus, occupation reflects a complex interplay of motives, habits and roles, and performance capacity and environmental conditions.

Volition, habituation, performance capacity, and environmental conditions always resonate together, creating conditions out of which our thoughts, feelings, and behavior emerge. The following are examples of such resonation:

◆ Anxiety from a lack of belief in skill interfering with performance
◆ Old habits interfering with new volitional choices
◆ The pull of values that keep a person going despite physical pain or environmental barriers

Values, interests, personal causation, roles, habits, performance capacity, and the physical and social context are always tethered together into a dynamic whole. What people do, think, and feel come out of that dynamic whole.

The second point underscores that humans require constant maintenance and reorganization, which is accomplished through the person's ongoing pattern of doing. The development, continued existence, and transformation of persons' characteristics depend on their ongoing acting, thinking, and feeling. Volition, habituation, and performance capacity are constituted, maintained, and changed through the very processes to which they are put to use.

Occupation is a dynamic process through which people maintain the organization of their bodies and minds. Engaging in work, play, and activities of daily living serves to organize the self (e.g., refines abilities, shapes thoughts and feelings about self, creates social identities, and forms habits).

Participation, Performance, and Skill

This model conceptualizes the doing of occupations at three levels:

◆ Participation
◆ Performance
◆ Skill

Participation

Occupational participation refers to engaging in work, play, or activities of daily living that are part of one's sociocultural context and that are desired and/or necessary to one's well-being. It is the broadest level at which doing can be examined. Examples of occupational participation are working in a full- or part-time job, routinely pursuing a hobby, maintaining one's home, and attending school.

Performance

Occupational performance refers to doing a specific occupational form. For example, when persons do things such as walking the dog, baking a cake, mopping the floor, balancing the checkbook, or mending a shirt, they are performing. Each area of participation is made up of a number of performances. For example, attending school may include

such occupational forms as reading a book, listening to a lecture and taking notes, writing a paper, and taking an examination.

Skill

Within their occupational performance, people carry out discrete purposeful actions. For example, making coffee is a culturally recognizable occupational form in many Western cultures. To do so, one engages in such purposeful actions as *gathering* together coffee, coffeemaker, and a cup; *handling* these materials and objects; and *sequencing* the steps necessary to brew and pour the coffee. These actions that make up occupational performance are referred to as skills. **Skills** are goal-directed actions that a person uses while performing (Fisher, 1999; Kielhofner, 2002). In contrast to performance capacity, which refers to underlying ability, skill refers to the discrete functional actions that make up actual performance. This model identifies three types of skills: **motor skills**, **process skills**, and **communication and interaction skills**. Detailed taxonomies of the skills that make up each of the three types of skills have been developed as part of creating assessments of skill. Fisher and colleagues have developed the taxonomies of motor and process skills that make up an Assessment of Motor and Process Skills (Doble, 1991; Fisher, 1993, Berspang & Fisher, 1995). Forsyth and her colleagues have developed a taxonomy of communication/interaction skills that make up the Assessment of Communication/Interaction Skills (Forsyth et al., 1998; Forsyth, Lai, & Kielhofner, 1999).

Occupational Adaptation, Identity, and Competence

This model defines **occupational adaptation** as the construction of a positive identity and achieving competence over time in the context of one's environment (Kielhofner, 2002). This definition acknowledges that occupational adaptation has two distinct and interrelated elements:

◆ Occupational identity
◆ Occupational competence

Occupational Identity

Occupational identity refers to the composite sense of who one is and wishes to become as an occupational being, which is generated from one's history of occupational participation. One's volition, habituation, and experience as a lived body are all integrated into occupational identity. Occupational identity reflects accumulated life experiences, which are then organized into an understanding of who one has been and a sense of desired and possible direction for one's future. Occupational identity serves both as a means of self-definition and as a blueprint for ongoing action.

Occupational Competence

Occupational competence is the degree to which one sustains a pattern of occupational participation that reflects one's occupational identity. Thus, while identity has to do with the subjective meaning of one's occupational life, competence has to do with putting that identity into action in an ongoing way. Competence appears to begin with organizing one's life to meet basic responsibilities and personal standards and extends to meeting role obligations and then achieving a satisfying and interesting life (Kielhofner & Forsyth, 2001).

Persons realize their occupational identity and competence over time as they develop and respond to life changes (including illness and impairment). Adaptation hinges on constructing identities that correspond to one's underlying capacities and environmental possibilities, which, therefore, can be put into effect in ongoing life.

Summary

The model incorporates a range of concepts related to the motivation, patterning, and performance of occupation and the influence of the environment on this process. As illustrated in Figure 10-1, p. 154, the model proposes that volition, habituation, and performance capacity represent the internal characteristics of the individual that influence occupation. These interact with the environment determining what the individual does. The model examines doing at three levels (skill, performance, and participation). Over time, the participation of the individual in work, play, and activities of daily living generates and sustains occupational identity and competence that together make up occupational adaptation.

 Problems and Challenges

When people's identities do not fit with their possibilities for enacting them, or when they become frayed by life circumstances, occupational adaptation is threatened. Most people will, at one time or another, experience a threat to or problems in occupational adaptation. Problems in occupational adaptation are explained in this model by the status of volition, habituation, performance capacity, and environmental factors.

> **When people's identities do not fit with their possibilities for enacting them or when they become frayed by life circumstances, occupational adaptation is threatened.**

The role of volition in disability may vary widely. Volition may lead to activities and occupational choices that are the sources of impairments. Acquired impairments may threaten and alter previously positive personal causation, interests, and

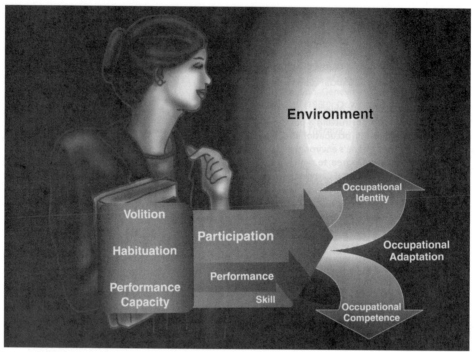

Figure 10-1. The process of occupational adaptation. (Reprinted from Kielhofner, G: Model of Human Occupation: Theory and Application, 3rd ed, Lippincott, Williams & Wilkins, Philadelphia, 2002)

values, leading to a breakdown of morale and motivation.

When habituation is affected by a disability, people can lose a great deal of what has given life familiarity, consistency, and relative ease. Impairments can invalidate established habits and require one to develop new habits for much of everyday life. New habits may be needed to accommodate to or manage the disability. Habits can also be eroded by long periods of enforced inactivity or destabilized by fluctuations or progressive deterioration of one's impairments. The onset of a disability may necessitate changing much of the manner of accomplishing the daily things that were at once taken for granted and familiar.

Persons with disabilities may lack opportunities to learn or enter occupational roles, while finding themselves assigned to marginal roles. Limitations of capacity can disrupt or terminate role performance or lead to major modifications in how one enacts the role.

One of the major tasks of living with disability is to construct for oneself a habituated pattern that allows one to live effectively and comfortably in accord with personal desires and needs. Reconstructing life following onset of a disability means moving from the known to the unknown. One must reencounter the world within one's altered condition in order to reconstruct a pattern of living represented in new or altered roles and habits.

New concepts of performance capacity that emphasize experience call attention to the unique experiences of having a particular disability that must be managed and used in dealing with the disability. Kielhofner et al. (2002) illustrate how disability and change can be illuminated by careful attention to the nature of the disability experience. Inasmuch as this approach is a radical departure from traditional ways of looking at performance capacity, it offers new ideas and innovative strategies for addressing impairments of performance capacity.

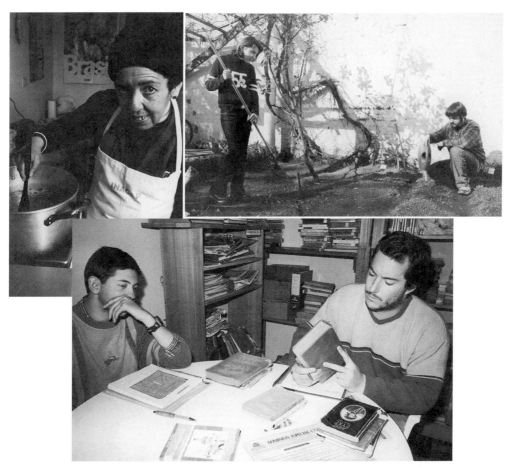

At Reencuentros, a community rehabilitation center in Chile, clients engage in preparing a noon meal, maintaining the center's library, and clearing the grounds. This MOHO-based program provides these and other real-life occupations as a means of enhancing clients' skills, habits, roles, and sense of meaning and efficacy.

This model also recognizes that physical and social environment can present significant barriers to occupational adaptation. Factors ranging form architectural barriers to social injustices can restrict the opportunity and place negative demands on persons with disabilities.

Just as this model views occupational adaptation to be a function of the interactive dynamics of volition, habituation, performance capacity, and environmental conditions, it recognizes that problems of adaptation are also a function the dynamic interaction of these factors. The model of human occupation thus recognizes occupational problems as multifactorial, involving motivation, the patterning of action, the experience of impairments, and physical and social contextual factors. Understanding occupational problems requires recognizing how these personal and environmental factors interrelate.

Therapeutic Intervention

The model of human occupation begins with the idea that all forms of intervention (even those with compensatory aims) involve change. For example, when individuals use a modification in the environment to compensate for permanent impairments, they must adjust their habits of performance and often revise their values and personal causation. Thus the concept of change and understanding the nature and process of change is central to this model's explanation of therapeutic intervention.

Chapter 18 (Kielhofner & Forsyth, 2002) of the most recent edition of *A Model of Human Occupation: Theory and Application* provides a detailed account of the process of change that occurs in therapy. It stresses that only clients can accomplish their own change. Volition, habituation, and performance capacity change are conceptualized as a function of the client's **occupational engagement** (i.e., the client's performance of one or more occupational forms and the attendant thoughts and feelings that occur as part of therapy). The concept of occupational engagement underscores two points:

> **The concept of change and understanding the nature and process of change is central to this model's explanation of therapeutic intervention.**

◆ For doing to be therapeutic, it must involve an actual occupational form, not a contrived activity.
◆ For the client to achieve change through doing, what is done must have relevance and meaning for the client.

The concepts of this model are also used to identify the kind of change that take place as a result of therapy. For example, the following are changes related to different aspects of the model:

◆ Enhance understanding of performance capacities (strengths and weaknesses)
◆ Develop emotional acceptance of limitations and pride in occupational abilities
◆ Acquisition of a new habit pattern that incorporates a new object
◆ Develop values that support positive occupational choices
◆ Improve awareness of responsibilities associated with success in various roles

◆ Increase participation in things of interest

The model also provides explanations for how a client's doing, thinking, and feeling propel the kinds of changes just noted. Kielhofner and Forsyth (2002) offer a taxonomy of client actions that occur in therapy and that drive such change. This taxonomy is designed to provide a more structured way for thinking about what clients do, think, and feel in therapy.

 # Technology for Application

The resources for applying this model include:

◆ A range of assessments
◆ A large number of documented case examples illustrating application of the model in assessment, treatment planning, and intervention
◆ Published papers and manuals that describe the implementation of programs based on the model

There are a variety of these resources for almost any area of practice.

Assessment Tools

To date, 19 assessments have been developed (including substantial empirical validation) for use with this model. Most of the assessments are explained in manuals that provide instructions for administration and interpretation supported by case examples. Each is briefly overviewed below. Table 10-1 summarizes some characteristics of these assessments.

TABLE 10-1. MOHO-BASED ASSESSMENTS

Assessment (Concepts addressed by the Assessment)	Occupational Adaptation		Volition			Habituation		Skills			Performance	Participation	Environment		Method of Data Gathering			Population			
	Identity	Competence	Personal Causation	Values	Interests	Roles	Habits	Motor	Process	Communication/Interaction			Physical	Social	Observation	Self-report	Interview	Children	Adolescents	Adults	Elderly
Assessment of Communication and Interaction Skills										X					X			X	X	X	X
Assessment of Motor and Process Skills								X	X						X			X	X	X	X
Assessment of Occupational Functioning			X	X	X	X	X	X	X	X								X	X	X	X
Child Occupational Self Assessment		X		X							X	X				X		X			
Interest Checklist					X											X			X	X	X
Model of Human Occupation Screening Tool			X	X	X	X	X	X	X	X	X				X				X	X	X
NIH Activity Record			X	X	X	X	X									X			X	X	X
Occupational Circumstances Assessment-Interview and Rating Scale		X	X	X	X	X	X				X	X	X	X			X		X	X	X
Occupational Performance History Interview-II	X		X	X	X	X	X				X	X	X	X			X		X	X	X
Occupational Questionnaire			X	X	X	X	X									X			X	X	X
Occupational Self Assessment		X	X	X	X	X	X				X	X	X	X		X			X	X	X
Occupational Therapy Psychosocial Assessment of Learning						X		X	X	X							X	X	X	X	
Pediatric Interest Profile					X											X		X	X		
Pediatric Volitional Questionnaire			X	X	X										X			X			
Role Checklist						X	X									X			X	X	X
School Setting Interview												X	X	X			X	X	X		
Volitional Questionnaire			X	X	X										X					X	X
Worker Role Interview			X	X	X	X	X						X	X			X			X	
Work Environment Impact Scale													X	X			X			X	

Observational Assessments

The Assessment of Communication and Interaction Skills (ACIS) (Forsyth et al, 1998) is an observational tool that measures an individual's skill in discourse and social exchange in the course of daily occupations. Observations, carried out in contexts that are meaningful and relevant to the clients' lives, are used to complete a rating form that consists of 20 items divided into 3 communication and interaction domains: physicality, information exchange, and relations. The Assessment of Motor and Process Skills (AMPS) (Fisher, 1999) is a structured, observational evaluation that measures motor and process skills exhibited in daily life tasks (i.e., persona and domestic activities of daily living). The client is rated on 16 motor skill items and process skill items. The results of both the AMPS and ACIS provide detailed information about why a person is having difficulty in performance.

The Volitional Questionnaire (VQ) (de las Heras et al., 2002) is an observational assessment that captures information on a client's volition and the influence of the environment on motivation. The VQ consists of 14 items that are rated according to the degree of spontaneity the client demonstrates. An environmental form captures relevant information on the influence of the context on motivation. The VQ provides information about the client's interests and values and the amount and kind of environmental support required to optimize the person's motivation. The Pediatric Volitional Questionnaire (PVQ) (Geist et al., 2002) is similar in format to the VQ but is designed for use with children between 2 and 6 years of age.

Self-Report Assessments

The Modified Interest Checklist (Kielhofner & Neville, 1983) is a self-report form that asks clients to indicate past and present interests and the degree of attraction clients express towards those interests. It also gathers information on clients' present and anticipated future participation in interests.

The NIH Activity Record (ACTRE) (Furst et al., 1987; Gerber & Furst, 1992) is a 24-hour log of activities that provides details on the impact of symptoms on task performance, individual perceptions of interest in and significance of daily activities, and daily habit patterns. Specific information gathered covers frequency and/or percentage of time spent in role activity and resting, frequency of rest periods during activity, frequency and/or percentage of time with pain and fatigue and time of day at or activity with which it occurs, plus volitional concerns such as interests, meaning, enjoyment, and perception of personal effectiveness.

The Occupational Questionnaire (OQ) (Smith, Kielhofner, & Watts, 1986) is a pen-and-paper self-report instrument that asks the client to indicate the activities he or she performs during each half hour on a typical weekday and weekend day. After listing the activities, the client indicates whether the activity is work, a daily living task, recreation, or rest and rates how well he or she does the activities, how important they are to him or her, and how much he or she enjoys doing them.

The Role Checklist (Oakley, Kielhofner, & Barris, 1985) is a self-report form on which the client first indicates, for each of 10 roles, whether they have been performed, are currently involved in, and/or plan to perform in the future. Clients are then asked to indicate how valuable each of the 10 roles is for them.

The Occupational Self Assessment (OSA) (Baron et al., 2002) is a two-part self-rating form. Section One includes a series of statements about occupational functioning to which the client responds by labeling each as an area of strength, adequate functioning, or weakness. The client then responds to these same statements, indicating the value he/she places on each item. Section Two includes a series of statements about the environments to which similar responses are given. Once clients have had an opportunity to assess their behavior and their environments, they review the items again in order to establish priorities for therapy, which can be translated into therapy goals. The Child Occupational Self Assessment (COSA) (Federico & Kielhofner, 2002) is similar to the OSA but includes content and format more suited to young respondents.

The Pediatric Interest Profiles (PIP) (Henry, 2000) are age-based profiles of play and leisure interests. These three profiles (The Kid Play Profile: 6-9 years; The Preteen Play Profile: 9-12 years; and the Adolescent Leisure Interest Profile: 12-21 years) were developed to assist therapists in identifying children with play-related problems and may also assist in identifying specific play interests to incorporate into intervention:

Interviews

The Occupational Performance History Interview (OPHI-II) (Kielhofner et al., 1997) gathers information about a client's past and present occupational performance. It is a three-part assessment that includes:

◆ A semistructured interview
◆ Three rating scales that provide a measure of the client's occupational identity, occupational competence, and the impact of the client's occupational settings
◆ A life history narrative that characterizes the client's occupational narrative

The Occupational Circumstances Assessment Interview and Rating scale (OCAIRS) (Haglund et al., 2001) is a briefer interview than the OPHI-II and focuses on an individual's occupational participation. After conducting the semistructured interview, the therapist completes an 11-item rating scale that includes items related to volition, habituation, skills, and readiness for change.

The Worker Role Interview (WRI) (Velozo, Kielhofner, & Fisher, 1998), is a semistructured interview that provides information about the psychosocial/environmental factors that impact work success. The interview is designed to have the client discuss various aspects of his or her life and job setting that have been associated with past work experiences. The WRI rating scale is composed of 16 items reflecting volition, habituation, and perceptions of the environment.

The Work Environment Impact Scale (WEIS) (Moore-Corner, Kielhofner, & Olson, 1998) is a semistructured interview designed to gather information about the impact of the work setting on a person's performance, satisfaction, and well-being. After the interview, the therapist completes a scale reflecting 17 environmental factors such as the physical space, social contacts and supports, temporal demands, objects utilized, and daily job functions.

The School Setting Interview (SSI) (Hoffman, Hemmingson, & Kielhofner, 2000) is a semistructured interview designed to identify the need for accommodations for students with disabilities in the schools setting. The SSI provides a picture of the child's functioning in 14 content areas including writing; reading; speaking; remembering things; doing mathematics; doing homework; taking examinations; going to art, gym, and music; getting around the classrooms; taking breaks; going on field trips; getting assistance; accessing the school; and interacting with staff.

Assessments Using Mixed Methods of Information Gathering

The Assessment of Occupational Functioning (AOF) (Watts et al., 1999) is administered as a semistructured interview or self-report form. It identifies strengths and limitations in personal causation, values, roles, habits, and skills. The occupational therapist scores the rating scale, which includes 20 items reflecting these concepts.

The Model of Human Occupation Screening Tool (MOHOST) (Parkinson & Forsyth, 2001) is a broad screening tool that provides an efficient overview of most of the model's concepts. It identifies client strengths and weaknesses in volition, habituation, skills, and environmental supports. The MOHOST is designed to be flexible in administration (using any combination of observation, discussion with the client, talking to ward/residential staff, and/or talking to relatives to gather information). The assessment enables clinicians to capture knowledge that they build up about a client from many sources and can be used at regular intervals to document baseline assessment and general progress. The MOHOST rating form objectifies the observations an occupational therapist would make as part of regular practice.

The Occupational Therapy Psychosocial Assessment of Learning (OT PAL) (Townsend et al., 2001) is an observational and descriptive assessment tool. It assesses a student's volition (ability to make choices), habituation (roles and routines), and environmental fit within the classroom setting. It gathers information from observation and brief interviews with the student, teacher, and a parent. A rating scale includes 21 items that address the major areas of making choices, habits/routine, and roles. The OT PAL allows the occupational therapist to determine the effectiveness of the fit between the student and the classroom environment and how that match impacts the student's performance in the classroom.

Formal Strategies for Intervention and Programs

A major emphasis in this model recently has been the delineation of specific strategies for its application. Kielhofner (2002) provides detailed information on the process of apply-

ing this model. Additionally, detailed manuals have been developed demonstrating application of the model (Braveman, 2001; de las Heras, Llerena, & Kielhofner, 2003; Olson, 1998). Another resource for application is the multiple case examples of applying the model that can be found in the literature. The second half of the current edition includes 13 chapters presenting cases that represent application of this model with diverse clients in a variety of settings, and many case examples can be found in published papers.

A wide range of programs using the model of human occupation has been described in the literature. These include, for example, programs for such diverse client groups as those with chronic pain (Gusich, 1984; Padilla & Bianchi, 1990), traumatic brain injury (DePoy, 1990), Alzheimer's dementia (Oakley, 1987; Olin, 1985), AIDS (Pizzi, 1990; Schindler, 1990), and borderline personality disorder (Salz, 1983). The model has guided programs for persons who are homeless and mentally ill (Kavanaugh & Fares, 1995), for battle-fatigued soldiers (Gerardi, 1996), for emotionally disturbed children and adolescents (Reekmans & Kielhofner, 1998; Sholle-Martin, 1987; Weissenberg & Giladi, 1989), and for children with attention deficit hyperactivity disorder (Woodrum, 1993). Moreover, the literature describes many programs based on the model of human occupation. These programs are designed for specific contexts, such as a day hospital (Gusich & Silverman, 1991), a work rehabilitation program (Mentrup, Niehaus, & Kielhofner, 1999), prison and correctional settings (Michael, 1991; Schindler, 1990), and early intervention settings (Schaaf & Mulrooney, 1989).

Research

Over 80 studies based on this model have been published (see Kielhofner and Iyenger, 2002 for a review). These include both basic research designed to test the theory and applied research that examine its utility in practice. Basic research on the model includes the following kinds of studies:

◆ Construct validity studies that seek to verify concepts (e.g., Doble, 1991; Mallinson, Kielhofner, & Mattingly, 1996; Oakley et al., 1986; Pan & Fisher, 1994)
◆ Correlative studies that examine the accuracy of relationships between constructs proposed in the theory (e.g., Barris, Dickie, & Baron, 1988; Duellman, Barris, & Kielhofner, 1986; Neville-Jan, 1994; Peterson et al., 1999)
◆ Studies comparing groups of concepts from the theory to test whether they explain group differences (Barris et al., 1986; Davies et al., 1994; Ebb, Coster, & Duncombe, 1989; Lederer, Kielhofner, & Watts, 1985)
◆ Prospective studies that examine the potential of the model's concepts and propositions to predict future behavior or states (Chen et al., 1999; Henry, 1994; Rust, Barris, & Hooper, 1987)
◆ Qualitative studies that explore the model's concepts and propositions in depth (e.g., Jonsson, Josephsson, & Kielhofner, 2000; Jonsson, Josephsson, & Kielhofner, 2001; Jonsson, Kielhofner, & Borell, 1997)

Applied research based on this model falls in the following categories:

◆ Psychometric studies leading to development of assessments (e.g., Brollier et al., 1989; Forsyth, Lai, & Kielhofner, 1999; Fossey, 1996; Viik et al., 1990)
◆ Studies of how the model's concepts influence therapeutic reasoning and practice (e.g., Muñoz, Lawlor, & Kielhofner, 1993; Oakley, Kielhofner, & Barris, 1985)
◆ Studies that examine what happens in therapy (e.g., Helfrich & Kielhofner, 1994; Kielhofner & Barrett, 1998)

◆ Studies that examine the outcomes of services based on the model (Josephsson et al., 1995; Kielhofner & Brinson, 1989)

Over time, research on this model has grown more sophisticated and rigorous. Many of the earlier and continuing studies have focused on validation of model of human occupation concepts and assessments. Studies that examine the therapy process and the outcomes of therapy are less well represented in the body of research, although there is a growing emphasis on such studies related to this model.

🌿 Discussion

Because of its broad focus, the model of human occupation is widely used, and many people have contributed to its development. Consequently, a substantial literature on this model exists and much technology for application has been developed. Over 80 articles and chapters discussing theoretical, applied, or research aspects of the model have been published in English. A current bibliography of literature on the model can be found on the Website: http://www.uic.edu/ahp/OT/MOHOC/

At the same time, this model's broad focus means that a great deal of developmental work is needed to validate and create a technology for applying it. The technology for application is better in some areas of application than in others. For example, while the model has more assessments developed specifically for use with it than with other models, it requires still more assessments if it is to be applied across the range of circumstances for which it has potential. This model has a robust research tradition. As noted earlier, many of the studies are focused on testing the theory and developing assessments. Future research will need to more clearly document the outcomes of services based on this model. While much anecdotal data, including cases and programs of intervention, suggest that the model guides effective therapy, additional evidence is needed.

The model of human occupation is unique in some of the issues it addresses. For example, it is the only model to directly address the motivation for occupation and the only one that emphasizes roles and habits. It also provides a unique view of the environment. Because of its broad focus the model is recognized as a holistic and comprehensive model for practice (Hubbard, 1991). Finally, since the model was one of the first models to develop with a strong focus on occupation, many persons see it as a useful integrating framework for therapy and for explaining the unique focus of occupational therapy.

TERMS OF THE MODEL

Communication and interaction skills	Conveying intentions and needs and coordinating social behavior to act together with people
Environmental impact	Influence (in the form of opportunity, support, demand, or constraint) that environment has on a particular individual
Habits	Acquired tendencies to automatically respond and perform in certain, consistent ways in familiar environments or situations
Habituation	Internalized readiness to exhibit consistent patterns of behavior guided by habits and roles and fitted to characteristics of routine temporal, physical, and social environments
Interests	What one finds enjoyable or satisfying to do
Internalized role	Incorporation of a socially and/or personally defined status and a related cluster of attitudes and actions
Lived body	Experience of being and knowing the world through a particular body
Motor skills	Moving self or task objects
Occupational adaptation	Construction of a positive occupational identity and achieving occupational competence over time in the context of one's environment
Occupational competence	Degree to which one is able to sustain a pattern of occupational participation that reflects one's occupational identity
Occupational engagement	Performance of one or more occupational forms and attendant thoughts and feelings that occur as part of therapy
Occupational forms	Rule-bound sequences of action that are oriented to a purpose, sustained in collective knowledge, culturally recognizable, and named
Occupational identity	Composite sense of who one is and wishes to become as an occupational being, generated from one's history of occupational participation
Occupational participation	Engagement in work, play, or activities of daily living that are part of one's sociocultural context and that are desired and/or necessary to one's well-being

TERMS OF THE MODEL

Occupational performance	Doing an occupational form
Occupational settings	The unique configurations of spaces, objects, occupational forms, and/or social groups that cohere and constitute a meaningful context for performance
Performance capacity	Ability for doing things provided by the status of underlying objective physical and mental components and corresponding subjective experience
Personal causation	Sense of competence and effectiveness
Physical environment	The natural and human-made spaces (e.g., a forest, pond, classroom, theatre) and the objects within them (e.g., trees, rocks, books, cars, computers)
Process skills	Logically sequencing actions over time, selecting and using appropriate tools and materials, and adapting performance when encountering performance
Skills	Observable, goal-directed actions that a person uses while performing
Social environment	Groups of persons and the occupational forms that individuals belonging to those groups perform
Values	What one finds important and meaningful to do
Volition	Pattern of thoughts and feelings about oneself as an actor in one's world that occur as one anticipates, chooses, experiences, and interprets what one does

Summary

Focus

The model of human occupation is concerned with:

◆ Motivation for occupation
◆ Occcupational life pattern
◆ Subjective dimension of performance
◆ Influence of environment on occupation

This model is intended for use with any person experiencing problems in occupational life

Interdisciplinary Base

This model uses concepts from:

◆ Psychology and anthropology, concerning human needs and motives
◆ Sociology, social psychology, and early occupational therapy literature concerning the patterning of behavior
◆ Concepts related to performance from phenomenological philosophy
◆ Environmental concepts from psychology, sociology, and anthropology
◆ Systems theory to frame how these factors are organized together

Theory

The model conceptualizes humans as composed of three elements:

◆ Volition
◆ Habituation
◆ Performance capacity

Volition refers to the process by which persons are motivated toward and choose what they do

Habituation refers to a process whereby doing is organized into patterns and routines

Performance capacity refers both to the underlying objective mental and physical abilities and the lived experience that shapes performance

Volition

Includes a deep human drive for action combined with thoughts and feelings about doing things

Volitional thoughts and feelings include:

◆ Personal causation, which is awareness of one's abilities and the sense of how effective one is in achieving what one wants
◆ Values that define what is worth doing, how one ought to perform, and what goals or aspirations deserve commitment
◆ Interests, which are dispositions to enjoy different types of doing

Volitional thoughts and feelings are embedded in a cycle of anticipation, choice, experience while doing, and subsequent interpretation

Habituation

Habituation organizes one's doing into the recurrent patterns that make up much of daily routines

Habituated patterns of action are governed by habits and roles that give regularity, character, and order to what people do and how they do it

Habits:

◆ Learned ways of doing occupations that unfold automatically
◆ Regulate behavior by providing a manner of dealing with environmental contingencies

Habits locate people in unfolding events

and allow them to steer their behavior toward familiar and expected circumstances

Roles:

◆ Serve as a framework for looking out on the world and for acting
◆ Profoundly influence the sense of who one is

Habituation:

◆ Regulates the patterned, familiar, and routine, allowing people to automatically recognize and respond to features and situations in the environment
◆ Steers people through routine circumstances that are managed without having to attend to them reflectively

Performance Capacity
New theory:

◆ Offers a different but complementary way of understanding performance capacity that focuses on subjective experience and its role in how people perform
◆ Asserts that instead of being simply an artifact or consequence of doing, experience is central to how people perform

Environment
Provides:

◆ Opportunities
◆ Resources
◆ Demands
◆ Constraints

The unique influence of environment on each individual is referred to as environmental impact.

Physical and social environment impact on motivation for, patterning, and performance of occupation:

◆ Physical environment:
◆ Natural and human-made spaces

◆ Objects within them
◆ Social environment:
◆ Groups of persons
◆ Occupational forms

Occupational settings are composed of unique configurations of spaces, objects, occupational forms, and/or social groups

Systems Theory

Systems theory frames how volition, habituation, performance capacity, and environment are interrelated and organized over time, emphasizing that:

◆ Occupation is dynamic and context-dependent
◆ People shape who they are by what they do
◆ Conceptualizes the doing of occupations at three levels:
  1. Participation
  2. Performance
  3. Skill

Occupational Adaptation, Identity, and Competence

Occupational adaptation has two distinct and interrelated elements:

◆ Occupational identity
◆ Occupational competence

Persons realize their occupational identity and competence over time as they develop and respond to life changes

Problems and Challenges

Most people will, at one time or another, experience a threat to or problems in occupational adaptation

Problems in occupational adaptation:

◆ Explained by the status of volition, habituation, performance capacity, and environmental factors
◆ Are multifactorial, involving motivation, patterning of action, experience of impair-ments, and physical and social contextual factors

Therapeutic Intervention

Concept of change and understanding nature and process of change is central to this model's explanation of therapeutic intervention

Provides a detailed account of process of change that occurs in therapy

Stresses that only clients can accomplish their own change

Concept of occupational engagement underscores two points:

◆ For doing to be therapeutic, it must involve an actual occupational form, not a contrived activity
◆ For client to achieve change through doing, what is done must have relevance and meaning for client

Concepts of this model are also used to identify kind of change that take place as a result of therapy

Model also provides explanations for how a client's doing, thinking, and feeling propels changes just noted

Technology for Applicaton

The resources for applying this model include:

◆ A range of assessments
◆ Case examples
◆ Programs based on model

Assessment Tools

To date 19 assessments have been developed for use with this model (see Table 10-1 for summary):

Formal Strategies for Intervention and Programs

Major emphasis recently has been delineation of specific strategies for application

New text provides detailed information on process of applying this model

Detailed manuals have been developed demonstrating application of model

Multiple case examples are in literature

Wide range of programs using the model has been described in literature

Research

Over 80 studies based on this model have been published including:

◆ Construct validity studies that seek to verify concepts
◆ Correlative studies that examine accuracy of relationships between constructs proposed in the theory
◆ Studies comparing groups of concepts from the theory to test whether they explain group differences
◆ Prospective studies that examine the potential of concepts and propositions to predict future behavior or states
◆ Qualitative studies that explore concepts and propositions in depth
◆ Psychometric studies leading to development of assessments
◆ Studies of how model's concepts influence therapeutic reasoning and practice
◆ Studies that examine what happens in therapy
◆ Studies examining outcomes of services based on model
◆ Over time, research on model has grown more sophisticated and rigorous

Discussion

Because of its broad focus, the model of human occupation is widely used and many people have contributed to its development

Substantial literature on this model exists

Much technology for application has been developed

Model is unique in some of the issues it addresses

Because of its broad focus, model is recognized as holistic and comprehensive model for practice

References

Baron K, Kielhofner, G, Iyenger, A, et al. (2002). The Occupational Self Assessment (OSA) (Version 2.0). Chicago: Model of Human Occupation Clearinghouse, Department of Occupational Therapy, College of Applied Health Sciences, University of Illinois at Chicago.

Barris, R, Dickie, V, & Baron, K. (1988). A comparison of psychiatric patients and normal subjects based on the model of human occupation. Occupational Therapy Journal of Research, 8, 3-37. Commentary by Mann, W & Klyczek, J, in same issue. Response to commentary by Barris, R & Dickie, V, in same issue.

Barris, R, Kielhofner, G, Burch, RM, et al. (1986). Occupational function and dysfunction in three groups of adolescents. Occupational Therapy Journal of Research, 6, 301–317.

Bernspang, B & Fisher, AG. (1995). Differences between persons with right or left cerebral vascular accident on the Assessment of Motor and Process Skills. Archives of Physical Medicine and Rehabilitation, 76 (12), 1–1151.

Braveman, B. (2001). Development of a community-based return to work program for people living with AIDS. Occupational Therapy in Health Care, 13(3–4), 113–131.

Brollier, C, Watts, JH, Bauer, D, et al. (1989). A concurrent validity study of two occupational therapy evaluation instruments: The AOF and OCAIRS. Occupational Therapy in Mental Health, 8(4), 49–59.

Chen, C, Neufeld, PS, Feely, CA, et al. (1999). Factors influence compliance with home exercise programs among patients with upper-extremity impairment. American Journal of Occupational Therapy, 53(2), 171–180.

Davies Hallet, J, Zasler, N, Maurer, P et al. (1994). Role change after traumatic brain injury in adults. American Journal of Occupational Therapy, 48(3), 241–246.

Depoy, E. (1990). The TBIIM: An intervention for the treatment of individuals with traumatic brain injury. Occupational Therapy in Health Care, 7(1), 55–67.

Doble, SE. (1991). Test-retest and inter-rater reliability of a process skills assessment. Occupational Therapy Journal of Research, 11(1), 8–23.

Duellman, MK, Barris, R & Kielhofner, G. (1986). Organized activity and the adaptive status of nursing home residents. American Journal of Occupational Therapy, 40, 618–622.

Ebb, EW, Coster, W & Duncombe, L. (1989). Comparison of normal and psychosocially dysfunctional male adolescents. Occupational Therapy in Mental Health, 9(2), 53–74.

Federico, J, & Kielhofner, G. (2002). The Child Occupational Self Assessment (COSA) (Version 1.0). Chicago: Model of Human Occupation Clearinghouse, Department of Occupational Therapy, College of Applied Health Sciences, University of Illinois at Chicago.

Fisher, AG. (1993). The assessment of IADL motor skills: An application of many-faceted Rasch analysis, American Journal of Occupational Therapy, 47 (4), 319–329.

Fisher, AG. (1999). The assessment of motor process skills (AMPS), 3rd ed. Ft. Collins, CO: Three Stars Press.

Forsyth, K, Lai, J-S & Kielhofner, G. (1999). The Assessment of Communication and Interaction Skills (ACIS): Measurement properties. British Journal of Occupational Therapy, 62(2), 69–74.

Forsyth, K, Salamy, M, Simon, S, et al. (1998). The Assessment of Communication and Interaction Skills (ACIS) (Version 4.0). Chicago: Department of Occupational Therapy, University of Illinois at Chicago.

Fossey, E. (1996). Using the occupational performance history interview (OPHI): Therapists' reflections. British Journal of Occupational Therapy, (5), 59, 223–228.

Furst, G, Gerber, L, Smith, C, et al. (1987). A program for improving energy conservation behaviors in adults with rheumatoid arthritis. American Journal of Occupational Therapy, 41, 102–111.

Geist, R, Kielhofner, G, Basu, S, et al. (2002). The Pediatric Volitional Questionnaire (PVQ) (Version 2.0). Chicago: Model of Human Occupation Clearinghouse, Department of Occu-

pational Therapy, College of Applied Health Sciences, University of Illinois at Chicago.

Gerardi, SM. (1996). The management of battle-fatigued soldiers: An occupational therapy model. Military Medicine, 161(8), 483–488.

Gerber, L & Furst, G. (1992). Validation of the NIH Activity Record: A quantitative measure of life activities. Arthritis Care and Research, 5, 81–86.

Gusich, R. (1984). Occupational therapy for chronic pain: A clinical application of the model of human occupation. Occupational Therapy in Mental Health, 4, (3), 59–73.

Gusich, RL & Silverman, AL. (1991). Basava day clinic: The model of human occupation as applied to psychiatric day hospitalization. Occupational Therapy in Mental Health, 11(2/3), 113–134.

Haglund, L, Henriksson, C, Crisp, M, et al. (2001). The Occupational Circumstances Assessment-Interview and Rating Scale (OCAIRS) (Version 2.0). Chicago: Model of Human Occupation Clearinghouse, Department of Occupational Therapy, College of Applied Health Sciences, University of Illinois at Chicago.

Helfrich, C & Kielhofner, G. (1994). Volitional narratives and the meaning of occupational therapy. The American Journal of Occupational Therapy, 48, 319–332.

Henry, AD. (2000). The Pediatric Interest Profiles: Surveys of Play for Children and Adolescents. San Antonio, TX: Therapy Skill Builders.

Henry, A, Tohen, M, & Tickle-Degner, L. (1994). Predicting psychosocial functioning and symptomatic recovery of adolescents and young adults following a first psychotic episode. Paper presented at the Joint Annual Conference of the American Occupational Therapy Association and the Canadian Association of Occupational Therapists, Boston.

de las Heras, CG, Geist, R, Kielhofner, G, et al. (2002). The Volitional Questionnaire (VQ) (Version 4.0). Chicago: Model of Human Occupation Clearinghouse, Department of Occupational Therapy, College of Applied Health Sciences, University of Illinois at Chicago.

de las Heras, CG, Llerena, V & Kielhofner, G. (2003). The remotivation process: Progressive intervention for individuals with severe volitional challenges (Version 1.0). Chicago: Model of Human Occupation Clearinghouse, Department of Occupational Therapy, College of Applied Health Sciences, University of Illinois at Chicago.

Hoffman, OR, Hemmingson, H & Kielhofner, G. (2000). A user's manual for the School Setting Interview (SSI) (Version 1.0). Chicago: Model of Human Occupation Clearinghouse, Department of Occupational Therapy, College of Applied Health Sciences, University of Illinois at Chicago.

Hubbard, S. (1991). Towards a truly holistic approach to occupational therapy. British Journal of Occupational Therapy, 54(11), 415–418.

Jonsson, H, Josephsson, S & Kielhofner, G. (2000). Evolving narratives in the course of retirement: A longitudinal study. American Journal of Occupational Therapy, 54(5), 463–470.

Jonsson, H, Josephsson, S & Kielhofner, G. (2001). Narratives and experience in an occupational transition: A longitudinal study of the retirement process. American Journal of Occupational Therapy, 55(4), 424–432.

Jonsson, H, Kielhofner, G & Borell, B. (1997). Anticipating retirement: The formation of narratives concerning an occupational transition. American Journal of Occupational Therapy, 51(1), 49–56.

Josephsson, S, Backman, L, Borell, L, et al. (1995). Effectiveness of an intervention to improve occupational performance in dementia. Occupational Therapy Journal of Research, 15, 36–49.

Kavanaugh, J & Fares, J. (1995). Using the model of human occupation with homeless mentally ill patients. British Journal of Occupational Therapy, 58(10), 419–422.

Kielhofner, G. (1980a). A model of human occupation, Part two: Ontogenesis from the perspective of temporal adaptation. American Journal of Occupational Therapy, 34, 657–663.

Kielhofner, G. (1980b). A model of human occupation, Part three: Benign and vicious cycles. American Journal of Occupational Therapy, 34, 731–737.

Kielhofner, G. (2002). A Model of Human Occupation: Theory and Application, 3rd ed. Baltimore: Lippincott, Williams & Wilkins.

Kielhofner, G & Barrett, L. (1998). Meaning and

misunderstanding in occupational forms: A study of therapeutic goal setting. American Journal of Occupational Therapy, 52(5), 345–353.

Kielhofner, G, Braveman, B, Finlayson, M, et al: Outcomes of vocational programs for persons with AIDS. American Journal of Occupational Therapy, in press.

Kielhofner, G & Brinson, M. (1989). Development and evaluation of an aftercare program for young and chronic psychiatrically disabled adults. Occupational Therapy in Mental Health, 9(2), 1–25.

Kielhofner, G, & Burke, J. (1980). A model of human occupation, Part one: Conceptual framework and content. American Journal of Occupational Therapy, 34, 572–581.

Kielhofner, G, Burke, J & Heard-Igi, C. (1980). A model of human occupation, Part four: Assessment and intervention. American Journal of Occupational Therapy, 34, 777–788.

Kielhofner, G & Forsyth, K. (2001). Measurement properties of a client self-report for treatment planning and documenting therapy outcomes. Scandinavian Journal of Occupational Therapy, 8 (3), 131–139.

Kielhofner, G, & Forsyth, K. (2002). Therapeutic strategies for enabling change. In Kielhofner, G: A Model of Human Occupation: Theory and Application, 3rd ed, pp 296–308. Baltimore: Lippincott, Williams & Wilkins.

Kielhofner, G & Iyenger, A. (2002). Research: Investigating MOHO. In Kielhofner, G: A Model of Human Occupation: Theory and Application, 3rd ed, pp 520–545. Baltimore: Lippincott, Williams & Wilkins.

Kielhofner, G, Mallinson, T, Crawford, C, et al. (1997). A user's guide to the Occupational Performance History Interview-II (OPHI-II) (Version 2.0). Chicago: Model of Human Occupation Clearinghouse, Department of Occupational Therapy, College of Applied Health Sciences, University of Illinois at Chicago.

Kielhofner, G & Neville, A. (1983). The modified interest checklist. Chicago: Model of Human Occupation Clearinghouse, Department of Occupational Therapy, College of Applied Health Sciences, University of Illinois at Chicago.

Kielhofner, G, Tham, K, Baz, T, et al. (2002). Performance capacity and the lived body. In Kielhofner, G: A Model of Human Occupation: Theory and Application, 3rd ed. Baltimore: Lippincott, Williams & Wilkins.

Lederer, J, Kielhofner, G & Watts, J. (1985). Values, personal causation and skills of delinquents and nondelinquents. Occupational Therapy in Mental Health, 5(2), 59–77.

Mallinson, T, Kielhofner, G & Mattingly, C. (1996). Metaphor and meaning in a clinical interview. American Journal of Occupational Therapy, 50, 338–346.

Mentrup, C, Niehaus, A & Kielhofner, G. (1999). Applying the model of human occupation in work-focused rehabilitation: A case illustration. Work, 12(1), 61–70.

Michael, PS. (1991). Occupational therapy in a prison? You must be kidding! Mental Health Special Interest Section Newsletter, 14, 3–4.

Moore-Corner, R, Kielhofner, G & Olson, L. (1998). The Work Environment Impact Scale (WEIS) (Version 2.0). Chicago: Model of Human Occupation Clearinghouse, Department of Occupational Therapy, College of Applied Health Sciences, University of Illinois at Chicago.

Muñoz, JP., Lawlor, M & Kielhofner, G. (1993). Use of the model of human occupation: A survey of therapists in psychiatric practice. Occupational Therapy Journal of Research, 13 (2), 117–139.

Neville-Jan, A. (1994). The relationship of volition to adaptive occupational behavior among individuals with varying degrees of depression. Occupational Therapy in Mental Health, 12(4), 1–18.

Oakley, F. (1987). Clinical application of the model of human occupation in dementia of the Alzheimer's type. Occupational Therapy in Mental Health, 7(4), 397–450.

Oakley, F, Kielhofner, G & Barris, R. (1985). An occupational therapy approach to assessing psychiatric patients' adaptive functioning. American Journal of Occupational Therapy, 39, 147–154.

Oakley, F, Kielhofner, G, Barris, R, et al. (1986). The role checklist: Development and empirical assessment of reliability. Occupational Therapy Journal of Research, 6, 157–170.

Olin, D. (1985). Assessing and assisting the person with dementia: An occupational behavior perspective. Physical & Occupational Therapy in Geriatrics, 3(4), 25–32.

Olsen, LM. (1998). Word Readiness: Day Treatment for Persons with Chronic Disabilities. Chicago: Model of Human Occupation Clearinghouse, Department of Occupational Therapy, College of Applied Health Sciences, University of Illinois at Chicago.

Padilla, R & Bianchi, EM. (1990). Occupational therapy for chronic pain: Applying the model of human occupation to clinical practice. Occupational Therapy Practice, 1(3), 47–52.

Pan, AW & Fisher, A. (1994). The assessment of motor and process skills of persons with psychiatric disorders. American Journal of Occupational Therapy, 48, 775–780.

Parkinson, S & Forsyth, K. (2001). A user's manual for the Model of Human Occupation Screening Tool (MOHOST) (Version 1.0). Unpublished manuscript. UK: MOHO CORE, University of London.

Peterson, E, Howland, J, Kielhofner, G, et al. (1999). Falls self-efficacy and occupational adaptation among elders. Physical and Occupational Therapy in Geriatrics, 16(1/2), 1–16.

Pizzi, MA. (1990). The model of human occupation and adults with HIV infection and AIDS. American Journal of Occupational Therapy, 44, 257–264.

Reekmans, M & Kielhofner, G. (1998). Defining occupational therapy services in child psychiatry: An application of the model of human occupation. Ergotherapie, 5, 6–13.

Rust, K, Barris, R & Hooper, F. (1987). Use of the model of human occupation to predict women's exercise behavior. Occupational Therapy Journal of Research, 7, 23–35.

Salz, C. (1983). A theoretical approach to the treatment of work difficulties in borderline personalities. Occupational Therapy in Mental Health, 3(3), 33–46.

Schaaf, RC & Mulrooney, LL. (1989). Occupational therapy in early intervention: A family-centered approach. American Journal of Occupational Therapy, 43, 745–754.

Schindler, VP. (1990). AIDS in a correctional setting. Occupational Therapy in Health Care, 7(2/3/4), 171–183.

Sholle-Martin, S. (1987). Application of the model

of human occupation: Assessment in child and adolescent psychiatry. Occupational Therapy in Mental Health, 7(2), 3–22.

Smith, N, Kielhofner, G & Watts, J. (1986). The relationship between volition, activity pattern and life satisfaction in the elderly. American Journal of Occupational Therapy, 40, 278–283.

Townsend, SC, Carey, PD, Hollins, NL, et al. (2001). The Occupational Therapy Psychosocial Assessment of Learning (OT PAL) (Version 1.0). Chicago: Model of Human Occupation Clearinghouse, Department of Occupational Therapy, College of Applied Health Sciences, University of Illinois at Chicago.

Velozo, C, Kielhofner, G, & Fisher, G. (1998). A user's guide to the Worker Role Interview (WRI) (Version 9.0). Chicago: Model of Human Occu-

pation Clearinghouse, Department of Occupational Therapy, College of Applied Health Sciences, University of Illinois at Chicago.

Viik, MK, Watts, JH, Madigan, MJ, et al. (1990). Preliminary validation of the Assessment of Occupational Functioning with an alcoholic population. Occupational Therapy in Mental Health, 10(2), 19–33.

Weissenberg, R & Giladi, W. (1989). Home economics day: A program for disturbed adolescents to promote acquisition of habits and skills. Occupational Therapy in Mental Health, 9(2), 89–103.

Woodrum, SC. (1993). A treatment approach for attention deficit hyperactivity disorder using the model of human occupation. Developmental Disabilities Special Interest Section Newsletter, 16 (1), 1–2.

Chapter 11

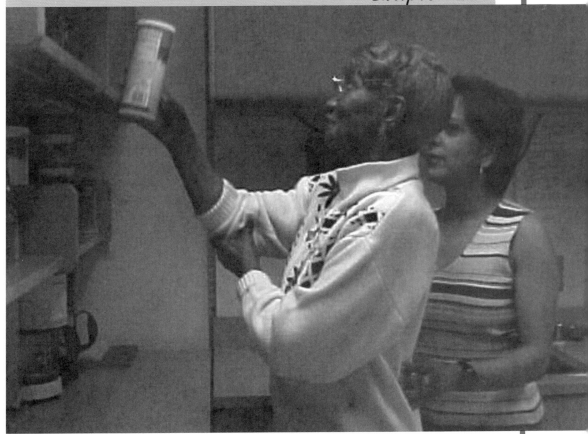

The Motor Control Model

A client who recently experienced shoulder dislocation secondary to reflex sympathetic dystrophy is engaged in a cooking activity. As the client does the various tasks required (e.g., reaching for ingredients on a shelf), the occupational therapist carefully observes her motor actions, at the same time giving her physical support to stabilize her standing. The therapist will facilitate the client's discovery of the most functional way she can go about accomplishing this necessary everyday activity while also noting how modifications in the physical environment and the way the client does the cooking tasks can increase her client's effectiveness. This combination of strategies for enabling the client to successfully complete a meal is reflective of the motor control model as it is practiced today.

Four treatment approaches of similar origin and with similar concepts and techniques have traditionally been used in occupational therapy for persons with brain trauma resulting in difficulty controlling movement. These are:

♦ The Rood approach
♦ Bobaths' neurodevelopmental therapy
♦ Brunnstrom's movement therapy
♦ Proprioceptive neuromuscular facilitation

These approaches share similar concepts and techniques (Trombly & Radomski, 2002). They are referred to collectively as neurodevelopmental approaches because they are based on a view of the nervous system and emphasize its developmental nature. All four neurodevelopmental approaches share the goal of improving **motor control;** that is, the ability to use one's body effectively while performing an occupation. Motor control includes such diverse components as generating and coordinating movement patterns of the head, limbs, and trunk, and maintaining balance during occupational performance.

As a group, these approaches have sought to explain motor impairment and to specify strategies of intervention aimed at improving motor control. These approaches address motor problems that occur as a result of damage to the central nervous system (CNS). With CNS damage, neural communication to muscles is often preserved but impaired because of the insult to central processing components of the brain.

The neurodevelopmental approaches are often taught and used together not only because they share concepts, but also because they draw upon much the same interdisciplinary knowledge. More recently, interdisciplinary conceptualizations of how humans achieve motor control have changed dramatically (Mathiowetz & Bass-Haugen, 1994). As a consequence, occupational therapists have developed a new conceptualiza-

tion of motor control that challenges some of the most basic assumptions of the neurodevelopmental approaches and replaces them with a new, modified view of how persons control movement in the context of occupations.

While offering a distinctly different conceptualization of how humans control movement, the contemporary motor control model, nevertheless, has evolved from the traditional neurodevelopmental approaches. Hence, it is important to consider the concepts and techniques of these neurodevelopmental approaches and how they are reconceptualized in the current motor control model.

 # Interdisciplinary Base

The traditional neurodevelopmental approaches as well as the current motor control model are based on interdisciplinary concepts about how motor control is developed and learned. These concepts come from neurophysiology, neuropsychology, human development, psychology, and human movement science (Trombly & Radomski, 2002). The neurodevelopmental approaches are based on older knowledge, whereas the motor control concepts represent recent concepts of motor control and motor development.

Traditional Interdisciplinary Concepts

Although the interdisciplinary base is complex, the following concepts are common to the neurodevelopmental approaches. Originally, normal movement was presumed to emanate from "genetically wired configurations of neurons" (Trombly, 1989, p. 78). These biologically determined movement patterns, which occur in response to sensory stimuli, are referred to as **reflexes.** Different reflex patterns emerge as the nervous system matures in the course of normal development. Movement patterns associated with the spinal cord and lower brain centers appear first, followed by those associated with higher brain centers. The emphasis on reflexes originates from the earliest interdisciplinary ideas about motor control dating back to the beginning of the last century. This approach suggested that movement was achieved through collective action of multiple reflexes (Mathiowetz & Bass-Haugen, 1994, 2002).

Later research and concepts showed the reflex model to be insufficient to explain motor control. This led to the concept of **hierarchical control,** which argued that movements are controlled from the top down. According to this argument, higher centers in the nervous system exert control over lower-level parts of the nervous system that organize reflexes (Mathiowetz & Bass-Haugen, 1994, 2002). The higher centers acquire and store motor programs that act as instructions for movement. So, for example, the theory holds that the pattern of movement required for reaching to grasp an object is stored in a CNS generalized motor program acquired from previous experiences of reaching and grasping. The program, an abstract representation of the sequence, duration, speed, and direction of movements, is required to effect the movements and postural adjustments necessary for reaching.

According to this hierarchical explanation, reflex patterns are integrated into voluntary movement and, therefore, come under higher-level control. Both the emergence of reflexes and their eventual integration into hierarchically controlled patterns of voluntary movement are considered to be the result of ongoing development and reorganization in the CNS. As the nervous system is considered the highest executive system involved in

> While offering a distinctly different conceptualization of how humans control movement, the contemporary motor control model, nevertheless, has evolved from the traditional neurodevelopmental approaches.

motor control, all abilities for and problems of motor control emanate from that system. Thus, the integrity of the CNS and its organization are considered the foundations of motor control.

Other important concepts derived from the earlier interdisciplinary literature were related to development (Mathiowetz & Bass-Haugen, 1995). Neurodevelopmental concepts stress that there is an invariant sequence of development. Motor control develops from head to foot **(cephalocaudal)** and from the middle of the body to the distant limbs **(proximodistal).** This sequence of development was believed to be driven by maturation of the CNS and to represent the gradual development of control of higher centers over lower centers. In this conceptualization, the environment did not have a direct role in influencing motor control. Rather, the organization of the CNS determined movement patterns, and changes in the CNS produced changes in motor performance.

A final concept common to all four approaches is the **plasticity** of the nervous system. The neurodevelopmental approaches all assume that the CNS is a flexible system with potential for organization and reorganization as the result of experience. Drawing upon the concept of neuroplasticity, the neurodevelopmental approaches argue that, since the experience of controlling movement is necessary to brain organization, such experience can be utilized in therapy to achieve organization or reorganization of the brain.

Contemporary Interdisciplinary Concepts

Newer interdisciplinary concepts have criticized and sought to replace concepts on which the neurodevelopmental approaches are based (Kamm, Thelen, & Jensen, 1990; Mathiowetz & Bass-Haugen, 1994, 2002).

The most important criticism of the idea of hierarchical control of movement is the observation that an almost infinite number of motor programs would be required to specify the necessary detail for even a simple task to be performed in variable contexts. Briefly stated, the argument goes as follows. The various muscles and joints involved in motion can be used and combined in a very large number of ways (these possibilities are referred to as degrees of freedom). If each of these degrees was controlled directly by a central mechanism, the instructions the central mechanism would have to store would be so complex as to be impossible. Hence, hierarchical conceptualization of motor control is recognized as implausible.

In its place, a new conceptualization based on dynamical systems concepts has been proposed (Kamm, Thelen, & Jensen, 1990; Mathiowetz & Bass-Haugen, 1994, 2002). This conceptualization focuses on the interaction of the human nervous and musculoskeletal systems with the environment. Moreover, the components of central nervous and musculoskeletal systems are considered to work together heterarchically, that is, cooperating together toward the production of movement but without central executive control. Finally, the context and the task the person is performing are understood to have a major role in the organization of motor control. This idea of multiple personal and environmental factors co-contributing to organize movement is referred to as **heterarchical control.**

Within the dynamical systems framework, this problem is addressed through the concept of **coordinative structures**, which are groups of muscles acting over many joints but constrained to behave together as a single functional unit to achieve a purposeful action. An example is natural tenodesis. Long flexor and extensor muscles acting over the wrist and finger joints coordinate to produce wrist extension and finger flexion as a single functional pattern for grasping. Such coordinative structures compress the available degrees of freedom (e.g., all the possible planes of movement of the wrist and finger joints) into a single pattern, eliminating the need for detailed central instructions for all the muscles involved. The dynamics for this process are provided locally as an emergent feature of the joints and muscles in action. Hence, coordinative structures do not require hierarchical control of all the details of movement.

When persons perform routine tasks they use certain preferred movement patterns out of the many patterns that are possible for accomplishing that particular task. These preferred patterns of doing a task, such as reaching for an object, are conceptualized as **attractor states**. These attractor states do not require centralized instructions (i.e., motor programs), which have pre-coded all the necessary movement patterns. Rather, the patterns of movement come together as a synergy during actual performance. That is, the movement pattern emerges from the dynamic interaction of the nervous and musculoskeletal systems with the environment and the task being performed.

The dynamical systems perspective argues that motor control is distributed among many components. These components include the CNS, components of the musculoskeletal system, goal of the task, and relevant conditions in the environment (e.g., the size, shape, weight, and location of an object to be grasped and lifted). Any one of these variables, whose change can shift a pattern of motor behavior into another pattern, is considered a **control parameter.**

Dynamical systems theory views motor control as an emergent phenomenon, arising out of the dynamics of all these components as they interact. Hence, the systems explanation does not view the CNS as the central executor of movement and eliminates the need for pre-coded instructions that specify all the details of movement ahead of time. Rather than depending on a motor program that contains all the necessary information for movement, the control of movement depends on the dynamic conditions of interacting systems. The dynamical systems view emphasizes that the parts of the CNS cooperate together to achieve performance rather than being hierarchically organized with higher centers controlling lower centers. Consequently, dynamical systems theory envisions all parts of the human system coming together in a functionally related and context-dependent way rather than in a fixed and centrally instructed way (Kamm, Thelen, & Jensen, 1990; Mathiowetz & Bass-Haugen, 1994, 2002).

The systems view also emphasizes that development is influenced not only by changes in the CNS but also by changes in all the elements involved in motor control (e.g., environment, task, CNS, and musculoskeletal system). Rather than being a fixed sequence of motor changes, development is a variable process of learning to find individual optimal solutions to **motor problems** (i.e., motor challenges such as learning to reach out and grasp an object) (Mathiowetz & Bass-Haugen, 1994, 2002).

From this discussion, it should be clear that the interdisciplinary concepts on which occupational therapy approaches to motor control have been founded have changed dramatically. Hence, it is not surprising that the conceptual practice model of motor control has changed. We will first examine occupational therapy's four neurodevelopmental approaches, which are based in the earlier reflex-hierarchical concepts, before going on to contrast these approaches with the current dynamical systems–based approach.

 # Theory and Technology for Application of the Neurodevelopmental Approaches

This section highlights the main theory and overviews the technology for application of the four neurodevelopment treatment approaches. While these approaches are founded on much the same interdisciplinary base and overlap substantially, they are discussed separately since they have different emphases and somewhat different arguments about movement problems and recovery of motor control.

The Rood Approach

This approach is named for its originator, Margaret Rood, an occupational therapist and physical therapist. She originally developed this approach for the treatment of persons with cerebral palsy, but it has since been applied to a wide variety of motor control problems.

Organization

According to Rood, normal motor control emerges from the use of reflex patterns present at birth. As these patterns are used and generate sensory stimuli in purposeful activities, they support voluntary control at a conscious (cortical) level. However, the patterns themselves are believed to be under unconscious (subcortical) control. Basic movement patterns do not require conscious attention, which instead can be directed to the goal or purpose of the task. This subconscious organization of motor control makes for efficiency in motor tasks. An additional observation of this approach is that different muscles have different responsibilities in the body; that is, they perform different kinds of work. Accordingly, Rood classified muscles into light-work muscles (muscles whose function is primarily movement) and heavy-work muscles (those whose function is primarily stabilization). These two types of muscles are under different types of nervous system control (i.e., heavy-work muscles tend to be more reflexively controlled, light-work muscles more voluntarily controlled), and they respond differently to sensory stimulation.

Motor Problems

Rood (1956) observed that, with CNS damage, the normal sequence of reflex development and learned voluntary motor control did not occur. Moreover, abnormal muscle tone was often present. **Muscle tone** refers to the state of stiffness or tension in muscle. Muscle tension is necessary to maintain postural states. A muscle that is sufficiently stiff is ready to be called on to contract appropriately when required. Muscle tone is maintained by the CNS in response to ongoing sensory information. When the CNS is impaired, muscles may not be adequately tense (hypotonic) or may be too tense (hypertonic).

Therapeutic Intervention

Underlying this approach is the hypothesis that appropriate sensory stimulation can elicit specific motor responses (McCormack & Feuchter, 1996). The therapeutic approach includes four strategies:

◆ Normalizing muscle tone by using sensory stimuli to evoke an appropriate muscle response
◆ Beginning with the person's current developmental level and progressing through the normal sequence of motor development
◆ Focusing attention on the goal or purpose of an activity
◆ Providing opportunities for repetition to reinforce learning

Much of Rood's technique centers on pro-viding appropriate sensory inputs to evoke muscle response (Rood, 1956). Sensory stimuli (e.g., applying ice, brushing, and stroking the area over muscles) and proprioceptive stimuli (e.g., manual joint compression, quick stretching, tapping, pressure applied by the therapist, resistance to movement) are used to facilitate muscles. Sensory stimuli such as slow rhythmic movement, neutral warmth, and maintained stretching are used by the therapist to inhibit muscles. Olfactory, gustatory, auditory, and visual stimuli are also used to facilitate or inhibit responses. These latter sensory stimuli are used when voluntary control is minimal and where abnormal tone and reflexes are present.

Treatment progresses sequentially, from evoking muscle response with sensory stimuli to using obtained responses in developmentally appropriate patterns of movement to purposeful use of the movements in activities. Rood identified a normal developmental sequence of motor behavior to be followed in treatment. Ideally, the various techniques of sensory stimulation are used in occupational therapy to assist the client to move voluntarily and to prepare the client for active participation in purposeful activities (McCormack & Feuchter, 1996).

Technology for Application

Within the Rood approach, therapists first identify the highest developmental motor pattern that the person can manage with ease. Treatment then begins with the next level, at which the person must struggle. Sensory stimulation and manual assistance may be used to help the person perform the movement until the person is able to achieve satisfactory voluntary control of the movement.

Rood's work initiated interest in occupational therapy concerning the role of sensory stimulation in recovery of motor control. However, information from neuroscience suggests that the way in which sensory stimulation affects motor responses is more complex than the approach suggested (Brunnstrom, 1970). For example, there is evidence that the physical response to sensory stimulation is mediated or modulated by psychological factors, such as the individual's emotional state and the perceived significance of sensory stimulation (e.g., touch). Hence, the relationship between sensory stimulation and motor response is not a simple linear one as assumed in the traditional therapeutic use of sensory stimulation.

Bobaths' Neurodevelopmental Treatment

The Bobaths, a neurologist and physiotherapist team, originally developed the neurodevelopmental treatment (NDT) approach for persons with cerebral palsy (Bobath, 1978). This approach is also believed to be effective for any person with abnormal movement due to a CNS deficit. For example, this approach is frequently included in the treatment of adult hemiplegia (Trombly & Radomski, 2002).

Organization

NDT is based on the following premises:

◆ Motor control involves learning the sensations of movement (not the movement per se)
◆ Basic postural movements are learned first, later elaborated on, and integrated into functional skills
◆ Every activity has postural control as its underlying foundation

Motor Problems

Motor problems following brain damage involve abnormal muscle tone (e.g., spasticity) and abnormal patterns of posture and movement that interfere with everyday functional activity. Moreover, when posture and movement are abnormal, the individual's sensation reflects these abnormal patterns and provides incorrect information to the CNS.

Therefore, the person is unable to experience and learn or relearn normal movement.

Therapeutic Intervention

Treatment requires that abnormal patterns be inhibited and replaced with the normal movement patterns that will provide appropriate sensory information for motor learning. Abnormal patterns are inhibited and normal ones are elicited by providing appropriate sensory stimuli. When persons are enabled to perform correct patterns of movement, the sensory information about movement that they generate for themselves enables the learning of motor control. Thus, the basis of this approach is for the client to learn how appropriate movement feels

Technology for Application

Evaluation consists of determining the highest developmental level at which the person can consistently perform. Evaluation also aims to describe muscle tone when the body is in various developmental positions and how tone changes in response to external stimulation or voluntary effort. The evaluation identifies, for example, whether a person is arrested at a particular developmental level of motor control or whether motor abilities are scattered across developmental levels with gaps in between. Thus, the evaluation provides an individualized picture of the person's development of motor control.

Treatment follows the developmental progression and emphasizes the correct **handling** of the person to inhibit abnormal distribution of tone or postures while stimulating and encouraging active motor performance at the next developmental level. Handling is based on the principle that there are key points of control for movement (usually, but not always, proximal areas, such as the shoulder girdle). The therapist handles these points to inhibit abnormal movement and facilitate normal movement (Trombly & Radomski, 2002). Handling can take place in association with voluntary efforts of the client; its aim is to facilitate more normal movement.

Sensory stimulation, such as physically tapping muscles, may also be used. Once normal responses are elicited, they are repeated, and the person is given the opportunity to practice the movement in purposeful tasks. The thrust of therapy is to encourage voluntary control over normal responses. The underlying belief of the NDT approach is that once a person is able to control a particular developmental motor pattern voluntarily, that person will be able to integrate it into skilled activities. The goal of treatment is to prepare the person for functional performance. However, direct involvement in tasks that significantly challenge capacities are considered contraindicated because they may elicit and reinforce maladaptive muscle tone and motor patterns.

The NDT approach has been used in occupational therapy to support and facilitate normal movement in the context of purposeful activities (Trombly & Radomski, 2002). Therapeutic activities can be adapted for clients with hemiplegia to follow the principles of this approach. Additionally, principles are incorporated into training adults with hemiplegia to perform daily living activities (e.g., teaching a person to inhibit abnormal muscle tone in his or her own body when such tone would otherwise interfere with dressing) (Trombly & Radomski, 2002).

Brunnstrom's Movement Therapy

Brunnstrom developed movement therapy as an approach to the treatment of motor control problems in persons with hemiplegia following cerebrovascular accident (Brunnstrom, 1970).

Organization

The view of organization is based on the observation that normal development involves progression of reflex development. Moreover, reflexes are modified, and their components are rearranged into purposeful movement. This is accomplished as higher centers in the brain take over.

Motor Problems

Brunnstrom observed that persons who experienced cerebrovascular accidents exhibited lower levels of motor function (i.e., reflex behavior) (Brunnstrom, 1970). She identified and categorized stereotypical limb movement patterns that occur sequentially in recovery from hemiplegia. She referred to these patterns as limb synergies. These synergies are patterned flexion or extension movements of the entire limb that are evoked by attempts to move the limb voluntarily, by efforts to move the unaffected limb, and/or by other sensory stimuli. Brunnstrom reasoned that because each of these reflex patterns was normal at some stage in the course of development, they could be considered normal when they appeared in persons with hemiplegia resulting from brain damage. The occurrence of these patterns was simply evidence that the function of the damaged CNS had reverted to an earlier developmental stage.

Therapeutic Intervention

Brunnstrom's therapeutic approach begins with eliciting reflex synergies and using them as the basis for progressively learning more mature voluntary movement, much as it is learned in normal development. This approach stresses using the motor patterns that are available to the client in order to progress through the recovery stages (Pedretti & Zoltan, 2001).

Technology for Application

In this approach, evaluation involves determining the person's sensory status (since the ability to sense and recognize patterns of movement is important to treatment), which reflexes are present, and the current level of recovery. Brunnstrom (1970) identified six levels of recovery from hemiplegia:

1. Flaccidity with no voluntary movement
2. Movement synergies beginning to appear
3. Voluntary control of synergies
4. Voluntary movements deviating from synergies
5. Voluntary independence from basic synergies
6. Voluntary isolated joint movements with near-normal coordination

Treatment is based on the following principles:

♦ Using the developmental recovery sequence
♦ Facilitating movement through sensory stimulation when no voluntary movement is present
♦ Encouraging volitional control over stimulated movements
♦ Reinforcing emerging synergies by asking the client to hold positions and move voluntarily
♦ Employing synergies that are under control in functional activities

The occupational therapy application of this approach centers on the use of controlled movements in purposeful activities. In stages 3 and 4 of recovery, when the client has some voluntary control, activities can be adapted to make use of these motor behaviors. Sometimes this involves using the affected extremity to stabilize objects while the unaffected arm is used in the task. Activities can be adapted to promote the use of existing synergies and to elicit motor behaviors that break out of, or combine, synergies and thus accomplish even greater volitional control of movement (Pedretti & Zoltan, 2001).

Brunnstrom's approach differs from the Bobath approach. The Bobaths maintained that motor patterns appearing after brain damage should not be used in retraining motor control. However, Brunnstrom argued that in the early stages of recovery, when only reflex activity is present, such activity must be used. Brunnstrom did agree, however, that reflex activity should be inhibited in the later stages of recovery.

Proprioceptive Neuromuscular Facilitation

Proprioceptive neuromuscular facilitation (PNF) is defined as "a method of promoting or hastening the response of the neuromuscular mechanism through stimulation of the proprioceptor" (Voss, Ionta, & Meyers, 1985, p. xvii). This approach is somewhat broader and more eclectic than the other three.

Organization

Several principles define the organization held by this approach (Meyers, 1995). According to this view, normal motor development proceeds cephalocaudally and proximodistally. Reflexes dominate early motor behavior and, with maturity, are integrated into voluntary motor behavior. Motor behavior is cyclic (alternating between flexion and extension phases). Normal goal-directed behavior is made up of reversing movements (e.g., flexing, then extending) and depends on a balance between antagonistic muscles (e.g., flexors and extensors). Motor behavior develops in an orderly sequence of total movement patterns. This development is not stepwise; instead, there is overlap between successive stages of motor development.

Increases in motor abilities require learning. This learning often involves acquiring a chain or series of steps and later integrating them into the task. Frequent stimulation and motor repetition support retention of learned motor abilities. A final, important principle is that motor learning requires multisensory information. Auditory, visual, and tactile systems provide sensory data along with proprioceptive information to program the learning of movement.

Motor Problems

In terms of this approach, impairment is any difficulty with motor control. PNF was originally developed for the treatment of persons with cerebral palsy and multiple sclerosis, but it has found application with a wide range of clients, including persons whose motor limitations are not of CNS origin.

Therapeutic Intervention

The therapeutic approach of PNF is multisensory. The kinds of sensory stimulation used include physical contact by the therapist, visual cues, and verbal commands. The central feature of treatment is the use of diagonal patterns of movement (i.e., moving extremities in a plane diagonal to the body midline) for recovery of motor function. Diagonal patterns are considered the treatment of choice because they involve natural movements that are part of normal development and require integration of both sides of the body.

Technology for Application

Evaluation is broad-based and may include determination of the developmental postures and movement patterns of which the individual is capable and of the person's ability to use these capacities in functional activities. The goal of evaluation is to gather a comprehensive picture of the strengths and challenges of the client's capacity for movement and to identify these in sufficient detail so that appropriate techniques for intervention can be selected.

Several techniques are used to encourage the client's engaging in natural diagonal patterns of movement. One method is irradiation, which seeks to facilitate specific muscle action by using stronger muscle groups to stimulate activity of weaker groups. Another technique, successive induction, aims to facilitate one voluntary motion by using another. A third technique, reciprocal innervation, uses voluntary motion to inhibit reflexes. Other techniques include appropriate positioning, use of manual contact for positioning or stimulation, and verbal commands and instructions for movement. Other

sensory stimulation, such as stretching muscles and providing resistance to movement, are also employed. Goal-directed movements combined with facilitation techniques are believed to be the most effective means of treatment.

Summary of Neurodevelopmental Approaches

Although the previous discussion illustrates the different emphases of the four neurodevelopmental approaches, the approaches have common views. By summarizing the common views of these four, the approaches can be collectively compared with the contemporary motor control approach in occupational therapy.

Organization

The neurodevelopmental approaches all share the following view of motor control (Mathiowetz & Bass-Haugen, 1994, 2002). They assert that the CNS is hierarchically organized (i.e., higher centers control lower centers) and that movement is controlled by sensory input to lower centers and through the encoded motor programs of higher centers. Development and learning occur because of maturational or experientially driven changes in the CNS. Essentially, motor control occurs because the human being learns to master movements and then uses those movements to accomplish tasks. Fixed sequences of motor learning and development are viewed as necessary consequences of how the system hierarchically builds on and modifies lower-level movement patterns (e.g. voluntary movement builds on reflex-driven postural control).

Motor Problems

According to the neurodevelopmental approaches, abnormal patterns of movement result directly from disorganization in the CNS. Damage to the CNS disrupts or interferes with sensory/perceptual inputs, motor programs, and the normal hierarchical organization of motor control. This, in turn, produces abnormal muscle tone, reflexes, and movement patterns.

Therapeutic Intervention

The neurodevelopmental approaches focus exclusively on understanding and remediating motor control deficits that are believed to result directly from the nature of damage to or disorganization in the CNS. The most basic concepts underlying the approach to intervention focus on:

◆ Inhibiting with sensory stimuli abnormal muscle tone, reflexes, and movement patterns
◆ Facilitating with sensory stimuli normal muscle tone and movement patterns

Underlying this focus is the assumption that all observed changes in the dynamics of muscle and movement are directly related to changes achieved in CNS organization.

The neurodevelopmental approaches em-phasize learning through task repetition with constant assistance (e.g. handling, positioning, instructions) and feedback from the therapist. They also emphasize a developmental progression from learning parts of a task to proceeding to combine the parts into a whole.

Recovery and treatment are expected to follow normal developmental sequences from reflex to voluntary control, from gross to discrete movements, and from proximal to distal control. Consequently, these approaches emphasize using movements that are normal or that follow recovery sequences. The perceived importance of these sequences is based on the assumption that they are "hard-wired" in the CNS.

Technology for Application

In the neurodevelopmental approaches, evaluation focuses on:

◆ Determining the status of muscle tone, sensation and perception, and postural control

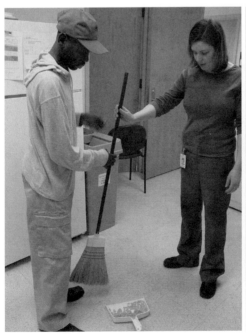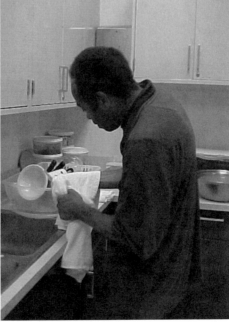

Everyday tasks are used as a context for evaluation and intervention in the model of motor control.

◆ Identifying abnormal reflexes and movement patterns

◆ Ascertaining the developmental level of existing motor control patterns

The technology for treatment relies heavily on the use of external sensory stimulation and handling to elicit correct patterns of movement. Moreover, these approaches emphasize practicing and mastering movement patterns with the assumption that, once normal movement patterns are mastered, they will generalize to functional motor control in occupational performance. Participation in occupation is not emphasized. When occupations are used, they are chosen because they are thought to elicit the appropriate movement patterns. Sometimes the use of occupational activities have been discouraged because they are seen as developing isolated splinter skills. Such splinter skills are viewed as specific to the task performed and hence not generalizable to other areas of performance. In general, occupation does not play a central role in the remediation of motor control deficits in the neurodevelopmental approaches.

Theory and Technology for Application of the Contemporary Motor Control Approach

The contemporary motor control approach is in the process of being more fully articulated in occupational therapy. While a number of authors have begun to refer to and make use of current motor control concepts, Mathiowetz and Bass-Haugen (1994, 1995, 2002) and Trombly and Radomski (2002) have offered the most systematic articulation to date in the occupational therapy literature.

Theory

The theory of this approach is strongly tied to the contemporary interdisciplinary conceptualization of motor control. While only recently elucidated in occupational therapy, it constitutes a coherent explanation of organization, problems and challenges, and intervention as it concerns the control of movement in occupational performance.

Organization

Motor control is viewed as emerging from the interaction of the human (CNS and musculoskeletal components) with environmental and task variables. Movement is a self-organizing phenomenon that depends on this dynamic interaction; it is not dependent solely on the CNS. The CNS is viewed as a heterarchically organized system with higher and lower centers interacting cooperatively with each other and with the musculoskeletal system.

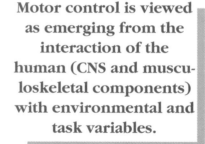

> Motor control is viewed as emerging from the interaction of the human (CNS and musculoskeletal components) with environmental and task variables.

Movement patterns are not invariant sequences "pre-wired" into the CNS. Instead, they are stable (or preferred) ways to accomplish occupational performance, given the unique characteristics of the human being and certain environmental conditions. These preferred patterns of movement can be perturbed by changes in any of the participating systems or in the environment.

Motor control is learned through a process in which the person seeks optimal solutions for accomplishing an occupation. Hence, learning is dependent on the characteristics of the performer, the context, and the goal of the occupation being performed. Patterns of movement become attractor states when they are practiced. When they are practiced under a wider range of conditions, they are more stable than when learned under narrow conditions. Changes in the environmental conditions, the occupation being performed, or the person can result in a disintegration or a qualitative shift in the preferred pattern of movement.

A variable whose change can shift the motor behavior into another pattern is referred to as a control parameter. Control parameters may be changes in variables within the musculoskeletal system, the task or the environment, or the CNS. For example, changes in strength, CNS maturation, size or weight of an object being handled, or the speed of action required for the task can be control parameters that change motor behavior patterns.

The contemporary model of motor control in occupational therapy emphasizes the role of the occupation being performed and the occupational context in which it is performed. Occupational form, which refers to goal and procedures of the occupational activity being performed, is recognized as having an important influence on all motor control. Within this model, motor control is viewed as behavior that self-organizes specifically in the context of performing a given occupational form (Lin, Wu, & Trombly, 1998; Trombly, 1995; Wu, Trombly, & Lin, 1994).

Finally, the contemporary motor control model does not emphasize a fixed developmental sequence. Developmental pathways depend both on the unique characteristics of the individual and on variations in the environment in which motor control is learned.

Problems and Challenges

When persons have CNS damage, problems of motor behavior result from the attempt to compensate for the damage while performing a specific occupational form in a given context. If the occupation or the environment in which the person is performing changes, the kind of motor behavior the person exhibits may also change (Mathiowetz &

Bass-Haugen, 1994, 1995; Trombly, 1995). Hence, while impairment of movement is related to deficits in the CNS, it is not directly caused by those deficits. Rather, movement patterns are a consequence of the dynamics that occur between a person with specific abilities and limitations (as represented in both the CNS and the musculoskeletal system) and the occupational and environmental demands faced in performing. Thus, for example, an abnormal movement pattern may be jointly influenced by CNS impairment and muscle weakness but may be present only under certain occupational and environmental conditions.

Therapeutic Intervention

A central premise of the task-oriented approach is that "functional tasks help organize behavior" (Mathiowetz & Bass-Haugen, 2002, p. 139). According to Mathiowetz and Bass-Haugen, therapy begins by identifying those tasks that are difficult to perform and by noting the preferred movement patterns the person uses for these tasks. The therapist then determines the personal and environmental systems that either support optimal performance or contribute to ineffective performance. This provides an identification of the supporting and limiting factors in motor control and serves as a basis for determining intervention. The therapist also seeks to determine the stability or instability of motor behaviors across occupational and environmental conditions. In this way, the range of conditions in which functional and impaired movement patterns are manifest can be determined. This reveals how strong an attractor state a particular movement pattern is and, therefore, how easily it can be disturbed or shifted to another pattern.

Depending on what evaluation reveals, intervention can differ. For example, if a person's motor behavior is unstable, the therapist may help the client find the optimal motor solution and practice it so that it becomes more stable. If the client is using a motor control strategy that accomplishes the goal of the task but that is not the most efficient or safe, the therapist may help the client to find and stabilize different strategies of movement.

The contemporary motor control approach stresses learning the entire occupation rather than discrete parts. This approach also emphasizes allowing persons to find their own optimal solutions to motor problems rather than relying on instructions and constant feedback. Persons are allowed to experiment and problem-solve in the context of occupational performance. Feedback on the overall consequences of performance is considered more useful than discrete feedback about parts of the performance.

> **The contemporary motor control approach stresses learning the entire occupation rather than discrete parts.**

The goals of treatment in this approach focus on:

◆ Accomplishing necessary and desired occupational forms in the most efficient way, given the client's characteristics
◆ Allowing the person to practice in varying and natural contexts so the learned motor behaviors are more stable
◆ Maximizing personal and environmental characteristics that enhance performance
◆ Enhancing problem-solving abilities of clients so they will more readily find solutions to challenges encountered in new environments beyond the treatment setting

Overall, this approach stresses a collaborative and client-centered approach that considers the client's roles and motives.

Technology for Application

Since the contemporary motor control approach is in an early stage of development, its technology is still being further developed and refined. The approach to evaluation is client-centered and task-oriented, emphasizing the observation of a person's attempts to perform meaningful occupational tasks in context. Evaluation methods incorporate both quantitative and qualitative data-gathering that examines how motor control varies in different occupational forms and contexts (Mathiowetz & Bass-Haugen, 2002; Trombly, 1995). Evaluation begins with observation of occupational performance and proceeds to examine underlying systems only when further understanding of how those systems are constraining performance is needed. For example, the therapist would not begin with evaluation of reflexes and muscle tone. Rather, the therapist would begin with examination of whether and how the persons performed necessary occupational forms. Then, when difficulties are noted, the therapist might proceed to identify whether and how muscle tone and abnormal reflexes contribute (along with the environment and the occupational form) to difficulties in performance. Consequently, the focus of evaluation is on occupational performance, not on the underlying general motor abilities.

This also means that the therapist begins by learning what occupational forms are necessary for the role performance of the client. When therapists examine human systems to determine how they are contributing to difficulties in performance, the CNS is recognized as important but only as one among several factors that co-determine performance. There are not yet validated standard methods of evaluation. However, principles of assessment and ways of incorporating existing assessments into the approach have been identified (Mathiowetz & Bass-Haugen, 2002). Because this model emphasizes the use of client-centered occupational forms, natural environments, and a process of active experimentation for optimal motor solutions, its techniques cannot be as readily specified as those of the neurodevelopmental approaches. These traditional approaches assumed that motor control was driven by a single system, the CNS. Hence, techniques were quite specific. This approach identifies multiple factors that influence motor control and argues that their relative importance and influence on a client's performance are situationally dependent. Hence, the actual techniques used in therapy require an individualized understanding of the client's situation across many dimensions. For those accustomed to the much more standardized approaches of the neurodevelopmental approaches, the motor control approach may, at first, appear much less prescriptive and specific. Bass-Haugen, Mathiowetz, and Flinn (2002) outline a number of principles of this approach. For example, under the general approach using an occupation-based focus, they note that the therapist should:

◆ Use functional tasks as the focus in treatment
◆ Select tasks that are meaningful and important in the client's roles
◆ Analyze the characteristics of the tasks selected for treatment
◆ Describe the movements used for the task performance
◆ Determine whether the movement patterns are stable or in transition
◆ Analyze the movement patterns and functional outcomes of task performance

Additionally, Sabari (1991), Flinn (1995, 1999), and Tse and Spaulding (1998) have outlined the implications of this approach for treatment of persons with specific impairments such as hemiplegia and Parkinson's disease. As principles and strategies of evaluation and intervention such as these are articulated and accompanied by case examples, the technology of this model should become more readily accessible.

Summary and Comparison of the Neurodevelopmental and the Contemporary Motor Control Approaches

In the previous sections, I overviewed the traditional neurodevelopmental and the contemporary motor control approaches. In general, the contemporary motor control approach replaces the more mechanistic explanation of movement with a more dynamic and holistic viewpoint. In contrast to the neurodevelopmental approaches, which de-emphasized the role of the environment and of occupation in motor control and in the remediation of motor control deficits, the contemporary model places a great deal of emphasis on both these elements.

Research

The Bobath NDT approach is the most studied of the four, although the studies tend to be methodologically weak (Levit, 2002). The studies do not clearly show that NDT therapy is an effective treatment. One study suggested that nonspecific play activities were as effective in producing motor behavior gain (parenthetically, the findings of this study appear more compatible with the theory of the contemporary motor control approach). There are no published studies of the effectiveness of NDT with persons who have hemiplegia. Research concerning the PNF approach is limited and focuses primarily on normal populations (Trombly & Radomski, 2002). Usually, each of these studies examined an isolated aspect of PNF, and the results from these studies are mixed. Overall, no systematic body of occupational therapy research has accumulated on the neurodevelopmental approaches.

While the contemporary motor control

approach is relatively new, studies (Math-iowetz & Bass-Haugen, 1994; Wu, Trombly, & Lin, 1994) have begun to provide support for the theory of this model. In summary of research, Ma and Trombly (2002) and Trombly and Ma (2002) note that 15 studies have examined the impact of occupational therapy on coordinated movement. Those studies concluded that among factors associated with positive outcomes are the use of meaningful objects and goal-oriented activities. These studies provide some support for the new motor control model, but it is noted that more research is needed.

Because both the traditional neurodevelopmental and contemporary motor control approaches are heavily based on interdisciplinary research, it is worth considering this research. Clearly, interdisciplinary researchers have strong evidence that contradicts many traditional concepts of motor control. Moreover, a robust research literature is developing that supports the dynamical systems approach. Hence, interdisciplinary studies suggest strongly that the traditional neurodevelopmental approaches need to be reconsidered, incorporated into, and/or replaced with the contemporary motor control approach.

🌿 Discussion

The transition from traditional neurodevelopmental approaches to a contemporary motor control approach raises a number of major challenges. Consideration will need to be given to which concepts and techniques from the traditional approach are still valid and useful in a contemporary framework. Moreover, further articulation of the theory and a great deal of work to develop a technology for application of the contemporary motor control model are needed.

The transition from traditional practice to practice based on the contemporary motor control model is likely to be somewhat uneven. The use of traditional neurodevelopmental approaches is widespread and characterized by strong allegiance of therapists to one or more approaches. Confusion about traditional versus new ideas is also a problem as some of the traditional approaches have attempted to incorporate new motor control ideas while implicitly retaining many of their original tenets.

These circumstances have already led to some disagreements between those who espouse traditional methods and those who are discussing the contemporary motor control approach and its explicit criticism of the traditional neurodevelopmental approaches. A good example of these disagreements is a letter to the editor published in the February 1995 issue of the *American Journal of Occupational Therapy*. A number of therapists strongly objected to a paper by Mathiowetz and Bass-Haugen that introduced new concepts of motor control that implicitly criticized the NDT approach (Cammisa et al., 1995). These therapists argued that NDT has been updated to incorporate new concepts of motor control. However, in response to this letter, the authors of the original article point out that the new concepts of motor control require more than updating NDT (Mathiowetz & Bass-Haugen, 1995). They argue that the new concepts call for a paradigm shift and even question the appropriateness of the term neurodevelopmental as it implies a view of motor control (i.e., a nervous system–driven model of motor control and a fixed developmental sequence) that is not in line with current understanding of motor control. This dialogue has continued in the literature (Burgess, 1989; Cohen, 1989).

Since the four neurodevelopmental approaches are long-standing occupational therapy approaches with significant following by practitioners, the change to a new model based on ideas that not only build on but also criticize and call for replacement and reorganization of the older concepts and techniques will no doubt be controversial for some time. Also, until a new motor control model is more fully articulated and supported with technology for application, therapists will no doubt find it challenging to begin to alter their practices. As when any major transformation in a model of practice occurs, the change it calls for will occur unevenly in practice and will take place over a period of time.

Nonetheless, the kinds of changes in conceptualization and application that are called for by the contemporary motor control approach are very promising. First, they parallel a transformation in thinking about human performance that cuts across many disciplines. Second, they reaffirm many traditional occupational therapy ideas that emphasize the importance of occupation in learning motor skills and restoring motor capacity. The neurodevelopmental approaches were very much founded in the paradigm of inner mechanisms described in Chapter 3. The reorganization of these approaches into a more contemporary motor control model signals the transformation of practice that emanated from that older paradigm to practice consistent with the current paradigm of occupational therapy.

TERMS OF THE MODEL	
Attractor states	Preferred movement patterns that emerge from the dynamic interaction of the person with the environment without centralized instructions
Cephalocaudal	Refers to sequence of motor development from the head downward
Control parameter	A variable whose change can shift a pattern of motor behavior into another pattern
Coordinative structures	Groups of muscles acting over many joints and constrained to behave together as a single functional unit to achieve a purposeful action
Handling	Therapist manipulation of the client's body
Heterarchical control	Conceptualization that argues that movements are controlled by systems cooperating toward the production of movement but without central executive control
Hierarchical control	Conceptualization that argues that movements are controlled from the top down (i.e., higher brain centers control lower ones)
Motor control	The ability to use one's body effectively in interacting with the environment
Motor problems	Challenges for movement such as learning to reach out and grasp an object
Muscle tone	The state of stiffness or tension in muscle
Plasticity	The nervous system's potential for organization and re-organization as the result of experience
Proximodistal	Refers to the sequence of motor development from the middle of the body to the distant limbs
Reflexes	Biologically determined movement patterns not under volitional control

MOTOR CONTROL MODEL

FOCUS

◆ Concerned with problems of movement following brain damage

◆ Consists of four traditional treatment approaches and a contemporary motor control model

INTERDISCIPLINARY BASE

◆ Concepts from neurophysiology, neuropsychology, cognitive psychology, and movement science

COMPARISION OF EACH OF THE MOTOR CONTROL APPROACHES

The Rood Approach	Bobaths' Neurodevelopmental Treatment	Brunnstrom's Movement Therapy	Proprioceptive Neuromuscular Facilitation
Organization	Motor control involves learning the sensations of movement. Basic postural movements are learned first, later elaborated, and integrated into functional skills.	Normal development involves a progression of reflexes that are modified and components of which are rearranged into purposeful movement as higher centers in the brain take over.	Development of motor behavior is cyclic—i.e., made up of reversing movements (e.g., flexing, then extending) and depends on a balance between "antagonistic" muscles (e.g., flexors and extensors).
Normal motor control emerges from the use of subcortically controlled reflex patterns present at birth; they support voluntary control at a conscious (cortical) level.			
Different muscles perform different work:			Motor behavior develops in an orderly sequence of total movement patterns with overlap between successive stages of motor development.
Light-work muscles primarily provide movement and are more voluntarily controlled. Heavy-work muscles primarily stabilize and are more reflexively controlled.			Motor learning involves acquiring a chain or series of steps and later integrating them into the task through stimulation and motor repetition.

MOTOR CONTROL MODEL

The Rood Approach	Bobaths' Neurodevelopmental Treatment	Brunnstrom's Movement Therapy	Proprioceptive Neuromuscular Facilitation
Problems and Challenges			
With CNS damage the normal sequence of reflex development and learning of voluntary motor control are impaired, and abnormal muscle tone is often present.	Brain damage results in spasticity and abnormal patterns of posture and movement that interfere with everyday functional activity.	Cerebrovascular accident (and other brain damage) leads to regression to lower levels of motor function (i.e., reflex behavior).	Motor learning requires multi-sensory information (i.e., auditory, visual, tactile, and proprioceptive).
	When posture and movement are abnormal, sensation provides incorrect information to the CNS, preventing learning or relearning of normal movement.	Stereotypical limb flexion or extension movement patterns occur sequentially in recovery from hemiplegia (limb synergies).	CNS damage and orthopedic problems can interfere with normal patterns of movement, reducing capacity for functional activity.

(Continued)

MOTOR CONTROL MODEL (*Continued*)

The Rood Approach	Bobaths' Neurodevelopmental Treatment	Brunnstrom's Movement Therapy	Proprioceptive Neuromuscular Facilitation
Therapeutic Intervention Progress from appropriate sensory inputs to evoke muscle response when voluntary control is minimal and abnormal tone and reflexes are present, to using obtained responses in developmentally appropriate patterns of movement, to purposeful use of the movements in activities	Abnormal patterns are inhibited and normal ones elicited by sensory stimuli. When persons perform normal patterns of movement, sensory information about movement allows learning of motor control.	Reflex patterns (normal at various stages in the course of development) elicited by brain damage can be built upon for relearning of motor control (thus, they should be initially facilitated and later inhibited).	Multisensory stimulation (including physical contact, verbal commands and visual cues). Employment of natural diagonal patterns of movement (i.e., moving extremities in a plane diagonal to the body midline).
Technology for Application Identify the highest developmental motor pattern that the person can do with ease Use sensory stimuli to normalize muscle tone Begin with current developmental level and progress through normal sequence of motor development. Focus attention on the goal or purpose of an activity. Provide opportunities for repetition to reinforce learning.	Determine the highest developmental level at which the person can consistently perform, distribution of muscle tone when the body is in various developmental positions, and how tone changes in response to external stimulation or voluntary effort.	Identify person's sensory status (sensation to recognize patterns of movement is important to treatment). Identify which reflexes are present, and determine level of recovery as manifest in reflex synergies of movement. Elicit reflex synergies of movement, and use them as the basis for learning progressively more mature voluntary movement.	Determine available developmental postures and movement patterns and ability to use them in functional activities to generate a comprehensive picture of capacity for movement Stimulate diagonal patterns for recovery of motor function through:

MOTOR CONTROL MODEL

The Rood Approach	Bobaths' Neurodevelopmental Treatment	Brunnstrom's Movement Therapy	Proprioceptive Neuromuscular Facilitation
	Abnormal patterns stopped (inhibited through sensory stimuli) and replaced with normal movement patterns (elicited through sensory stimuli) to provide appropriate sensory information for motor learning in developmental sequence.	Employment of developmental recovery sequence: Facilitate movement through sensory stimulation	Facilitating specific muscle action by using stronger muscle groups to stimulate activity of weaker groups (irradiation).
		Encourage volitional control over stimulated movements	Facilitating one voluntary motion by using another (successive induction) and inhibiting reflexes by voluntary motion (reciprocal innervation).
	Handling of the person to inhibit abnormal distribution of tone or postures while stimulating and encouraging active motor performance at the next developmental level.	Reinforce emerging synergies through voluntary use in functional activities	
		Elicit motor behaviors in purposeful tasks that break out of, or combine, synergies for greater volitional control of movement	Appropriate positioning, using manual contact to position or stimulate the individual.
	Practice new abilities in purposeful tasks to encourage voluntary control over normal responses in purposeful activities.		Giving verbal commands and instructions for movement.
			Sensory stimulation such as stretching muscles and providing resistance to movement.
			Goal-directed activities combined with facilitation techniques.

(Continued)

COMPARISON OF NEURODEVELOPMENTAL APPROACHES AND MOTOR CONTROL APPROACHES

Traditional Neurodevelopmental Approaches (Common Features)	Contemporary Motor Control Approach
Organization	
CNS is hierarchically organized (i.e., higher centers control lower centers).	Motor control is a self-organizing phenomenon that emerges from the interaction of the human system (CNS and musculoskeletal components) with environmental and occupational variables.
Movement is controlled by sensory input to lower centers and through the encoded motor programs of higher centers.	CNS is a heterarchically organized system with higher and lower centers interacting cooperatively and with the musculoskeletal system.
Development and learning result from changes in the CNS.	Movement patterns are stable/preferred ways to accomplish occupational performance (attractor states) given the unique characteristics of the human being and environmental conditions.
Fixed sequences of motor learning and development.	Motor control is learned when the person seeks optimal solutions for accomplishing an occupation and depends on the characteristics of the performer, the context, and the goal of the occupation being performed.
	Developmental pathways depend on unique characteristics of the individual and on variations in the environment.
Problems and Challenges	
Abnormal muscle tone, reflexes and patterns of movement result directly from disorganization in the CNS.	Motor impairment is a consequence of the dynamics that occur between a person with specific abilities and limitations (as represented in both the CNS and the musculoskeletal system) and the occupational and environmental demands faced in trying to perform.

Therapeutic Intervention

Inhibition of abnormal muscle tone, reflexes, and movement patterns with sensory stimuli.

Facilitation of normal muscle tone and movement patterns with sensory stimuli.

Learning through task repetition with constant assistance (e.g. handling, positioning, instructions) and feedback from the therapist.

Progression from learning parts of a task to combining the parts into a whole.

Progression of recovery and treatment through developmental sequence (reflex to voluntary control, gross to discrete movements, and proximal to distal control).

Using movements that are normal or which follow recovery sequences.

Technology for Application

Determine status of muscle tone, sensation and perception, and postural control.

Identifying abnormal reflexes and movement patterns.

Ascertaining the developmental level of existing motor control patterns.

External sensory stimulation and handling to elicit correct patterns of movement.

Practicing and mastering movement patterns.

Participation in occupational forms is not emphasized.

Research

Research on neurodevelopmental approaches is limited.

Preliminary studies have begun to provide support for the theory of contemporary motor control approach.

Emphasizes person's attempts to perform meaningful occupational tasks in context.

Intervention depends on:

Identification of those tasks that are difficult to perform, noting the preferred movement patterns for these tasks and their degree of stability/instability.

Determination of personal and environmental systems that either support optimal performance or contribute to ineffective performance.

Emphasizes:

Learning the entire occupation rather than discrete parts.

Allowing persons to find their own optimal solutions to motor problems.

Examines occupational performance and proceeds to examine underlying systems when further understanding of how those systems are constraining performance is needed.

Emphasizes the use of client-centered occupational forms, natural environments, and a process of active experimentation for optimal motor solutions.

Techniques used in therapy require an individualized understanding of the client's situation across many dimensions.

References

Bass-Haugen, JB, Mathiowetz, V & Flinn, N. (2002). Optimizing motor behavior using the occupational therapy task-oriented approach. In Trombly, CA & Radomski, MV (eds.): Occupational Therapy for Physical Dysfunction, 5th ed, pp 481–499). Philadelphia: Lippincott, Williams, & Wilkins.

Bobath, B. (1978). Adult Hemiplegia: Evaluation and Treatment, 2nd ed. London: William Heinnemann Medical Books.

Brunnstrom, S. (1970). Movement therapy in hemiplegia. New York: Harper & Row.

Burgess, MK (1989). Motor control and the role of occupational therapy: Past, present & future. American Journal of Occupational Therapy, 43, 345–348.

Cohen, H. (1989). Occupational therapy and motor control. American Journal of Occupational Therapy, 43, 289–290.

Cammisa, K, Calabrese, D, Meyers, M, et al. (1995). NDT theory has been updated. American Journal of Occupational Therapy, 49, 176.

Flinn, N. (1995). A task-oriented approach to the treatment of a client with hemiplegia. American Journal of Occupational Therapy, 49, 560–569.

Flinn, N. (1999). Clinical interpretation of "Effect of rehabilitation tasks on organization of movement after stroke." American Journal of Occupational Therapy, 53, 345–347.

Kamm, K, Thelen, E & Jensen, JL. (1990). A dynamical systems approach to motor development. Physical Therapy, 70, 763–775.

Levit, K. (2002). Optimizing motor behavior using the Bobath approach. In Trombly, CA & Radomski, MV (eds.): Occupational Therapy for Physical Dysfunction, 5th ed, pp 521–541). Philadelphia: Lippincott, Williams, & Wilkins.

Lin, K, Wu, C, & Trombly, CA. (1998). Effects of task goal on movement kinematics and line bisection performance in adults without disabilities. American Journal of Occupational Therapy, 52, 179–187.

Ma, H, & Trombly, CA. (2002). A synthesis of the effects of occupational therapy for persons with stroke, part II: Remediation of impairments. American Journal of Occupational Therapy, 56, 260–274.

Mathiowetz, V & Bass-Haugen, J. (1994). Motor behavior research: Implications for therapeutic approaches to central nervous system dysfunction. American Journal of Occupational Therapy, 48, 733–745.

Mathiowetz, V & Bass-Haugen, J. (1995). Authors response (to NDT Theory has been updated). American Journal of Occupational Therapy 49, 176.

Mathiowetz, V, & Bass-Haugen, J. (2002). Assessing abilities and capacities: Motor behavior. In Trombly, CA & Radomski, MV (eds.): Occupational Therapy for Physical Dysfunction, 5th ed, pp 137–159. Philadelphia: Lippincott, Williams, & Wilkins.

McCormack, GL & Feuchter, F. (1996). Neurophysiology of sensorimotor approaches to treatment. In Pedretti, LW (ed.): Occupational Therapy: Practice Skills for Physical Dysfunction, 4th ed, pp 351–376. St. Louis: CV Mosby.

Meyers, BJ. (1995). Proprioceptive neuromuscular facilitation (PNF) approach. In Trombly, K (ed.): Occupational Therapy for Physical Dysfunction, 4th ed, pp 474–498. Baltimore: Williams & Wilkins.

Pedretti, LW & Zoltan, B. (eds.) (2001). Occupational Therapy Practice Skills for Physical Dysfunction, 5th ed. St Louis: CV Mosby Co.

Rood, M. (1956). Neurophysiological mechanisms utilized in the treatment of neuromuscular dysfunction. American Journal of Occupational Therapy, 10, 220–224.

Sabari, JS. (1991). Motor learning concepts applied to activity-based intervention with adults with hemiplegia. American Journal of Occupational Therapy, 45, 523–530.

Trombly, CA. (1989). Motor control therapy. In Trombly, CA (ed.): Occupational Therapy for Physical Dysfunction, 3rd ed, pp 72–95. Baltimore: Williams & Wilkins.

Trombly, CA. (1995). Occupation: Purposefulness and meaningfulness as therapeutic mechanisms. American Journal of Occupational Therapy, 49(10), 960–972.

Trombly, CA & Ma, H. (2002). A synthesis of the effects of occupational therapy for persons with stroke, Part I: Restoration of roles, tasks, and activities. American Journal of Occupational Therapy, 56, 250–259.

Trombly, CA & Radomski, M. (2002). Occupation therapy for physical dysfunction, 5th ed. Philadelphia: Lippincott, Williams, & Wilkins.

Tse, D & Spaulding, S. (1998). Review of motor control and motor learning: Implications for occupational therapy with individuals with Parkinson's disease. Physical & Occupational Therapy in Geriatrics, 15(3), 19–38.

Voss, DE, Ionta, MK & Meyers, BJ. (1985). Proprioceptive Neuromuscular Facilitation: Patterns and Techniques, 3rd ed. New York: Harper & Row.

Wu, C-Y, Trombly, C & Lin, K-C. (1994). The relationship between occupational form and occupational performance: A kinematic perspective. American Journal of Occupational Therapy, 48, 679–687.

Chapter 12

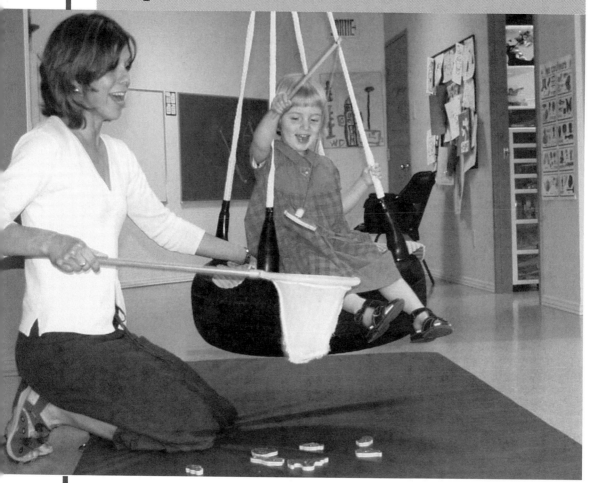

The Sensory Integration Model

An occupational therapist engages a young client in a pretend game of fishing as the client sits on a suspended swing. While on the surface the activity looks simply like play, the occupational therapist has carefully selected the activity to give the child opportunity to develop better control of her posture and arm movements while dealing with the various sensations of moving her body, feeling the sway of the swing, and watching her targets. This kind of experience, which emphasizes helping a client integrate and use a number of sources of **sensory information** in the midst of accomplishing a pleasurable task, is typical of the sensory integration model.

The sensory integration model was originated by A. Jean Ayres as she studied the relationship between children's learning disabilities and their problems in interpreting sensation from the body and environment. Ayres published two books, *Sensory Integration and Learning Disabilities* (Ayres, 1972) and *Sensory Integration and the Child* (Ayres, 1979). Numerous publications by other authors have presented clinical application and research related to this model of practice. The most recent texts concerning this model are the first and second editions of *Sensory Integration: Theory and Practice* (Bundy, Lane, & Murray, 2002; Fisher, Murray, & Bundy, 1991). These texts provide comprehensive reviews of concepts, research, and clinical applications of this model. Another recent text, *Sensory Integration and Self-Regulation in Infants and Toddlers* (Williamson & Anzalone, 2001) also provides resources for applying this model to children age 1–3 years.

This model grew out of Ayres' observation that a subgroup of children with learning disabilities had difficulty interpreting sensory information from their bodies and the environment. She also observed that sensory processing problems were often related to deficits in motor and academic learning. Sensory integration is based on a conceptualization of how the brain functions as an organizer and interpreter of sensory information. It is concerned with failures of the brain to become properly organized for processing and integrating sensory information.

The sensory integration model is generally considered most relevant for persons with mild to moderate problems in learning and behavior who do not have frank neurological damage. The model addresses problems of sensory organization in the brain, but not outright physical damage to the central nervous system (CNS) such as occurs in stroke, cerebral palsy, and spina bifida. Accordingly, sensory integrative impairment is recognized when the brain fails to organize properly in the absence of clear neurological damage to the CNS or peripheral sensory pathways. The model was originally designed for application with children, but it is applied to adults who continue to demonstrate problems that were present in childhood (Bundy & Murray, 2002).

Ayres believed that all children with learning disabilities were not homogeneous. Rather, she suspected that they would manifest different types of sensory integrative problems. To pursue this line of reasoning, she constructed tests to study the behavioral manifestations of sensory processing problems. Findings from a series of studies comparing normal children and children with sensory integrative problems were analyzed to identify patterns of sensory integrative impairment. The identified patterns were interpreted in light of what was known about functional neurology and neuropsychology. Thus, the model provides empirical support for the existence of collections of problems and for the neurological explanations for those problems.

Interdisciplinary Base

The sensory integration model is based on experimental neuroscience literature (Bundy & Murray, 2002), on normal development studies, and on investigations with children who have learning disabilities (Clark et al., 1989). In its early stages of development, the model was influenced by the neurodevelopmental approaches (see Chapter 11). Since understanding of the brain is central to this model, new information from the neurosciences is incorporated in the model and used to revise its theory. The most recent texts (Bundy et al., 2002; Fisher et al., 1991) introduced systems concepts and concepts related to play from psychology and the social sciences.

🌿 Theory

Ayres (1972) defined sensory integration as the "neurological process that organizes sensation from one's own body and from the environment and makes it possible to use the body effectively within the environment" (p. 11). Sensory integration theory is based on five assumptions (Bundy et al., 2002). The first assumption is that of **neural plasticity,** which is the ability of the brain to change or be modified as a result of ongoing experiences of sensory processing. The second assumption is that there is a developmental sequence of sensory integrative capacities. This sequence unfolds as a result of the interaction between normal brain maturation and accumulation of sensory experiences. While the brain's developmental sequence is considered to be biologically determined, the brain is also dependent on sensory processing to organize its biological potential in the course of development. The third assumption is that the brain functions as an integrated hierarchical whole in which higher levels take control over and are controlled by level functions. The fourth assumption is that brain organization and adaptive behavior are interactive; that is, brain organization makes possible adaptive behavior, and adaptive behavior (which involves the processing of sensory information) impacts brain organization. The fifth assumption is that persons have an inner drive to participate in sensory motor activities. These assumptions are reflected in the theory of the model.

The model proposes a number of constructs related to sensory processing and identifies and hypothesizes relationships between those constructs.

> **The model proposes that this ability to organize sensory information and to use it to learn and perform develops as the child interacts with normal environmental challenges.**

Organization

The basic view of sensory integration concerning how persons normally come to organize and use sensory information is that (Bundy et al., 2002):

> Learning is dependent on the ability to take in and process sensation from movement and the environment and to use it to plan and organize behavior. (p. 5)

The model proposes that this ability to organize sensory information and to use it to learn and perform develops as the child interacts with normal environmental challenges. The processing of sensory information in the brain results in development of new neural interconnections that allow sensory information to flow through appropriate channels and be interrelated with other sensory data. Sensory integration results in formation of a meaningful picture of self and the world, which guides performance. For example, learning new motor skills, such as riding a bicycle, involves the generation of an image of one's own body as well as a sense of the body's movements in relation to the bicycle, to the forces of gravity, and so forth. To be able to ride a bicycle is to have an appreciation of all these factors and to know how it feels to integrate them into the performance. Thus, the integration of sensory data also involves interpreting and making sense of that data (Bundy et al., 2002; Pratt, Florey, & Clark, 1989).

Sensory integration is a process in which sensory intake, sensory integration and organization, and adaptive occupational behavior result in a spiral of development (Bundy & Murray, 2002). The child's adaptive use of sensory information in the context of sensory motor activities further develops the sensory integrative capacity of the brain. This enhanced capacity provides the basis for further intake of sensory information in future sensory motor activities. Thus, the spiral continues, with the child building on each new level of brain organization achieved as a result of previous adaptive behavior. According to the model, play is the major arena in which sensory motor behavior takes place.

The sensory integration model was originally based on an evolutionary view of the brain, which emphasized that "as the brain evolved, higher and newer structures like the cerebral cortex remained dependent on adequate functioning of older structures" (Pratt, Florey, & Clark, 1989, p. 45). More recently, the model stresses that the brain functions as a whole, with important connections between cortical and subcortical functions. The higher cortical processes require that sensory integration occur at lower subcortical levels. Moreover, lower subcortical levels depend on cortical functions for processing sensory information (Bundy & Murray, 2002). Nonetheless, the focus of sensory integration is on those sensory processes that are mostly subcortical and that profoundly affect higher cortical processes. Because these sensory integrative processes are so fundamental, they are thought to affect a wide variety of emotional and behavioral aspects of a child's behavior as well as the ability to learn academic skills.

Areas of Sensory Functioning

The sensory integration model is concerned with multimodal sensory processing (i.e., integrating at least two sources of sensory information). Most attention has been directed to tactile, **vestibular,** and proprioceptive sensory information, but auditory and visual sensory information has also been considered (Bundy & Murray, 2002). Ayres, in particular, emphasized vestibular sensation (sensory awareness of one's position in rela-

tion to gravity) as a basis for sensory organization in the brain. She indicated that the experience of gravity and the use of the body in relationship to gravity is a ubiquitous feature of human action (Ayres, 1972). For example, the pervasive challenge that infants face in movement is the struggle to rise against gravity.

Proprioception is the perception of joint and body movement and of the position of the body and its segments in space. Proprioception depends on sensory information from the muscles and joints about their states. Proprioception also involves information via an important efferent feedback loop. This loop, associated with motor planning, allows sensory data about the position of body parts to be integrated with data about the motor effort exerted to effect placement or movement of the body parts. This feedback allows one to differentiate between active (voluntary) and passive (involuntary) movement and to form an image of the effects of one's efforts in placing and moving body parts (Fisher, 1991).

Together, vestibular and proprioceptive (vestibular-proprioceptive) sensation consists of "inputs derived from active movements of one's own body" (Fisher, 1991, p. 71). Vestibular receptors (located in the inner ear) detect movement of the head and elicit compensatory head, trunk, and limb movements, which correct for any movement of the head, trunk, or limb. These receptors are also connected with eye muscles and enable the eyes to move in order to compensate for movement of the head.

The vestibular-proprioceptive system provides a consistent frame of reference from which other sensory data are interpreted. That is, the knowledge of one's position in space and the position of one's body parts provides a constant backdrop of awareness against which other sensory data can be understood. In particular, vestibular-proprioceptive sensory data serve as a reference point for monitoring and controlling movement. Tactile data provide information to the individual concerning physical contact with the external world. Visual and auditory data also provide information emanating from the external environment. Sensory integration is the process whereby all sensory data are organized and processed in the brain, converted to meaningful information, and used to plan and execute motor behavior.

Inner Drive, Play, Mind-Brain-Body Relations

Ayres argued that children had an inner drive to seek out organizing sensations (Ayres, 1979). This drive is manifest in sensory-motor and play activities, and these activities are critical to the development of sensory integration in the child (Bundy, 2002b). This drive begins with the self-organizing tendency of the brain, which requires the processing of sensory informa-

tion, and is manifest in a subjective urge for exploration and mastery (Pratt, Florey, & Clark, 1989).

The model further proposes that the mind and brain are interrelated (Kielhofner & Fisher, 1991). Their interdependence requires that children have positive experience in using their bodies for the brain to be properly oriented to receive and organize sensory information and for the child to be motivated to seek out appropriate sensory experiences. Thus, experience and motivation are viewed as necessary elements of the process of sensory integration.

In the course of play, children fulfill their needs for action. As Bundy and Koomar (2002) point out, play is the primary medium of sensory integrative experiences. In the occupation of play, the child is properly oriented to generate and process sensory information.

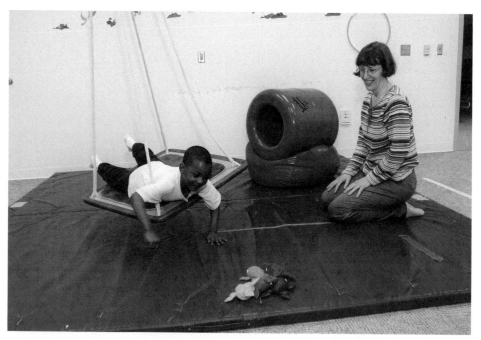

A young boy uses proprioceptive and vestibular sensory input to reach for beanbag animals and help them "find their home" inside the barrel.

The Spiral Process of Self-Actualization

The various components of the view of order are combined into an overall schema, which the authors (Bundy et al., 2002) refer to as the spiral process of self-actualization. This conceptualization reflects an integration of many ideas developed over the years within the sensory integration model. As Bundy, Lane, and Murray (2002) note, it also reflects an attempt to synthesize sensory integration concepts with the conceptualization of motivation from the model of human occupation (see Chapter 10). Traditionally, sensory integration theory noted that the motivation of the child was important, but the main emphasis in concepts and arguments was on the neurological structures and processes involved in sensory processing and organization. This conceptualization provides a clearer account of the nature and role of motivation in sensory integration. Figure 12-1, p. 204, illustrates the process. As represented in the lower, gray band, the inner drive leads the individual to seek out and engage in sensorimotor activities that provide opportunities for sensory intake (Bundy & Murray, 2002). Through a process of sensory integration, the central nervous system (CNS) must process, organize, and modulate sensory intake from the body and the environment (Bundy & Murray, 2002). Furthermore, the individual must organize and plan adaptive behaviors (which include both postural and motor skills). Neuronal models (i.e., neurologically encoded memories of what to do and how to do it) can be used to plan new and more complex behaviors. This is represented in the second loop (the dark line), which shows neuronal models being generated from sensory integrative

experiences and leading to the organization and planning of new adaptive behaviors. Thus, neuronal models develop from sensory feedback generated by the planning, active performance, and outcomes of an adaptive behavior (Bundy & Murray, 2002).

The upper white band of the spiral shows how sensory integration is part of the occupational behavior of the child. Volitional state (the innate drive to participate in occupation and the belief in skill) also influences the selection of sensorimotor action. The child's occupational behavior generates feedback on the production and outcome of action. This feedback influences the child's sense of mastery, control, and confidence as well as the experience of meaning and satisfaction in the behavior. This provides the basis for further motivation and self-direction, which in turn influences the ongoing processes of adaptive behavior, sensory integration, and occupational behavior.

Problems and Challenges

As noted, an important component of this model has been the identification, through research, of the types of sensory integrative impairments and the explanation of these in light of existing knowledge about nervous system function. The basic view of impairment in the sensory integration model is as follows. When individuals have deficits in processing and integrating sensory inputs, they also experience difficulty in planning and producing behavior that, in turn, interferes with conceptual and motor learning (Bundy et al., 2002). The delineation of sensory integrative impairments has changed over time with new research findings. According to Bundy and Murray (2002, p. 6) "sensory integrative impairment

> **When individuals have deficits in processing and integrating sensory inputs, they also experience difficulty in planning and producing behavior that, in turn, interferes with conceptual and motor learning.**

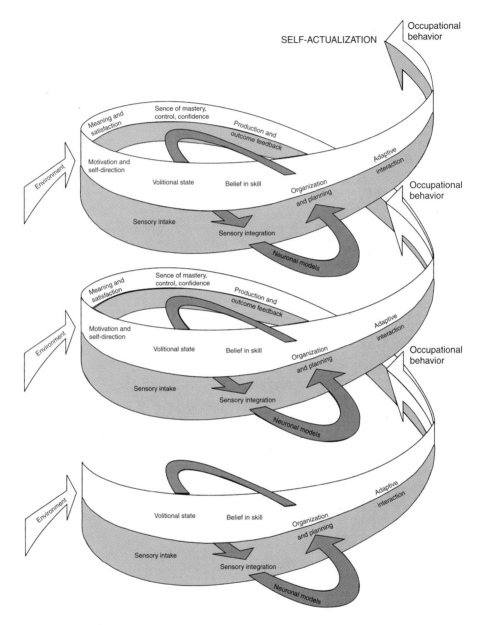

Figure 12-1. Spiral process of sensory integration. (From Bundy et al, Sensory Integration: Theory and Practice, 2nd ed. FA Davis, Philadelphia, 2002 with permission.)

manifests itself in two major ways: poor modulation and poor praxis." They go on to note that individuals can evidence one or both types of sensory integrative impairment.

Dyspraxia

Praxis refers to the capacity to plan new movements. Dyspraxia related to sensory integrative problems "have their bases in poor sensory processing" (Reeves & Cermak, 2002, p. 71). Persons with dyspraxia have difficulty with motor planning, which is manifest as clumsiness (Reeves & Cermak, 2002). Dyspraxia is not a problem of motor coordination (i.e., execution of motor behavior) but rather is related to difficulty in forming a plan of action. Praxis involves knowing how to execute an action. Dyspraxia is mostly seen in difficulty with learning how to perform a new task. Once the person with dyspraxia learns and practices a task, the person can usually perform it adequately. However, for the person with dyspraxia, learning a particular skill does not seem to result in more basic learning that generalizes to other, similar types of performances. Dyspraxia is often manifest in childhood as clumsiness and through difficulty with ordinary tasks such as buttoning, tying shoe laces, and handwriting. While it is recognized that not all persons with dyspraxia have sensory integrative impairment, it is hypothesized that some forms of dyspraxia are related to deficits in sensory integration. Two types of dyspraxia related to sensory integration are recognized:

♦ Somatodyspraxia, which is thought to be a result of poor processing of tactile and (also likely) vestibular and proprioceptive sensation and is considered a more severe form of dyspraxia (Fisher and Bundy, 1991; Lai et al., 1996).
♦ Deficits in **bilateral integration** (using the two sides of the body in a coordinated fashion) and sequencing of motor actions, which is proposed to be related to deficits in vestibular and proprioceptive processing (Reeves & Cermak, 2002). Impairments of bilateral integration and sequencing praxis include poor coordination of the two sides of the body, confusion of right and left, the tendency to avoid moving one's arms past the body's midline to the other side of the body, and difficulty in planning and sequencing movements, especially those involving both sides of the body.

Underlying and related to these two types of dyspraxia are deficits in posture, tactile discrimination. Postural deficits are thought to

contribute to deficits in bilateral integration and sometimes to somatodyspraxia. Children are considered to have postural deficits when they exhibit meaningful clusters of indicators that include such things as extensor muscle tone, proximal stability, and equilibrium. Deficits in tactile discrimination are thought to be a basis of somatodyspraxia. Persons are considered to have these deficits based on testing that indicates problems identifying the characteristics of touch.

Sensory Modulation Impairments

Modulation refers to the nervous system's regulation of its own activity (Bundy & Murray, 2002). Traditionally, problems of sensory modulation have been less clearly demonstrated in research. However, recent research (Dunn, 1999; McIntosh et al., 1999) has helped clarify the nature of these impairments. Sensory modulation impairments refer, then, to the tendency to underreact or overreact to sensation and include four types of impairments:

♦ **Sensory defensiveness** (including tactile), which is a fight-or-flight reaction (e.g., aggressiveness or withdrawal) to sensation that others would not consider noxious
♦ Gravitational insecurity, which is a "fear of movement, being out of an upright position, or having one's feet off the ground (Bundy & Murray, 2002)
♦ Aversive responses to movement that would not be considered noxious by others
♦ Underresponsiveness to sensation, which refers to children behaving as though they do not notice sensation or react less intensively than others would

In sum, persons with **sensory modulation impairments** have difficulty maintaining normal limits of registering and responding to sensations. They tend to excessively overreact or underreact to **sensory information** or to shift between the two extremes (Lane, 2002).

One of the important characteristics of the identified sensory integrative problems is the extent to which their categorization and existence is based on research. Another important element of how these problems are conceptualized is the theory concerning their basis in disturbance in underlying brain functions. A great deal of effort has gone into documenting and explaining the patterns of sensory integrative-related behaviors observed in children.

Therapeutic Intervention

As noted earlier, the authors view sensory integration as a process in which ongoing experiences of engaging in adaptive behavior

result in further brain organization, making possible even more complex adaptive behaviors. When a person's brain fails to organize and process sensory information adequately, a disruption of this normal cycle of sensory integration is recognized.

Strictly speaking, therapy based on the sensory integration model aims at remediation of the sensory integrative problem. Thus, the goal of sensory integrative therapy is to improve the ability to integrate sensory information. This involves changes in the organization of the brain. Sensory integrative approaches are based on the argument that provision of opportunities for enhanced **sensory intake,** provided within the context of a meaningful activity and the planning and organizing of an adaptive behavior, will improve the ability of the CNS to process and integrate sensory inputs and, through this

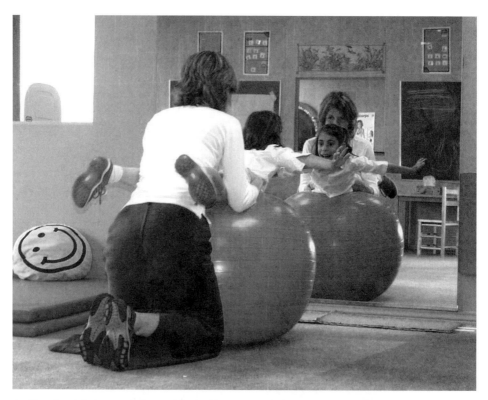

A girl pretends to be an airplane while working on muscle tone and vestibular processing. This activity is used to assess the capacity to take and maintain a position against gravity.

process, enhance conceptual and motor learning (Fisher & Murray, 1991).

Sensory integration–based therapy emphasizes the integration of vestibular, proprioceptive, and tactile sensations and not just the motor response. For this reason, using suspended equipment is a hallmark of sensory integration therapy (Parham and Mailloux, 2001).

Technology for Application

The sensory integrative model has enjoyed a well-developed technology for application. Assessment and intervention procedures have been thoroughly developed and clearly outlined. Nonetheless, a number of factors including questions about the efficacy of sensory integration treatment, time limitations and other conditions under which services can be given as well as new views of neuromotor rehabilitation have led to some reformulation of what is considered sensory integration best practice (Bundy and Murray, 2002). This section will first discuss the traditional technology for application and then go on to examine a contemporary perspective on application.

Assessment

Assessment procedures in this model traditionally included include the use of a formalized battery of tests, informal observation of performance, and data gathered from caregivers and other sources. Informal data, along with the formal test battery results, are used to arrive at an assessment of whether a person has a sensory integrative impairment and, if possible, to specify the nature of that impairment. Bundy (2002a) offers a comprehensive discussion of assessment that emphasizes the need to begin assessment with a top-down approach that first examines the ability of clients to carry out daily life tasks. Her discussion also recommends alternatives to the

more time-consuming formal testing that was traditionally part of sensory integrative assessment.

The Sensory Integration and Praxis Tests (SIPT) are a battery of tests designed to help the therapist identify and understand sensory integrative impairments in children 4 through 8 years of age. The battery tests the relationships among tactile processing, vestibular-proprioceptive processing, visual perception, and practice ability. The tests are conceptualized as assessing the major behavioral manifestations of sensory integrative deficits. The tests are grouped in four overlapping areas (Bundy, 2002a):

◆ Form and space, visual-motor coordination, and constructional ability
◆ Tactile discrimination
◆ Praxis
◆ Vestibular and proprioceptive processing

The SIPT include 17 individually administered tests, which can be completed in about 90 minutes. All the tasks on the test are performance-oriented. They range from the Finger Identification Test, which asks the child to point to the finger(s) previously touched by an examiner, through the Standing and Walking Balance Test, to Design Copying, a test in which the child is asked to copy designs.

The tests are computer-scored. The company that does the scoring produces a report that includes statistical comparisons between the tested child and those observed in samples of normal and disabled children who were used to develop the tests. The SIPT were developed over nearly three decades, during which clinical experiences and research have been used to determine which testing procedures were the most meaningful to include. Statistical analysis of the items most useful in identifying impairment was used to develop and refine test items and testing procedures. Statistical studies, which have identified patterns of scores that indicate types of impairment, are the basis for interpretation of the test results.

Interpretation of the SIPT scores is based on meaningful clusters of scores. Research has shown that a particular pattern of low scores is indicative of a particular kind of problem. Thus, interpretation begins with examination of test scores to see if any such pattern exists (Bundy, 2002a).

The SIPT are the mainstay of sensory integrative assessment, but because of the restricted age range (4 to 9 years of age), other tests of motor, cognitive-perceptual, and sensory-processing capacity may be used. Additionally, as Bundy (2002a) notes, evaluation with the SIPT should be complemented with the following kinds of information:

◆ Developmental pattern, intellectual capacity, and diagnoses
◆ Observations, especially those of postural responses
◆ Assessment of sensory modulation through observation and history-taking or the use of new assessments such as the Sensory Profile (Dunn, 1999)

Sensory integrative treatment is meant to have a broad impact on behavior; thus, observations of neuromotor status and behavioral organization are also relevant to monitoring progress (Clark et al., 1989).

Treatment Approach

Any discussion of the application of this model in practice must begin with a recognition that sensory integrative procedures have been applied to a wide range of populations beyond the children with learning disabilities for which the model was originally developed. For example, the model has been applied to adults, persons with frank brain damage, persons with schizophrenia, and individuals with mental retardation (Arendt,

MacLean, & Baumeister, 1988; King, 1974). There has been considerable controversy over whether such individuals are appropriate candidates for sensory integrative approaches. Additionally, many persons have been criticized for using techniques from sensory integration without a systematic application of its principles. While they may refer to the resulting therapy as sensory integration, it is in fact not so. The text, *Sensory Integration: Theory and Practice* (Bundy et al., 2002), took a conservative approach; arguing for a clear identification of the presence of sensory integrative problems before the sensory integrative approaches are used. The authors of the text believe that the model has application with adults and may have potential for people with problems other than learning disability. The text outlines the authors' rationales for application of the model.

Traditional Treatment Guidelines

The sensory integrative model provides specific guidelines for the kind of sensory integrative experiences hypothesized to be of most benefit to a child. Treatment planning is based on identification of the child's problems and the underlying reasons for those problems; that is, the particular difficulty with processing sensory information. Understanding the difficulty requires understanding of the structure and function of sensory systems and how they are implicated in sensory integration problems (Lane, 2002). The vestibular-proprioceptive system provides a good example of the logic of intervention. Knowledge of the anatomy and physiology of the vestibular-proprioceptive system is used to determine what kind of sensory experience would most effectively stimulate vestibular organs and proprioceptors and elicit particular **postural reactions.** In this case, understanding neurological structures provides the logic for determining which therapeutic procedures should have particular impacts on the sensory system. The following quote from a discussion of treatment planning for a child, Steven, further illustrates the kind of specificity that can be achieved in choosing appropriate sensory integrative therapy (Bundy, 1991):

> Sensory integration theory suggests that Steven's difficulties with postural stability and bilateral integration and sequencing of projected limb movements should be addressed by activities that provide opportunities for him to take in enhanced vestibular-proprioceptive information. More specifically, the theory suggests that opportunities to take in linear vestibular-proprioceptive information in the context of activities that demand sustained postural control (in a variety of positions) and coordinated use of both sides of the body will be most appropriate. (p. 342)

Sensory integration theory does not yet present a complete picture of the various problems children manifest, nor does it explain all the underlying mechanisms. Thus, there are some gaps in information about how best to proceed in therapy. In such cases, the therapist uses all available information about the child to determine a prudent course of therapy.

Play as the Media

This model emphasizes that the child must actively choose the actions that occur in therapy. In play, the child is given control and the enticement to choose appropriate sensory motor behaviors. Bundy (2002b) emphasizes the importance of play as the vehicle for therapy based on the sensory integrative model.

> **This model emphasizes that the child must actively choose the actions that occur in therapy.**

She points out three factors that are critical for maintaining a playful approach to intervention:

◆ Perception of internal control
◆ Intrinsic motivation
◆ Freedom from the constraints of reality (Bundy, 2002b)

Bundy (2002b) also recommends careful assessment of play, using such instruments as the Test of Playfulness (Bundy, 2000). She notes that play can result in improvements in sensory integration and that the most important by-product of therapy may be improving the client's ability to play.

Equipment

Because of the special needs for sensory experiences (especially vestibular), sensory integration treatment has come to be associated with a variety of specially designed suspended equipment (trapezes, hammocks, and swings) and scooter boards. Such equipment, which is commercially available, provides the means of achieving desired sensory experiences in the context of play.

Contemporary Guidelines for Application of This Model

As noted at the beginning of this chapter, a number of factors have led to some rethinking of how to best deliver sensory integrative therapy. Bundy and Murray (2002) propose a number of principles that reflect current thinking about use of this model in practice. Some of the guidelines, which reflect an appreciation of the more limited time for therapy, include such approaches as setting objectives that can be accomplished in the short term and that are understood by clients and caregivers and that involve clients and caregivers in implementing aspects of intervention. Also related to changes in the context of services is the role of the occupational therapist as a consultant to family members or other professionals. An important component of this role is often to help these persons reframe their understanding of the person with sensory integrative problems (e.g., helping a teacher understand that sitting still may actually interfere with rather than improve a child's ability to pay attention in the classroom).

Other guidelines reflect new ideas from the task-oriented approach (see Chapter 11), which emphasize attention to how the task and environment might contribute to observed difficulties in performance and include appropriate interventions directed at these issues. Overall, there is a shift in orientation from an exclusive focus on remediating the underlying problem in the client to focusing on how the problem interacts with external conditions that interfere with everyday performance and deciding on the most efficacious strategy of intervention.

🌿 Research

The sensory integration model has been the subject of a great deal of research. Ongoing research has contributed to the development of the SIPT (Bundy, 2002a) and, concurrently, to the validation of underlying sensory integration constructs. Pivotal studies in this area are the factor analytic studies, which identified meaningful clusters of test scores (Bundy 2002a). These studies demonstrated that poor performance in a particular cluster of tests was typical of a child with a particular kind of sensory integrative problem. Based on this research, it is thought that test score patterns can be indicative of whether and of what type of sensory integrative problem a person may have.

A second area of research includes studies of the effectiveness of sensory integrative therapy. Examining studies completed between 1972 and 1981, Ottenbacher (1991) conducted a meta-analysis (a method of using data from several studies to determine whether there is evidence of a treatment effect) and concluded that there was evidence of treatment effectiveness. Hoehn and Baumeister (1994) criticized some of the studies Ottenbacher included as lacking sufficient rigor. Vargas and Camilli (1999) later used meta-analysis to examine studies reported between 1983 and 1993 and found very little evidence for treatment effectiveness, which is not surprising as many studies conducted in the last two decades failed to demonstrate positive outcomes of treatment. Bundy, Lane, and Murray (2002) conclude that evidence concerning the effectiveness of sensory integration–based therapy is "mixed at best and downright negative at worst" (p. 22). They also note that despite the lack of evidence for treatment effectiveness, parents and therapists are enthusiastic about their first-hand experience with sensory integration–based therapy. One possibility is that the therapy produces positive outcomes but not for the reasons specified by sensory integration theory and measured in studies (Kaplan et al., 1993). For example, it is hypothesized that the relationship between the therapist and child may account for outcomes or that sensory integration principles are used to reframe how problems are perceived by others in the child's environment, leading to positive outcomes.

Tickle-Degnen (1988) noted that studies have not yet examined mediating factors that might explain better when and how sensory integration–based therapy works and for what types of individuals. The fact that research on sensory integration has been so extensively discussed and critiqued reflects the fact that there is a body of research upon which meaningful discussion and critique can be based.

 # Discussion

The sensory integration model is the most extensively researched and developed model of practice in occupational therapy. Nonetheless, the use of the model in practice has been subject to some criticism and controversy. Therapists have applied this model to populations that others deemed inappropriate for sensory integration treatment. Others have borrowed ideas and techniques from the model incompletely, resulting in clinical practices not justified by the theory.

Moreover, it is sometimes confused with other related approaches. For example, Bundy, Lane, and Murray (2002) noted that sensory integration treatment should be differentiated from sensorimotor approaches in that the latter emphasize specific motor responses, whereas the concern of the former is specifically with how the child processes sensation. They also differentiate sensory integration from sensory stimulation programs in that the latter apply sensation to the child whereas in the sensory integrative approaches, the child seeks out the sensation.

This highly complex and well-developed model is both attractive to therapists and challenging to master. However, as noted, application of the model has not always been systematic. Clark et al. (1989) note that "entry level therapists should not expect to be able to provide sensory integrative procedures upon graduation" (p. 484). They point out considerable skill is required for use of this practice model. Therapists who wish to administer the SIPT must become certified either through approved graduate or continuing education courses and an examination process. The model represents an area of specialty practice in occupational therapy that requires training and experience beyond that of the generically trained therapist.

TERMS OF THE MODEL	
Bilateral integration	Using the two sides of the body together
Dyspraxia	Difficulty with volitional action directed to the environment
Neural plasticity	The ability of the brain to change or be modified
Postural reactions	Changes in one's body position to maintain equilibrium
Praxis	Planning of motor action; involves knowing how to do an action
Proprioception	Perception of joint and body movement and of the position of the body and its segments in space
Sensory defensiveness	Hypersensitivity to sensation resulting in a disorganized output
Sensory information	Sensations (e.g., from touch, movement)
Sensory intake	Taking in of sensations from the environment or internally from the body
Sensory modulation impairment	Tendency to underreact or overreact to sensation
Vestibular sensation	Sensory awareness of one's bodily position in relation to gravity

Summary: The Sensory Integration Model

Focus

◆ Organization of sensory information in the CNS and its use in guiding adaptive motor behaviors that make up occupational performance

Interdisciplinary Base

◆ Experimental neuroscience (brain structures and processes)
◆ Normal development studies
◆ Systems concepts
◆ Concepts related to play from psychology

Theory
Organization

◆ Sensory integration is a process in which sensory intake, sensory integration and organization, and adaptive occupational behavior result in a spiral of development The brain functions as a whole
◆ Sensory integration is multi-modal sensory processing (i.e., integrating at least two sources of sensory information) in which sensory data are organized and processed in the brain, converted to meaningful information, and used to plan and execute motor behavior
◆ Children have an inner drive to seek out organizing sensations
◆ Mind and brain are interrelated; subjective experience is a necessary part of the adaptive spiral of sensory integration

Problems and Challenges

◆ When individuals have deficits in processing and integrating sensory inputs, deficits in planning and producing behavior occur that interfere with conceptual and motor learning
◆ There are two major types of sensory integrative impairments:

1. Poor modulation
2. Poor praxis

Dyspraxia

◆ Dyspraxia is related to difficulty in forming a plan of action
◆ Two types of dyspraxia related to sensory integration are recognized:
   1. Somatodyspraxia
   2. Deficits in bilateral integration
◆ Sensory modulation impairments refer to the tendency to underreact or overreact to sensation and include four types of impairments:
   1. Sensory defensiveness
   2. Gravitational insecurity
   3. Aversive responses to movement
   4. Underresponsiveness to sensation

Therapeutic Intervention

◆ Aimed at remediation (change) of the sensory integrative problem
◆ Goal is to improve ability to integrate sensory information by changing organization of the brain
◆ Enhanced sensory intake, which occurs when a child plans and organizes adaptive behavior in a meaningful activity, improves ability of the CNS to process and integrate sensory inputs

Technology for Application

◆ Assessment procedures include a formalized battery of tests (Sensory Integration and Praxis Tests), informal observation of performance, and data gathered from caretakers and other sources
◆ Data are used to arrive at an assessment of whether a person has a sensory integrative impairment and, if possible, to specify the nature of that impairment
◆ Sensory integrative experiences selected to benefit a child are derived from identification of the child's deficits and the theory

concerning the underlying reasons for those deficits; i.e., the particular difficulty processing sensory information

◆ Play is a vehicle for therapy; environmental demands are matched to the persons' capacity and challenge them to engage in new sensory-motor action; in play the child is given control and enticement to choose appropriate sensory motor behaviors

◆ New applications of the approach emphasize:

1. Consideration of how task and environment affect performance and addressing these issues
2. Short-term goals
3. Consultation with parent, teacher, and others

Research

◆ Ongoing research has contributed to the development of the Sensory Integration and Praxis Tests and validation of underlying sensory integration constructs

◆ Studies of the effectiveness of sensory integrative therapy have provided mixed and increasingly negative evidence of treatment effectiveness

References

Arendt, RE, MacLean, WE & Baumeister, A. (1988). Critique of sensory integration therapy and its application in mental retardation. American Journal on Mental Retardation, 92, 401–411.

Ayres, AJ. (1972). Sensory Integration and Learning Disabilities. Los Angeles: Western Psychological Services.

Ayres, AJ. (1979). Sensory Integration and the Child. Los Angeles: Western Psychological Services.

Bundy, AC. (1991). The process of planning and implementing intervention. In Fisher, AG, Murray, EA & Bundy, AC (eds.): Sensory Integration: Theory and Practice, pp 333–353. Philadelphia: FA Davis.

Bundy, AC. (2000). Test of playfulness manual (Version 3). Ft. Collins, CO: Colorado State University.

Bundy, AC. (2002a). Assessing sensory integrative dysfunction. In Bundy, AC, Lane, SJ & Murray, EA (eds.): Sensory Integration: Theory and Practice, 2nd ed, pp 169–198. Philadelphia: FA Davis.

Bundy, A.C. (2002b). Play theory and sensory integration. In Bundy, AC, Lane, SJ & Murray, EA (eds.): Sensory Integration: Theory and Practice, 2nd ed, pp 227–240. Philadelphia: FA Davis.

Bundy, AC & Koomar, JA. (2002). Orchestrating intervention: The art of practice. In Bundy, AC, Lane, SJ & Murray, EA (eds.): Sensory Integration: Theory and Practice, 2nd ed, pp 241–260. Philadelphia: FA Davis.

Bundy, AC, Lane, SJ, & Murray, EA. (eds.) (2002). Sensory Integration: Theory and Practice, 2nd ed. Philadelphia: FA Davis.

Bundy, AC & Murray, EA. (2002). Introduction to sensory integration theory. In Bundy, AC, Lane, SJ & Murray, EA (eds.): Sensory Integration: Theory and Practice, 2nd ed, pp 3–33. Philadelphia: FA Davis.

Clark, F, Mailloux, Z, Parham, D, et al. (1989). Sensory integration and children with learning disabilities. In Clark, PN & Allen, AS (eds.): Occupational Therapy for Children, 2nd ed, pp 457–509. St. Louis: CV Mosby.

Dunn, W. (1999). Sensory profile: User's manual. San Antonio: Psychological Corporation.

Fisher, AG. (1991). Vestibular-proprioceptive processing and bilateral integration and sequencing deficits. In Bundy, AC, Lane, SJ & Murray, EA (eds.): Sensory Integration: Theory and Practice, pp 71–107. Philadelphia: FA Davis.

Fisher, AG & Bundy, AC. (1991). The interpretation process. In Bundy, AC, Lane, SJ & Murray, EA (eds.): Sensory Integration: Theory and Practice, pp 234–250. Philadelphia: FA Davis.

Fisher, AG & Murray, EA (1991). Introduction to sensory integration theory. In Fisher, AG, Murray, EA & Bundy, AC (eds.): Sensory Integration: Theory and Practice, pp 3–26. Philadelphia: FA Davis.

Fisher, AG, Murray, EA, & Bundy, AC. (eds.)

(1991). Sensory Integration: Theory and Practice. Philadelphia: FA Davis Company.

Hoehn, TP & Baumeister, A (1994). A critique of the application of sensory integration therapy to children with learning disabilities. Journal of Learning Disabilities, 27, 338– 350.

Kaplan, BJ, Polatajko, HJ, Wilson, BN, et al. (1993). Reexamination of sensory integration treatment: A combination of two efficacy studies. Journal of Learning Disabilities, 26, 342–347.

Kielhofner, G & Fisher, AG. (1991). Mind-brain-body relationships. In Fisher, AG, Murray, EA & Bundy, AC (eds.): Sensory Integration: Theory and Practice, pp 27–45. Philadelphia: FA Davis.

King, LJ (1974). A sensory-integrative approach to schizophrenia. American Journal of Occupational Therapy, 28, 529–536.

Lai, JS, Fisher, AG, Magalhaes, LC, et al. (1996). Construct validity of the Sensory Integration and Praxis Test. Occupational Therapy Journal of Research, 16, 75–97.

Lane, SJ. (2002). Sensory modulation. In Pratt, PN & Allen, AS (eds.): Occupational Therapy for Children, 2nd ed, pp 101–122. St Louis: CV Mosby.

McIntosh, DN, Miller, LJ, Shyu, V, et al. (1999). Sensory modulation and disruption, electrodermal responses, and functional behaviors. Developmental Medicine and Child Neurology, 41, 608–615.

Ottenbacher, K. (1991). Research in sensory integration: Empirical perceptions and progress. In Fisher, AG, Murray, EA & Bundy, AC (eds.): Sensory Integration Theory and practice, pp 388–389. Philadelphia: F.A. Davis.

Paraham, LD & Mailloux, Z. (2001). Sensory integration. In Case-Smith, J, Allen, AS & Pratt PN (eds.): Occupational Therapy for Children, 4th ed, pp 329–351. St. Louis: Mosby.

Pratt, PN, Florey, LA & Clark, F. (1989). Developmental principles and theories. In Pratt, PN & Allen, AS (eds.): Occupational Therapy for Children, 2nd ed, pp 19–47. St Louis: CV Mosby.

Reeves, GD & Cermak, SA. (2002). Disorders of praxis. In Bundy, AC, Lane, SJ & Murray, EA (eds.): Sensory Integration: Theory and Practice, 2nd ed, pp 71–100. Philadelphia: FA Davis.

Tickle-Degnen, L. (1988). Perspectives on the status of sensory integration theory. American Journal of Occupational Therapy, 42, 427–433.

Vargas, S & Camilli, G. (1999). A meta-analysis of research on sensory integration treatment. American Journal of Occupational Therapy, 53 (2), 189–198.

Williamson, GG & Anzalone, ME. (2001). Sensory integration and self-regulation in infants and toddlers: Helping very young children interact with their environment. Washington, DC: Zero to Three.

Chapter 13

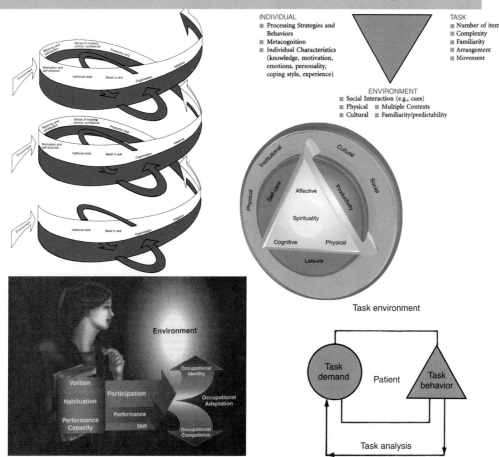

Conceptual Models of Practice: The State of the Art

The previous chapters presented seven contemporary conceptual practice models. This chapter will look across these models and identify the:

◆ Range of phenomena these models address
◆ Nature of client problems these models identify
◆ Vision and approach to therapy offered by the models
◆ Kind of theory the models offer
◆ Research basis of each model

The aim of this chapter is to characterize the state of the art in the development of models. It will discuss what they individually and collectively contribute to the conceptual foundations of the field.

Phenomena Addressed by the Models

Occupational therapy's overall concern is with how persons maintain adaptive (i.e., functional and satisfying) patterns of occupational participation in their contexts. As noted in Chapter 4, the field recognizes that many factors contribute to a person's success in occupational adaptation. These factors include such things as being physically able to do the necessary and desired occupations, having motivation for engaging in occupations, having acquired necessary habits, and having available the appropriate environmental supports. These and other such factors are the phenomena that must be understood in the field.

Each conceptual practice model focuses on one or more of these phenomena. No single model can address all of them, but it is important that the models of practice collectively provide an understanding of the range of personal and environmental phenomena that are involved in occupational participation.

As noted in Chapter 4, the field of occupational therapy recognizes that both person- and environment-related factors influence occupational participation. Consequently, models typically address both these elements in some way. In the first section that follows, we will first examine the phenomena related to the person addressed by each model. The second section will discuss how each model addresses phenomena related to the environment.

Phenomena Related to the Person

We can conceptualize the phenomena addressed by models on a continuum from physical to psychosocial aspects of the person. Consequently, models can be seen as distributed across this continuum, depending on what aspect of the person they address. Table 13-1, p. 215, illustrates the continuum of phenomena addressed by models and also indicates typical concepts with which the models address those phenomena.

The biomechanical and motor control models are both concerned with how humans produce the physical movements necessary to performing the occupations that make up their everyday lives. The biomechanical model addresses movement through concentrating on biomechanics (i.e., how the organization of bones, joints, and muscles influences the kinds of movements humans can produce) (Trombly & Radomski, 2002). Representative concepts from this model are strength and range of motion.

The motor control model is concerned with how movement is controlled (Mathiowetz & Bass-Haugen, 2002). Originally, this model was focused exclusively on the role of the central nervous system (CNS) in controlling movement. While this model has adopted a recent view that emphasizes the co-contributions of the CNS, task, and environment in organizing movement, it still retains a strong focus on the CNS. Thus, it offers such concepts as muscle tone and reflexes, which describe CNS influences on movement.

The sensory integration model focuses on how sensory information is processed in the nervous system and is used to plan and guide motor action (Bundy, Lane, & Murray, 2002). This model extensively considers processes involved in the reception, interpretation, and integration of sensations. The concept of sensory modulation, which addresses how persons respond to various sensory inputs, is

TABLE 13-1. THE CONTINUUM OF PHENOMENA

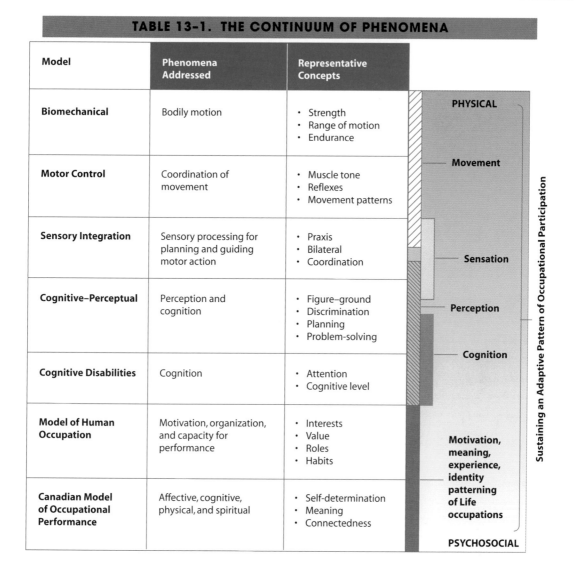

Model	Phenomena Addressed	Representative Concepts	
Biomechanical	Bodily motion	• Strength • Range of motion • Endurance	**PHYSICAL** Movement
Motor Control	Coordination of movement	• Muscle tone • Reflexes • Movement patterns	
Sensory Integration	Sensory processing for planning and guiding motor action	• Praxis • Bilateral • Coordination	Sensation
Cognitive–Perceptual	Perception and cognition	• Figure–ground • Discrimination • Planning • Problem-solving	Perception
Cognitive Disabilities	Cognition	• Attention • Cognitive level	Cognition
Model of Human Occupation	Motivation, organization, and capacity for performance	• Interests • Value • Roles • Habits	**Motivation, meaning, experience, identity patterning of Life occupations**
Canadian Model of Occupational Performance	Affective, cognitive, physical, and spiritual	• Self-determination • Meaning • Connectedness	**PSYCHOSOCIAL**

Sustaining an Adaptive Pattern of Occupational Participation

representative of this aspect of the sensory integration model. This model also has a major focus on how the processing of sensation affects motor action. The concept of praxis, which refers to the planning of movement, is representative of this aspect of the model. Finally, because this model considers how sensations are integrated and interpreted, it also makes contributions to understanding perception.

The cognitive-perceptual model (Katz, 1998; Toglia, 1998) addresses the dual phenomena of perception and cognition and the impact of these processes on performance. Figure-ground discrimination is a typical concept representing the focus on perception and cognition as well as such concepts as planning and problem-solving.

The cognitive disabilities model (Allen, 1992) focuses exclusively on cognition and its role in performance. The concept of attention is typical of how this model describes the cognitive process. The concept of cognitive level is central to how this model views cognition as existing on a continuum from higher to lower levels.

The model of human occupation addresses three phenomena (Kielhofner, 2002). First, it considers how persons are motivated to engage in occupations. The concepts of interests and values are part of how this model considers motivation. Second, this model considers how people organize their occupations into everyday patterns, offering the concepts of roles and habits. Third, the model considers how persons' experience of doing contributes to their performance capacity.

The Canadian model of occupational performance focuses on occupational performance (Canadian Association of Occupational Therapists, 1997). It identifies the personal factors influencing performance as including affective, cognitive, and physical components. It further identifies spirituality as being central to the person. Representative concepts related to spirituality are self-determination, meaning, and connectedness.

Phenomena Related to the Environment

Each of these models also addresses the environment in some way. In some models, the environment is only implicitly addressed. In other models, the environment is explicitly conceptualized as a factor in occupational

TABLE 13-2. ENVIRONMENTAL PHENOMENA

Model	Phenomena Addressed	Typical Concern
Biomechanical	Physical properties requiring motion	• Weight of objects
Motor Control	Properties of objects and tasks that create conditions for movement	• Object characteristics influencing how they can be handled • Task demands
Sensory Integration	Sensory characteristics of environment	• Tactile properties of objects
Cognitive–Perceptual	Social, physical, and cultural elements that influence the ability to process information	• Visual and verbal cues
Cognitive Disabilities	Cognitive demands of tasks and objects used	• Task complexity
Model of Human Occupation	Impact (resources, opportunities, constraints and demands) posed by • objects • spaces • occupational forms • social groups	• Meaning of objects • Social attitudes
Canadian Model of Occupational Performance	Institutional, physical, social, and cultural dimensions of context that elicit responses	• Social policy • Patterns of social relationships

participation. Table 13-2 shows the environmental phenomena addressed by each model and identifies its typical concerns with the environment.

The biomechanical model does not specifically address the environment in its concepts. However, implied in the model is how the physical environment poses demands for movement. This includes such things as the weight of objects or the requirements for climbing posted by stairs.

The motor control model has, in its more recent formulation (Mathiowetz & Bass-Haugen, 2002), specified that the properties of objects and tasks in the environment combine with personal characteristics to influence motor movement. Thus, this model considers such things as, for example, how the shape of objects used or the demands for movement of a particular task influence the coordination of movement.

Sensory integration theory does not focus specifically on conceptualizing the environment, but it is concerned with the sensory properties of the environment (Bundy, Lane, & Murray, 2002). Thus, this model is concerned with the tactile properties of and the potential of toys and objects (such as swings and scooters) to provide certain sensory experiences.

The cognitive-perceptual model in its most recent formulation considers how the social, physical, and cultural elements of the environment influence sensory processing (Katz, 1998). This model is concerned with such things as the visual and verbal cues available in the environment.

The cognitive disabilities model (Allen, 1992) does not explicitly address the environment, but its focus on environmental compensation and task analysis is implicitly concerned with the cognitive demands posted by objects and tasks in the environment. Thus, task complexity (e.g., the number of steps involved in a task) is a typical concern of this model.

The model of human occupation and the Canadian model of occupational performance both emphasize the inseparability of person and environment and the influence that the latter has on what a person does. Both models specifically conceptualize the nature of the environment and how it influences occupational participation.

The model of human occupation conceptualizes the environment as made up of objects, spaces, occupational forms, and social groups, whose properties impact on persons who interact with them (Kielhofner, 2002). The concept of impact stresses that the environment provides resources, opportunities, demands, and constraints, depending on the unique characteristics of the individual. Some typical concerns identified by this model are the meaning that objects hold for individuals and the way social attitudes influence people.

The Canadian model of occupational performance (Canadian Association of Occupational Therapists, 1997) conceptualizes the environment as made up of institutional, physical, social, and cultural dimensions. This model includes concerns for such things as patterns of social relationships and how they influence occupational performance. This model is also unique in that it explicitly identifies such macro-factors as social policy influencing the person (Townsend, 1998).

 ## Problems Identified and View of Therapy

Each conceptual practice model identifies and targets certain kinds of problems. Corresponding to these identified problems, each model offers a rationale for and approach to doing therapy. Table 13-3, p. 218, illustrates the problems and therapeutic rationale and approach associated with each model.

The biomechanical and motor control models address problems of movement (Trombly & Radomski, 2002; Mathiowetz &

TABLE 13-3. PROBLEMS ADDRESSED BY MODELS AND APPROACH TO INTERVENTIONS

Model	Problem Addressed	Representative Concepts
Biomechanical	Limited range of motion, strength, endurance	• Positioning, exercise, and conditioning to prevent impairment and improve capacity • Provide orthoses and prostheses, adapted equipment, and environmental modifications to compensate for impairments
Motor Control	Problems of motor coordination	• Use of sensory input and goal directed action to elicit and organize movement patterns • Modification of task and/or environment to elicit more effective movements
Sensory Integration	Problems with sensory processing and adaptive movement	• Support person to engage in adaptive movements to elicit sensory information and organize the brain • Educate caretakers and adapt environment to maximize functioning given sensory–integrative challenges
Cognitive–Perceptual	Perceptual and cognitive impairments	• Train in cognitive and perceptual capacities • Teach client ways to make allowances for limitations • Adapt task and/or environment
Cognitive Disabilities	Cognitive limitations	• Alter task/environment to match level of cognitive capacity • Educate caretakers about limitations
Model of Human Occupation	Personal and environmental problems influencing choice, organization, and performance of occupations	• Support client's occupational engagement to support/enhance motivation, adaptive patterning, and performance of occupations • Modify environment to support/enhance motivation, adaptive patterning, and performance of occupations
Canadian Model of Occupational Performance	Mismatch between person, environment, and occupation that restricts occupational performance	• Collaborate and involve clients (or their caretakers) in decision making and action to change personal, occupational, or environmental factors restricting performance

Bass-Haugen, 2002). The former is concerned with restrictions of movement that occur because of limitations in range of motion, strength, and endurance related primarily to the musculoskeletal system, the peripheral nervous system, and the cardiopulmonary system. The motor control model is concerned with problems of coordination due to CNS damage. The biomechanical model focuses on ways to prevent deformity and to improve movement capacity through such things as, for example, positioning and exercise. When limitations of movement are permanent, this model seeks to compensate for these problems by means of prostheses, orthoses, specialized equipment, and environmental modifications. The contemporary motor control model sees motor control as a function of CNS status, task, and environment. Consequently, it proposes therapy that improves control of movement either through enhancing CNS processes and or modifying the tasks and environment.

Sensory integration focuses on problems with sensory processing and adaptive movement. Traditionally, this model used an exclusively remediative strategy of supporting the client to engage in adaptive movements to elicit sensory information and organize the brain. More recently, this model (Bundy, Lane, & Murray, 2002) also includes strategies of educating caretakers such as teachers and parents to understand the needs of the client and modifying the environment to maximize functioning, given the person's sensory-integrative limitations.

The cognitive-perceptual model and the cognitive disabilities model focus on problems in the domain of perception and cognition. The cognitive-perceptual model (like the motor control model) employs a contemporary view that performance is influenced by the person's characteristics, the task, and the environment. Thus, this model combines strategies of training the person in capacities, teaching the person to make adaptations in how he/she goes about doing things to allow for limitations, and adapting the task and environment to enhance performance. The cognitive disabilities model does not recommend any remedial approaches and, therefore, proposes only altering the task and environment and advising caretakers about the client's limitations.

> **When the seven conceptual practice models are considered together, it becomes apparent that occupational therapy addresses a wide range of problems. To a significant degree, this is why occupational therapists tend to think of their practice as holistic.**

The model of human occupation focuses on both personal and environmental problems that negatively impact on how people choose, organize, and perform their occupations. Intervention based on this model supports or enhances motivation, adaptive patterning of occupation and performance. It also proposes modifications of the social and physical environment to achieve these same ends.

The Canadian model of occupational performance focuses on restrictions in occupational performance that emanate from a mismatch among the person, occupation, and environment. It proposes a collaborative approach that involves clients (or their caretakers) in decision-making and action to change personal, occupational, and/ or environmental factors to enhance performance.

When the seven conceptual practice models are considered together, it becomes apparent that occupational therapy addresses a wide range of problems. To a significant degree, this is why occupational therapists tend to think of their practice as holistic. However, no single model ordinarily encompasses all the problems that any single client experiences. Thus, in practice, therapists must combine models. Models are rarely sufficient, of themselves, to provide a holistic approach to practice or a comprehensive understanding of the range of problems that will be addressed in therapy.

The model of human occupation and the Canadian model of occupational performance can be distinguished from other models in that they focus more broadly on how other factors, such as motivation, organization of lifestyle, and personal self-determination, affect occupation. The remaining models are focused on reducing the extent or impact of impairments on performance. For this reason the two broader models are often used in combination with models that focus on impairments experienced by the client or client group.

🌿 Theory Offered by the Models

Theorizing includes description and explanation. Description is the more basic level of theorizing that provides an ordered way of thinking about phenomena. Thus, description involves naming or labeling phenomena and categorizing them into classes or types (i.e., creating taxonomies).

Explanation is a more advanced level of theorizing that provides an account of how some phenomena work. Explanation is critical to applied theories since it provides the basis for the two important processes of prediction and management. When a theory gives an accurate account of how phenomena work, it allows:

◆ Accurately anticipating what will happen under different circumstances (prediction)
◆ Systematically influencing or shaping circumstances or events to achieve desired outcomes (management)

Prediction and management are important in therapy. For example, therapists assess a client's capacities in order to anticipate (and help the client and/or the client's family to anticipate) the client's ability to function under certain circumstances (e.g., living independently) in the future. Therapists seek to manage phenomena when they alter the environment or engage the client in experiences that are aimed to achieve certain outcomes or changes. Therapists cannot accurately predict or manage phenomena without an explanation that provides the rationale for these processes.

Current models of practice fall into two categories based on the type of theory they provide:

◆ Models in which the theory is primarily descriptive
◆ Models that both describe and explain

Predominantly Descriptive Models

Two of the seven models are primarily descriptive: the cognitive disabilities model and the Canadian model of occupational performance. The cognitive disabilities model states that cognition underlies and influences performance and that the state of the brain determines cognition. However, this model does not offer any explanations of this process and refers to medical explanations of brain pathology that restrict cognition. The model focuses on describing the levels and components of cognition. Because this model is not concerned with producing change in cognition, it offers no explanation of the process of cognitive development.

As noted in Chapter 7, the Canadian model of occupational performance began as an attempt to specify guidelines for practice and describe occupational therapy's domain of concern. This model has remained largely descriptive in format. It provides taxonomies of the components of occupational performance, of the environment, and of the person. It also states a series of beliefs and values and specifies principles and guidelines for client-centered practice. However, the model offers only a few explanatory statements about how the phenomena named in the model actually work. The process of applying the model involves selecting theories that do provide explanations to guide the therapy process (Fearing & Clark, 2000).

Descriptive and Explanatory Models

The five models that offer explanations of phenomena in additional to description are characterized by statements about the relationships between phenomena. These statements explain how various qualities and processes are linked (e.g., that they co-vary, or that one causes the next). When several such statements are linked together, they constitute a network of explanation that accounts for how some phenomena work.

The biomechanical model offers detailed descriptions of the human musculoskeletal system. It also offers explanations of the factors underlying movement, such as how force is generated by muscles and how muscle strength changes with changes in exercise. Most of this theory was developed outside of occupational therapy, but it nonetheless provides critical knowledge for understanding the dynamics of how humans produce movement and for understanding and addressing impairments of movement.

The motor control model provides descriptions, such as the developmental sequence of reflexes and motor control. It also provides an explanation of how coordinated movement is produced. As noted in Chapter 11, the theoretical explanation of the production of movement has shifted from a focus on the CNS to a focus on how the CNS combines with the musculoskeletal system, the task, and the environment to influence movement. This explanation relies heavily on ideas developed outside occupational therapy. Nonetheless, writers within the field have contextualized these arguments in an occupational therapy framework (Mathiowetz & Bass-Haugen, 2002).

Sensory integration offers a descriptive taxonomy of sensory processes and provides one of the most sophisticated theories of the field. It seeks to explain how the sensation is organized and used for movement. Even though this model builds on theory developed in other fields, it clearly makes a unique theoretical argument developed within occupational therapy.

The cognitive-perceptual model has traditionally been very concerned with description (e.g., developing taxonomies of perceptual and cognitive functioning). However, as noted in Chapter 9, this model is now more concerned with providing explanations of the perceptual and cognitive process involved in occupational performance. This model is still developing and incorporates theoretical concepts developed into an occupational therapy framework.

The model of human occupation similarly provides a number of taxonomies, such as the categorization of process, motor, and communication/interaction skills. This model provides explanations for the motivation for occupation and of how persons manage to organize their occupational performance into everyday patterns. More recently, it has added a concern for explaining the role that experience plays in performance. This model draws concepts from a wide range of disciplines and integrates them into a theoretical framework that is unique to occupational therapy.

In summary, models that offer theoretical explanations give accounts for how phenomena work going beyond mere description or statements of beliefs or values. By doing so, these models provide an important understanding of the nature and workings of phenomena that must be addressed in practice. Moving from description to explanation is an important step in the development of models. Moreover, while all models borrow and build

> **Moving from description to explanation is an important step in the development of models.**

upon interdisciplinary concepts, it is important that the theoretical formulations offered by occupational therapy models are framed to address unique occupational therapy perspectives. As we saw here, models vary in the extent to which they have developed explanatory theory and the extent to which that theory has been uniquely developed as occupational therapy theory.

Research

As noted in Chapter 5, research is important for validating and improving the theory and the technology of models. The research underlying each model reflects, to a large extent, how that model has developed. In this section we will briefly compare the research underlying each model.

The biomechanical model is based on a wealth of research about the musculoskeletal system and how it can be modified (e.g., studies of how exercise affects muscle strength and studies examining the dynamic role of muscles and muscle groups in movement) and on the relationship between the capacity for motion and the ability to do things. This research has been conducted largely outside of occupational therapy.

A more limited body of research has examined this model within occupational therapy, such as studies of the relationship between musculoskeletal functioning and performance and studies examining muscle action and movement in actual task performance. Finally, a few studies have research that has examined the outcomes of biomechanical-based interventions.

The motor control model and the cognitive-perceptual model grew out interdisciplinary concepts and research on the CNS and its role in movement, perception, and cognition. A handful of studies have examined how differences in the environment and task have influenced perceptual, motor, or cognitive

aspects of performance. There is very little research that has examined the application and efficacy of the contemporary versions of these two models in practice. To an extent the limited research may reflect the fact that these two models have been reformulated and that approaches to studying the newer theory has yet to be worked out. It may also reflect the fact that there already exists substantial interdisciplinary research relevant to these models. For example, scientists from a number of fields have contributed substantial research related to the theory underlying the motor control model.

The cognitive disabilities model is a unique formulation developed within occupational therapy. Therefore all the research related to this model has been done in the field. This research is modest (fewer than 20 published studies could be found), mostly focused on development of the assessments associated with this model. Similarly, the Canadian model of occupational performance is unique to the field, and its body of research has been contributed by occupational therapists. This model is also supported by a modest body of research. Just over 20 published studies could be found. Most of the studies are focused on development of the Canadian Occupational Performance Measure.

Over 80 published studies conducted in occupational therapy have examined some aspect of the model of human occupation. These include a number of investigations that have tested the underlying theory. Many of the studies are related to developing assessments. Still other studies have examined the model's utility in practice and documented outcomes of services based on the model.

The sensory integration model is the most extensively researched model in the field. It is difficult to identify the exact number of studies related to this model, because many studies use concepts related to but not strictly based on the model. Nonetheless, numerous studies have examined and contributed to this model's conceptualization of sensory integrative problems and have examined the impact of this model in practice.

In summary, models vary tremendously in the extent and way they have been researched. As we saw, some models are built on interdisciplinary knowledge that includes substantial research. However, these models tend to have less empirical support for their formulation and use in occupational therapy. Other models developed and researched exclusively within occupational therapy tend to have a more modest research base. At this time, the model of human occupation and the sensory integrative model have the most substantial empirical scrutiny.

> **Models are always works in progress; thus, it is important to consider how a model is being developed.**

and some of the models have been in the making for half a century. Nonetheless, on the whole, these models are still in relatively early stages of development. Further theoretical clarification, development of technology for application, and research will be needed to augment each of these models.

The field's models constitute the major theory building and research of occupational therapy. Moreover, they provide the major corpus of the field's knowledge that guides the everyday practice of occupational therapists. In the final analysis, occupational therapy practice will only be as valuable as the conceptual models on which it is based.

 # Conclusion: Further Directions for Model Development

Chapter 5 argued that a conceptual practice model should have theory, technology for application in practice, and research to examine the theory and application. The seven conceptual practice models vary in how fully each of these elements are currently developed. By carefully considering these factors, readers of this text can and should draw their own conclusions about the relative merit of each model.

Models are always works in progress, so it is important to consider how a model is being developed. Also, because models develop over a long period, one must also take a long view on the impact of models in the field. Every one of the seven models has been around in some form for over two decades,

References:

Allen, C. (1992). Cognitive Disabilities. In Katz, N. (ed.): Cognitive Rehabilitation: Models for Intervention in Occupational Therapy, pp 1–21. Boston: Andover Medical Publishers.

Bundy, AC, Lane, SJ & Murray, EA. (2002). Sensory Integration: Theory and practice, 2nd ed. Philadelphia: FA Davis.

Fearing, VG & Clark, J. (2000). Individuals in Context: A Practical Guide to Client-Centered Practice. Thorofare, NJ: Slack.

Katz, N. (1998). Cognition and Occupation in Rehabilitation: Cognitive Models for Intervention in Occupational Therapy, pp 4–50. Bethesda, MD: American Occupational Therapy Association.

Kielhofner, G. (2002). A Model of Human Occupation: Theory and Application, 3rd ed. Baltimore: Lippincott, Williams & Wilkins.

Mathiowetz, V & Bass-Haugen, JB. (2002) Assessing abilities and capacities: Motor behavior. In Trombly, CA & Radomski, MV (eds.): Occupational Therapy for Physical Dysfunction, 5th ed, pp 137–159. Philadelphia: Lippincott, Williams & Wilkins.

Toglia, JP. (1998). A dynamical interactional model to cognitive rehabilitation. In Katz, N. (ed.): Cognition and Occupation in Rehabilitation: Cognitive Models for Intervention in Occupational Therapy, pp 4–50. Bethesda, MD: American Occupational Therapy Association.

Townsend, E. (ed.) (1997). Enabling Occupation: An Occupational Therapy Perspective. Ottawa, Ontario: CAOT Publications ACE.

Townsend, E. (1998). Using Canada's 1997 guidelines for enabling occupation. Australian Occupational Therapy Journal, 45, 1–6.

Trombly, CA & Radomski, M. (2002). Occupational Therapy for Physical Dysfunction, 5th ed. Philadelphia: Lippincott, Williams & Wilkins.

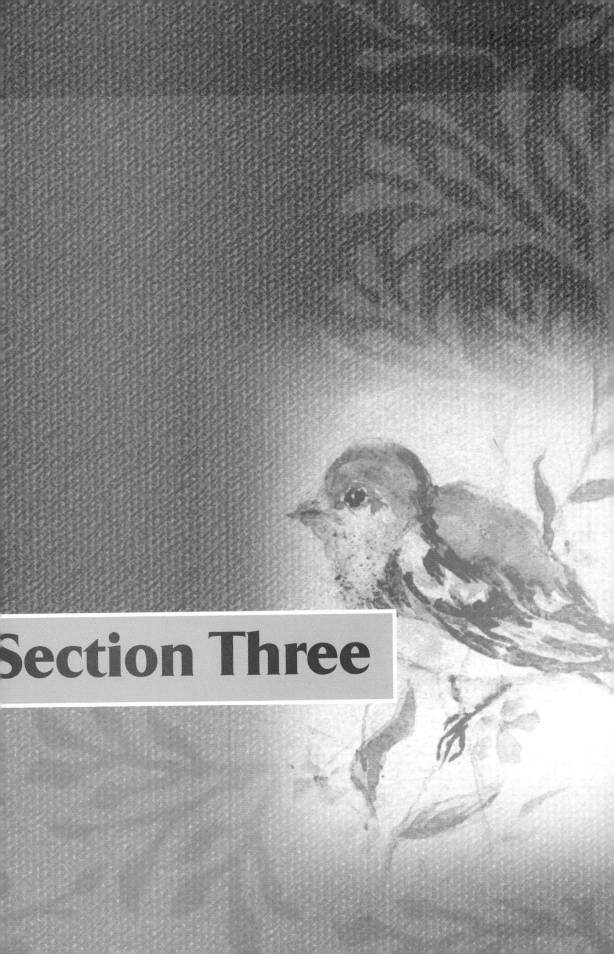

Section Three

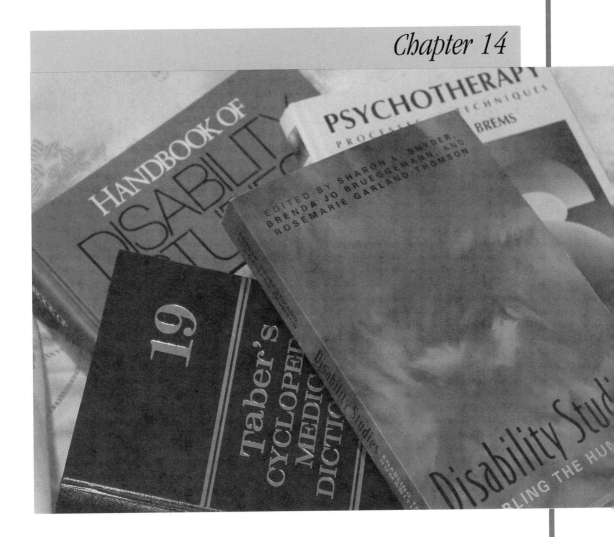

Chapter 14

The Nature and Use of Related Knowledge

I n Section Two, we examined seven conceptual practice models. These models provide much of the theory and technology that occupational therapists employ in practice. Nonetheless, therapists routinely need knowledge beyond that provided by these models. Therefore, therapists use knowledge developed in other fields. I refer to such knowledge as related knowledge since it does not belong to occupational therapy but is related to the concerns and practice of the profession.

Occupational therapists use related knowledge to supplement the conceptual practice models which define and guide the main elements of occupational therapy practice.

 ## Types of Related Knowledge

Two types of related knowledge are often used to supplement conceptual practice models:

◆ Foundational knowledge related to the interdisciplinary base of the models
◆ Applied knowledge addressing issues not addressed by models

Foundational knowledge is generally knowledge linked to basic sciences or disciplines. For instance, the biomechanical model builds upon the knowledge of anatomy (particularly musculoskeletal anatomy) and physiology, and the sensory integration and cognitive-perceptual models build on knowledge from the neurosciences. Other models, such as the model of human occupation, build on knowledge from psychology and the social sciences. In fact, many readers will recognize that these bodies of knowledge often make up what are considered prerequisites to courses that teach the conceptual practice models.

Applied knowledge is generally knowledge developed for application in other professions. One example is behaviorism, developed in psychology. This theory employs the concept of reinforcement (i.e., positive and negative consequences of behavior) to explain and manage the acquisition and relinquishing of behavior patterns. The following is an instance in which an occupational therapist might use a behavioral approach in combination with an occupational therapy model. Adolescent clients with behavioral problems may be engaged in occupations designed to allow them to explore, to pursue interests, and to develop a sense of efficacy, based on the model of human occupation. Those same adolescents may be informed that if they become verbally or physically aggressive, they may lose points in the token economy (i.e., a behavioral approach wherein clients may earn and lose points that can be cashed in for privileges and/or desired goods). In this instance, an occupational therapy model defines the major aspects of therapy, but knowledge and techniques drawn from behaviorism are used to manage behaviors interfering with participation in therapy.

 ## Three Exemplary Bodies of Related Knowledge

The potential bodies of knowledge that make up related knowledge for occupational therapy are very broad, so no comprehensive coverage of this information is possible. To illustrate how related knowledge is used in the field, I took the strategy of including three major bodies of knowledge that cut across almost any application of occupational therapy. Three bodies of knowledge discussed in this section are:

◆ The medical model
◆ Intra- and interpersonal theories
◆ Disabilities studies

The medical model is developed and used in medicine. It has always served as important related knowledge in occupational therapy. Knowledge is often borrowed from psychotherapeutic traditions of psychology and psychiatry to guide the therapeutic use of self in occupational therapy practice. The interdisciplinary field of disabilities studies emphasizes understanding disability from the perspective of persons who have disabilities. (Albrecht, Fitzpatrick, & Scrimshaw, 2000; Longmore, 1995; Oliver, 1996; Scotch, 2001;

Shapiro, 1993). Central to this perspective is the argument that many of the problems faced by persons with disabilities can be located more properly in the environment, in everything from physical barriers to stigmatizing attitudes to outright discrimination. Ideas from disability studies have many lessons to teach occupational therapists and therefore constitute important related knowledge.

The three bodies of related knowledge that I have chosen to discuss represent three distinct, sometimes opposing, and potentially complementary views of the condition of disability and how to go about changing it. The medical model locates the problem as a condition in the individual, which requires the ministrations of an authoritarian medical expert to remove or attenuate it. Psychotherapy locates the problem in an arrested process of development that must be refacilitated through an empathic relationship between the client and therapist. Disability studies locate the problem in social conditions that transform impairment into disability; it envisions social change and empowerment of disabled persons as groups. Each of these perspectives identifies what is likely a partial truth in the situation of any client and highlights the fact that different clients at different points in their journey will require a knowledgeable expert, a respectful advocate, and an empathetic collaborator.

> **Occupational therapists use related knowledge to supplement the conceptual practice models which define and guide the main elements of occupational therapy practice.**

 Discussion

In most instances, an occupational therapist could not be an effective practitioner without recourse to related knowledge. Therefore, the use of related knowledge is a basic characteristic of good practice. It is important to remember, however, that related knowledge is not unique to occupational therapy. Thus, it cannot serve as a source of professional identity or as the defining component of an occupational therapist's competence. Rather, related knowledge serves as adjunctive and complementary to the field's paradigm and conceptual practice models.

References

Albrecht, GL, Fitzpatrick, R & Scrimshaw, SC. (eds.). (2000). Handbook of Social Studies in Health and Medicine. London: Sage Publications.

Longmore, PK. (1995). The second phase: From disability rights to disability culture. The Disability Rag and ReSource, 16, 4–11.

Oliver, M. (1996). Understanding Disability: From Theory to Practice. New York: St. Martin's Press.

Scotch, RK. (2001). From Good Will to Civil Rights: Transforming Federal Disability Policy, 2nd ed. Philadelphia: Temple University Press.

Shapiro, JP. (1993). No Pity: People with Disabilities Forging a New Civil Rights Movement. New York: Random House.

Chapter 15

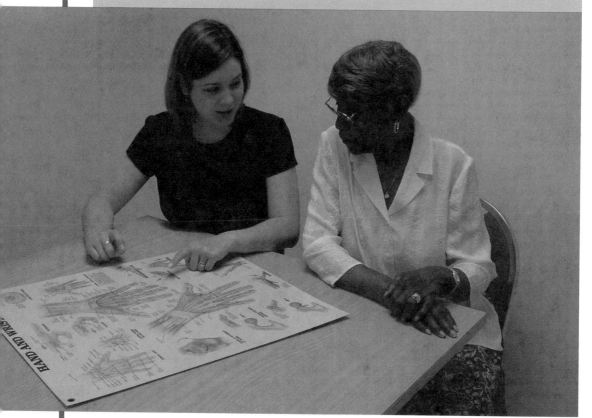

The Medical Model

An occupational therapist works with a client following an upper extremity injury that required surgery. As part of her approach, the therapist explains to the client the postsurgical healing process and its implications for safely engaging in occupations. In a wide range of circumstances, therapists must have an understanding of their clients' disease processes and prognoses, the expected side effects of medication, or the pathway of recovery from trauma and/or surgical procedures. In these instances, occupational therapists are drawing upon related knowledge from the medical model.

The medical model was developed in and for the practice of medicine, although aspects of it are used in many health disciplines, including occupational therapy. This model addresses disease and trauma that interrupt ordinary bodily function. The model has resulted in a steady growth of scientific knowledge concerning:

◆ Biochemical constituents of the human body and their cause-and-effect relationships
◆ The nature, causes, and management of disease and trauma (Dubos, 1959)

Practitioners using this model aim to eliminate or contain the effects of disease or trauma through manipulation or alteration of bodily structures and processes.

Interdisciplinary Base

Modern medical knowledge derives from several interdisciplinary sources. First, the medical model includes a set of beliefs about healing that has origins in the medical system of the ancient Greeks (Dubos, 1959). According to Grecian mythology, the god Asclepius was a healer who cured with medicinal plants and surgery. Asclepius wielded esoteric knowledge as part of his healing art. With absolute authority, he ministered to a passive and compliant recipient of the healing action. The idea of the physician as an authority and the client as a compliant recipient of care derives from this mythological divine healer (Siegler & Osmond, 1974).

With the advent of the 20th century, medicine increased its scientific base dramatically. At that time, scientists had made great strides in understanding the physical world through careful examination of the building blocks of nature and their interrelationships (Capra, 1982). Medicine emulated the intel-

lectual models of early physical sciences (Capra, 1982; Riley, 1977), adopting a view in which:

◆ The body was seen as a complex machine
◆ The task of medicine was conceived as repairing breakdowns in the machine (i.e., disease and trauma) (Capra, 1982)

Knowledge foundational to and incorporated into the medical model has been generated by many disciplines including basic sciences such as genetics, biochemistry, anatomy, and physiology, as well as applied sciences such as pharmacology, nutrition, and bioengineering (Bertalanffy, 1966; Capra, 1982).

Theory
Organization

Because the medical model is focused primarily on problems (i.e., disease and trauma), it has been less concerned with developing concepts illuminating the underlying order of the human body. In fact, medicine relies primarily on the work done in basic and applied biological and biochemical sciences for this information. However, medicine has implicitly, if not always explicitly, employed the concept of health to define organization in the human body. In the medical model, health is generally defined by three themes:

◆ The absence of disease
◆ Homeostasis
◆ Normative states

Because of its focus on illness, the medical model approach to defining health has been primarily to proceed "inductively by enumeration of examples [of disease] and then health is the absence of all of those states" (Brody, 1973, p. 75). Although some efforts have been made to define health as more than the mere absence of disease (e.g., concepts of wellness) (Berliner & Salmon, 1980), these efforts are largely outside of the traditional medical model.

The medical model also views order in terms of homeostasis, the notion that living systems try to maintain certain predetermined states (Bertalanffy, 1966). Examples of homeostatic processes are the maintenance of blood pressure and body temperature. An extension of the idea of homeostasis is how the body seeks to restore order when it has been disturbed by disease or trauma. Thus, for example, understanding of immunological processes by which the body fends off infections or the healing process following accidental or surgical trauma is important to medicine.

Finally, the study of anatomical and physiological dimensions of the body resulted in descriptions of what is normative. For example, the understanding of the organization of the musculoskeletal system has resulted in the idea of what constitutes the average body. Similarly, descriptions of physiological processes have resulted in descriptions of typical physiological states. These norms have become accepted as the standard for health, and deviation from these norms is the basis for identification of problems.

Problems and Challenges

The medical model identifies problems in terms of:

◆ Disease and trauma
◆ Disturbances in homeostasis
◆ Deviations from body norms

These three aspects of medically identified problems often overlap. Central to the medical model is the concept of disease. A critical step in the development of the medical model

> **A critical step in the development of the medical model was the conceptual separation of the person experiencing an illness from the underlying disease that is identified as residing within the person.**

was the conceptual separation of the person who is experiencing an illness from the underlying disease that is identified as residing within the person (Foucault, 1973). This abstraction is at the core of all medical thought and practice and allows the medical practitioner to define the disease, homeostatic disturbance, or bodily abnormality as a negative state that needs to be altered or eradicated. Disease is viewed as disrupting the homeostatic order of biological processes because it forces somatic functions beyond normative limits.

Critical to understanding disease are its:

◆ Syndromatic signs and symptoms
◆ Etiology
◆ Prognosis

Signs of disease refer to the cluster of physical indicators (e.g. swelling, fever, abnormal physiological values) that represent a deviation from bodily norms. Symptoms refer to individuals' experiences and complaints (e.g., pain, fatigue, and difficulties with bodily processes and functions). An important step in the understanding of any disease or trauma is identification of the attendant signs and symptoms.

Etiology refers to the underlying cause of the disease process. Careful description of the root source and unfolding of physical events that constitute each disease process is basic to the medical model. Typical causes of disease include:

◆ Infectious or noxious agents entering the body (e.g., viral infections, lead poisoning, exposure to asbestos)
◆ Genetic disorder (e.g., Down's syndrome)
◆ Externally imposed physical trauma to the body (e.g., spinal cord injury) or breakdown of the body due to wear and tear

(e.g., carpel tunnel syndrome or cere-brovascular accident)

Medical researchers originally sought to identify the single cause of a disease process; it is now recognized that many if not most diseases are a result of many contributing and interacting factors. Originally the medical model was only interested in biological factors that contributed to disease status (Blaney, 1975; Ludwig & Othmer, 1977; Siegler & Osmond, 1974). However, it is now recognized that biological factors need not be the sole cause of disease and that such factors as psychological stress contribute to some disease processes.

Prognosis refers to the natural course that a disease will take. Prognosis includes understanding both the underlying unfolding of the physiological processes and their consequences (e.g., impairment, pain, or death). Prognosis is important in making decisions about whether, when, and how to intervene. For example, the consequences of letting a disease take its natural course versus risking the side effects of medical procedures must sometimes be weighed. Also, identification of how far a disease has progressed along its natural course may also influence the type of medical intervention chosen.

Medicine has applied the basic approach of investigating the syndrome, etiology, and prognosis of disease to a vast number of disease and trauma states. Many of these are now well understood while others are still partly or poorly understood. Also, because of the emergence of new disease processes (AIDS being one example), medicine is constantly investigating and generating understanding of new problems.

🌿 Action Implications

Action derived from the medical model is guided by the germ theory of disease. That is, control of disease is best accomplished by attacking the causative agent or focusing treatment on that part of the body affected by disease (Dubos, 1959). The aim of medicine is to identify the appropriate therapeutic agents that could be applied to eradicate or arrest the disease process (Brody, 1973). Therapeutic agents include drugs and procedures (e.g., surgery, radiation) that attack the disease or remove or repair the diseased component (Ludwig & Othmer, 1977). This requires that the physician carefully collect data on the signs and symptoms manifest by the client in order to arrive at a correct diagnosis. When the disease is correctly identified, the physician, depending on the existing knowledge about the disease, will have some degree of ability to predict and control the course of illness. The diagnosis is critical in the medical model, because it predicts the path of the disease and indicates the appropriate treatment or treatment options.

Nonetheless, only in a limited number of diseases does medicine have sufficient knowledge to proceed in this fashion (Brody, 1973). In fact, there is a continuum from those diseases for which there is rather certain knowledge of etiology, course, and treatment to those about which little or nothing is known. Consequently, physicians often operate with only partial knowledge about a disease and its treatment. Even when there is fairly good knowledge about the efficacy of medical interventions, there will be substantial variation in how individual clients react to the treatments. For example, optimal dosage of medication and the experience of side effects is a matter of great variation among clients for certain conditions and their treatment. Thus, medication sometimes involves a trial-and-error period during which both the desired results and side effects are monitored in order to achieve correct prescription.

Often, treatment cannot be directed at underlying causes (which may not be known) and instead focuses on managing symptoms without affecting the underlying problem (Ludwig & Othmer, 1977). This means that medical model treatment may be curative, compensatory, syndromatic, or symptomatic (Mechanic, 1978). In curative treatment, causative agents are attacked, and the condition is reversed. Compensatory treatment aims to minimize further problems and maintain function, while syndromatic treatment manages major problems related to the disease without cure. Finally, symptomatic treatment simply alleviates some problems without altering basic causes or effects of the disease. Only a very small percentage of medical treatment is curative (Ludwig & Othmer, 1977).

 ## Research

Medical research includes ongoing research into basic physiological processes of the body; investigation of the nature, causes, and course of diseases; and investigation to develop and test therapies for various diseases. Biomedical research has yielded one of the largest scientific bodies of knowledge available to modern societies. In the 20th century, great strides were made in understanding the human body, the most notable of which was unraveling the human genome. Vast amounts of money are directed to the study of various disease processes and how they can be cured or attenuated. As a consequence, medical model knowledge continues to grow exponentially. Nonetheless, knowledge about diseases can range from those about which very little is still known or for which little can be done to those that are more completely understood and can be readily eradicated or

managed. This circumstance reflects the fact that new problems are always emerging and indicates the vast number of medical problems that must be investigated on an ongoing basis. It also reflects the fact that the medical model, for all its analytic power, is sometimes limited in its ability to appreciate the multifactorial nature of some disease processes.

 ## Discussion

The medical model is clearly the most influential and successful force in modern health care. The knowledge of this model underlies the successful management of a large range of illnesses and traumatic conditions. Many of the accomplishments of applying this model represent truly remarkable achievements that result in significant life-saving and the reduction of pain and suffering. As a technical achievement, the medical model is remarkable.

The medical model has both ideological and knowledge components. The ideological component of the medical model includes a set of beliefs about the physician's role as a healer with authority over clients. The knowledge component is a reductionist, biochemical body of information that explains disease as an interruption of normal physiological processes and yields procedures to eliminate disease through manipulation or alteration of somatic structures and processes. The medical model can thus be defined as the beliefs and knowledge that define physicians as authoritative healers and that enable them to cure, ameliorate, or arrest disease through recognition and alteration of its manifestation in bodily states. Despite its important accom-

> **The medical model can thus be defined as the beliefs and knowledge that define physicians as authoritative healers and that enable them to cure, ameliorate, or arrest disease through recognition and alteration of its manifestation in bodily states.**

plishments, a number of limitations and weaknesses of the medical model have been identified.

The idea of the physician as an authoritative healer and the client as a passive and compliant recipient of medical care has been criticized. Authors have called for a more egalitarian and collaborative model in which the client shares in the process of managing the disease and recovery. This becomes especially true in cases in which medicine cannot provide a cure or reverse the medical problem, and the client must have an active role in ongoing management of the disease process.

Engel (1962, 1977) criticizes the medical model for its lack of concern for factors other than the biomedical. He argues that the medical model has led to undesirable treatment practices, such as overuse of surgery and drugs and inappropriate use of diagnostic procedures. The value of diagnostic procedures is directly related to the certainty of etiological and therapeutic implications of the diagnosis. This requires that much be known about the disease, its course, its alterability, and the agents that have power to control the disease processes. Where knowledge is less certain, the physician's ability to effectively apply the medical model is limited. For example, many persons have criticized the use of the medical model in psychiatry, where many diagnoses do not approach the degree of knowledge and certainty needed for effective delineation of etiology, course (prognosis), and treatment (Goffman, 1961; Leifer, 1970; Szasz, 1961).

Another criticism of the medical model is its stance that disease is a negative state. In cases where disease can be identified and eradicated, this stance is largely unproblematic. However, this aspect of the medical model falters when a disease process is chronic, produces impairments, and cannot be eradicated by medical procedures. In such instances, the medical model stance on disease and impairment as negative can result in devaluing of the person (Gill, 2001; Leifer, 1970). Moreover, the negative identification of disease can be used to justify practices that amount to social control, as in the case of psychiatric illness (Leifer, 1970; Szasz, 1961).

Any discussion of the medical model must also recognize that in many instances occupational therapists work alongside physicians who derive their status and expertise from the medical model. Rogers (1982) points out cogently that there are critical differences between occupational therapy's approach to identifying problems and doing therapy and that of the medical model. Medicine is primarily concerned with eradicating disease. Siegler and Osmond (1974) go so far as to argue that the physician's role does not include addressing impairment. Occupational therapy seeks primarily to influence how people conduct their lives in the face of permanent impairments (Reilly, 1962). In that sense, the respective contributions of the medical model and occupational therapy can be complementary. Occupational therapists should be aware of both the strengths and limitations of the medical model. It is also important to recognize what while therapists use information from the medical model as related knowledge in practice, the overall approach and contributions of occupational therapy are different from those of the medical model.

🌿 Summary

The medical model:

◆ Concerns biochemical constituents of the human body and their cause-and-effect relationships

◆ Concerns the nature, causes, and management of disease and trauma

◆ Aims to eliminate or contain the effects of disease or trauma through manipulation or alteration of bodily structures and processes

Interdisciplinary Base

◆ Beliefs about healing that define the physician as an authority and the client as a compliant recipient of care derives from the Greek mythological divine healer, Asclepius
◆ Intellectual models of early physical sciences resulted in:
   1. The body being seen as a complex machine
   2. The task of medicine being conceived as repairing breakdowns in the machine
   3. Basic sciences, such as genetics, biochemistry, anatomy, and physiology
   4. Applied sciences, such as pharmacology, nutrition, and bioengineering

Theory
Organization
Health is defined by three themes:

◆ The absence of disease
◆ Homeostasis (the notion that living systems try to maintain certain predetermined states)
◆ Normative physiological states

Problems and Challenges
The medical model identifies problems in terms of:

◆ Disease and trauma
◆ Disturbances in homeostasis
◆ Deviations from body norms

Disease is viewed as disrupting the homeostatic order of biological processes because it forces somatic functions beyond normative limits

Critical to understanding disease is its:

◆ Syndromatic signs (physical indicators) and symptoms (individuals' experiences, complaints, and symptoms)
◆ Etiology (underlying cause of the disease process)
◆ Prognosis (natural course that a disease will take)

Action Implications

◆ Action derived from the medical model is somatic and guided by the germ theory of disease (attacking the causative agent or focusing treatment on that part of the body affected by disease)
◆ Diagnosis is critical in the medical model because it predicts the path of the disease and indicates the appropriate treatment or treatment options

Research

◆ Medical research includes ongoing research into basic physiological processes of the body; investigation of the nature, causes, and course of diseases; and investigation to develop and test therapies for various diseases
◆ Knowledge about diseases can range from those about which very little is still known, or for which little can be done, to those that are more completely understood and can be readily eradicated or managed

Discussion

◆ The medical model has both ideological and knowledge components
◆ The ideological component is a set of beliefs about the physician's role as a healer with authority over clients
◆ The knowledge component is a reductionist, biochemical body of information that explains disease as an interruption of

normal physiological processes and that yields procedures to eliminate disease

◆ Criticized for:

1. Lack of concern for factors other than biomedical

2. Undesirable treatment practices such as overuse of surgery and drugs and inappropriate use of diagnostic procedures

3. Its stance that disease is a negative state that can result in devaluing of the person and justifying practices that amount to social control

◆ There are critical differences between occupational therapy's approach to identifying problems and doing therapy and that of the medical model:

◆ Medicine is primarily concerned with eradicating disease and reducing the extent to which it results in impairments

◆ Occupational therapy seeks primarily to influence how people conduct their lives in the face of permanent impairments

References

Berliner, HS & Salmon, JW. (1980). The holistic alternative to scientific medicine: History and analysis. International Journal of Health Services, 10(2), 133–147.

von Bertalanffy, L. (1966).General systems theory and psychiatry. In Arieti, SR (ed.). American Handbook of Psychiatry, vol 3. New York: Basic Books.

Blaney, PH. (1975). Implications of the medical model and its alternatives. American Journal of Psychiatry, 132, 911–914.

Brody, H. (1973). The systems view of man: Implications for medicine, science, and ethics. Perspectives in Biology and Medicine, 17, 71–92.

Capra, F. (1982). The Turning Point: Science, Society, and the Rising Culture. New York: Simon & Schuster.

Dubos, R. (1959). The Mirage of Health. New York: Harper & Row.

Engel, GL. (1962). The nature of disease and the care of the patient: The challenge of humanism and science in medicine. Rhode Island Medical Journal, 65, 245–252.

Engel, GL. (1977).The need for a new medical model: A challenge for bio-medicine. Science, 196, 129–135.

Foucault, M. (1973). The Birth of the Clinic: An Archaeology of Medical Perception. New York: Vintage Books.

Gill, CJ. (2001). Divided understandings: The social experience of disability. In Albrecht, G, Seelman, K & Bury, M (eds.). Handbook of Disabilities Studies, pp 351–372). Thousand Oaks, CA: Sage.

Goffman, E. (1961). Asylums. New York: Doubleday.

Leifer, R. (1970). Medical model as ideology. International Journal of Psychiatry, 9, 13–34.

Ludwig, AM & Othmer, E. (1977). The medical basis of psychiatry. American Journal of Psychiatry, 134, 1087–1092.

Mechanic, D. (1978). The doctor's view of disease and the patient. In Mechanic D (ed.). Medical Sociology, 2nd ed. New York: Free Press.

Reilly, M. (1962). Occupational therapy can be one of the great ideas of 20th century medicine. American Journal of Occupational Therapy, 76, 1–9.

Riley, JN. (1977). Western medicine's attempt to become more scientific: Examples from the United States and Thailand. Social Science and Medicine, 11, 549–560.

Rogers, J. (1982). Order and disorder in medicine and occupational therapy. American Journal of Occupational Therapy, 36, 29–35.

Siegler, M & Osmond, H. (1974). Models of Madness, Models of Medicine. New York: Harper & Row.

Szasz, T. (1961). The Myth of Mental Illness: Foundations of a Theory of Personal Conduct. New York: Harper & Row.

Chapter 16

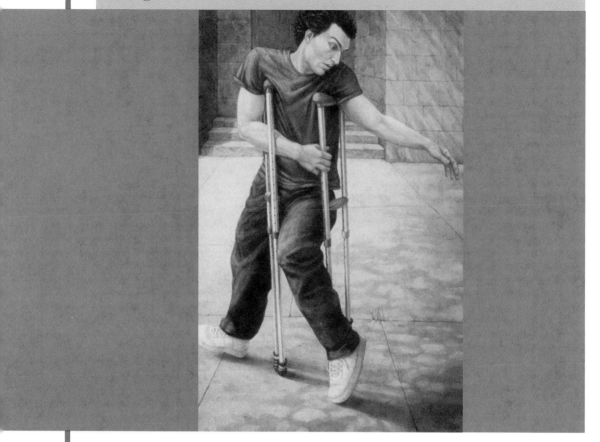

Disability Studies

The painting above is Riva Lehrer's portrait of William Shannon, alias "Crutchmaster," an accomplished dancer, choreographer, and video artist. Shannon's choreography is based on his body and its movements, as affected by severe osteoarthritis and Legg-Perthes disease. Visual and performing artists like Lehrer and Shannon strive to challenge non-disabled notions of beauty and contest stereotypical notions of disability. Their work is part of disability studies, a diverse body of scholarly, reflective work that seeks to reframe our understanding of disability and how to respond to it.

Disability studies addresses the issue of disability from a unique perspective. The field emerged in the 1970s and 1980s as a counterpoint to the then dominant view of disability (Scotch, 2001). The prevailing view of disability, which disability studies contravenes, can be summarized in three broad, interrelated themes.

First, disability was conceptualized by the medical model and related health professions as an abnormality or deficit requiring professional management (Linton, 1998; Nagi, 1991; Scotch, 2001; Zola, 1972). This framework considered disability synonymous with personal impairment, and its solution was to fix the disabled person* (Nagi, 1991; Rioux, 1997). The second viewpoint defining disability was an economic model. Disability was conceptualized in terms of disabled persons' inability to be self-sufficient and productive, thereby requiring economic and social support (Hahn, 1985; Oliver, 1990; Rioux, 1997). The third concept, a societal perspective, cast impairment as inherently negative, rendering disabled persons in a variety of images, from the malevolent deviant to the victim of a personal tragedy (Asch & Fine, 1988; Gill, 2001; Snyder, Brueggeman, & Garland-Thompson, 2002; Zola, 1972).

The medical and economic perspectives reflected and reinforced dominant cultural views that cast disability in negative terms. Furthermore, these professional and societal conceptualizations of disability have translated into public policies that have defined and shaped disabled persons' lives (Hahn, 1997; Scotch, 2001).

Disability studies has sought to challenge and correct these views of disability. Perhaps the most critical goal has been to identify the cause of disability as environmental barriers rather than as impairments and to relocate disability from residing in the individual to inhering in societal attitudes and actions. As disability studies has evolved, it has also retold the story of disability, challenging the standing assumptions not only about the causes but also about the very nature of disability. Finally, disability studies has sought to transform disability from an "individual or medical problem into a civil rights issue" (Paterson & Hughes, 2000, p. 30).

🌿 Interdisciplinary Base

Disability studies has attracted scholars from a range of disciplines. Many of the themes represented in the field were first articulated in the social sciences. Disability studies draws on political and economic concepts as well as gender and race studies in their articulation of how disabled persons are oppressed. It builds on concepts from the humanities in the examination of various ways disability is represented in popular culture, literature, and art. Especially important to disability studies is the social constructivist argument that both everyday and specialized (e.g., scientific) ways of knowing are not absolute and, instead, reflect historical, ideological, and cultural forces and biases (Jeffreys, 2002). This postmodern perspective has been used

> **As disability studies has evolved, it has also retold the story of disability, challenging the standing assumptions not only about the causes but also about the very nature of disability.**

---

*The matter of language is an important theme in disability studies. In considering how best to refer to persons who have impairments that result in disability I was guided by the many scholars today who prefer the term "disabled person."

as a platform from which to critique and deconstruct predominant cultural and professional conceptions of disability.

While disability studies has generally eschewed concepts of disability from professional literature because of its ideological base, some ideas from these fields, such as the concept of identity from psychology, have been used. In the end, disability studies includes a broad sweep of interdisciplinary perspectives.

 # Deconstructing and Reconstructing Conceptions of Disability

Disability studies is fundamentally different from the other typical bodies of knowledge occupational therapists encounter. Because its aim has been to critique and deconstruct the extant notion of disability, it has:

◆ Illuminated biases and fallacies in standing societal and professional conceptions and approaches to addressing disability
◆ Offered alternative conceptions and action implications of disability

Thus, it has sought to achieve a number of fundamental shifts in thinking about and taking action with reference to disability.

In this section I describe in detail the three traditional, dominant conceptions of disability. I examine how disability studies scholars have critiqued these perspectives. Finally, I present the alternative conceptualizations of disability.

Disability as a Medical Problem Rooted in Impairment

The medical model perspective developed by rehabilitation professionals generated a concept of disability as rooted in the disabled person's physical, emotional, sensory, or cognitive impairments that, in turn, were the consequence of some disease process or trauma (Longmore, 1995a; Longmore, 1995b; Wendell, 1996; Zola, 1993a). This approach firmly located disability in the person (Linton, 1998; Nagi, 1991; Rioux, 1997; Scotch, 2001). The disease/trauma, impairment, and disability were all considered the unfortunate property of the individual.

This perspective was reinforced by a positivist scientific approach that sought to describe and measure the disabled person's impairments and document their relationship to limitations in activities of daily living and work (Rioux, 1997; Zola, 1993a). Readers will recognize that this perspective reflects much of the scholarship underlying occupational therapy models described in Section Two of this text.

Because of its grounding in the medical model, rehabilitation's impairment approach to disability imputed the impairment and its underlying causes as problems (i.e., negative states to be eradicated or attenuated) and the rehabilitation enterprise emerged as an effort to prevent, minimize, and, to the extent possible, reduce the consequences of impairment (Zola, 1993a). The unquestioned assumption of rehabilitation has been that disability (defined as deviation from normative physical and psychological structures and processes) is undesirable to both the disabled person and to society at large. This perspective rationalizes and engenders efforts to prevent and reduce impairment (and if not the impairment itself, then its public appearance) (Linton, 1998; Nagi, 1991; Scotch, 2001; Zola, 1972). The emphasis of rehabilitation efforts has been to transform the disabled person toward a state that most approximated "normal" function and appearance. As noted in Chapter 15, the concept of bodily averages served as the measure of normal states and the "ideal" of outcomes from medically derived therapies.

The Impairment Model as a Tool of Social Control

The positive impact of many rehabilitation services notwithstanding, disability scholars have pointed out that rehabilitation perspectives and practices have had important downsides for disabled people. These include three interrelated elements. First, rehabilitation practices reinforce the idea that the disability is the disabled person's problem (to the relative omission of considerations of how environmental factors, especially the social environment, contributed to disability*) (Linton, 1998; Nagi, 1991; Scotch, 2001; Zola, 1972). Consequently, they "cannot account for, let alone combat ... bias and discrimination" (Longmore, 1995b, p. 6). Second, the rehabilitation professional is cast as the expert on the disabled person's condition, the implication being that the essence or meaning of disability is to be located in the objective descriptions of disability produced in professional classificatory and explanatory systems. Moreover, the disabled person is expected to be the compliant recipient of care (Zola, 1972). Third, rehabilitation efforts enforce a version of normalcy that pressures disabled persons to fit in by appearing and functioning as much like non-disabled persons as possible (Jeffreys, 2002; Scott, 1969; Zola, 1972).

A consequence of these three elements is that the rehabilitation enterprise has taken on the guise of administering social control. Thus, therapy can be construed as a process oriented to maintaining social norms rather than ameliorating individuals' problems. That is, therapy aims to eliminate clients' characteristics and traits that threaten the legitimacy of mainstream values, ideals, practices, and rules.

In a classic study, Scott (1969) documented how the rehabilitation of blind persons, contrary to aims of enabling them to be more functional, systematically socialized them into becoming compliant and dependent. The first stage in this process involves an invalidation of the disabled persons' understanding of their own disability. For instance, Scott (1969) notes that the blind person is "rewarded for showing insight and subtly reprimanded for continuing to adhere to earlier notions about his problems. He is led to think that he 'really' understands past and present experiences when he couches them in terms acceptable to his therapist" (p. 79). In this way, the disabled person's understanding of his own disability is invalidated and replaced with an official, professional definition. The blind person is persuaded to learn ways of behaving that follow the professional conception of the problem of blindness, however much the conceptions may contradict personal experience.

Another example of how rehabilitation efforts can impose definitions and solutions to problems to the detriment of the disabled persons' self-sufficiency is illustrated in Jeffreys' (2002) description of his brother, Jim, who did not have legs because of a congenital condition. He recalls Jim "swaying precariously in his custom-fitted bucket atop his latest pair of DuPont artificial legs, all their straps and plastics cloaked in slacks, the idea being to make him look as standardized as possible, even though the contraption imprisoned him" (p. 36).

---

*Most current concepts of disability in rehabilitation include consideration of how the environment contributes, along with impairment, to creating disability. To the extent that the current paradigm of rehabilitation does admit of the environmental dimension of disability, it has been influenced by disability scholars. Another feature that differentiates the current incorporation of environmental factors in the understanding of disability is the much stronger (if not exclusive) emphasis that disability studies puts on environmental factors (especially social, political, and economic aspects of the environment).

Contrast Jim's fate with McBryde Johnson's (2003) description of what happened when her muscle-wasting disease left her too weak to hold up her spine: "At 15, I threw away the back brace and let my spine reshape itself into a deep twisty s-curve.... Since my backbone found its own natural shape, I've been entirely comfortable in my own skin" (p. 51). The irony is that while her strategy resulted in a more comfortable physical existence, it clearly violated what would be considered medical good sense, as surgery and braces would have given her a more "normal" appearance and function.

McBryde Johnson's rejection of such medical advice and Jim's subsequent discarding of his prosthetic limbs not only violate what is considered appropriate medical counsel but also evoke negative social reactions. The dilemma they face is faced by many disabled people. They must either choose an uncomfortable mode of embodiment not suited to their actual physical selves or face the discomfort of others who cannot abide their disruption of physical norms (as defined medically and socially). To the extent that rehabilitation efforts shepherd disabled people toward conformity with social norms, they reinforce the dilemma (Jeffreys, 2002; Linton, 1998; Zola, 1972).

Disability as an Economic Problem

The perceived economic consequences of disability (i.e., the required resources for persons who could not care for themselves or work) (Albrecht & Verbrugge, 2000) have always been a matter of public and political concern. Although nations have addressed disability differently, depending on their social philosophies (Albrecht & Bury, 2001), the development of welfare policies globally has underscored the perception that disabled persons are essentially a negative factor in the economic marketplace (Longmore & Goldberger, 2000).

The development of rehabilitation services designed to reduce dependence on services and enhance entry into the workforce has been shaped by concern to reduce the perceived burden of disabled persons on a modern society (Albrecht, 1992; Albrecht & Bury, 2001; Albrecht & Verbrugge, 2000). The idea of independence that was threaded throughout rehabilitation literature carried a subtext that dependence was an undesirable human state that both reduced the dignity of the individual and, importantly, created a burden for others. Concern with the economic costs of disability is highlighted in the creation of disability as an administrative category (Stone, 1984). Indeed, a complex bureaucracy exists in the United States and elsewhere to determine who is properly classified as disabled and therefore deserving of disability services and public support.

As a consequence of how the public and politicians viewed disability, the image of the disabled person as possessing limitations that prevented them from being self-sufficient (i.e., able to care for themselves and contribute labor in the marketplace) was firmly ensconced. Moreover, the development of a rehabilitation enterprise that documented functional limitations and their relationship to self-care and work reinforced the image of the disabled person as productively incapable. Finally, in rehabilitation, practitioners become instruments of social oppression when they locate the problem in the client rather than in the environment. For example, Abberley (1995) documented that occupational therapists consistently attributed failures in therapy to client problems such as a lack of motivation rather than to economic problems such as lack of resources or opportunities. Conversely, they attributed successes to their expertise rather than to client efforts.

Disability studies scholars have sought to turn the prevailing economic perspective on its head. They argue that, instead of disabled persons being a drain on public resources,

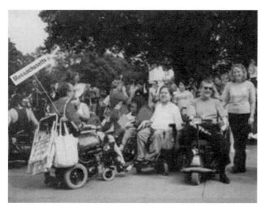

National activists participate in the Garrett Rally, held in October 2000, to demonstrate support to uphold the American with Disabilities Act (ADA) in the Supreme Court case Garrett vs. University of Alabama. Frustrating to disability rights advocates, the court ruled that Congress did not have the authority when it passed this act to allow individuals to sue states for employment discrimination. To the detriment of the disability community, the decision grants states immunity from damages as a result of lawsuits brought by their employees against states under the ADA. (Photo courtesy of Sharon Snyder and Suburban Access Squad)

people represent an oppressed minority group are data illustrating that these people fare much worse than non-disabled persons in housing, education, transportation, and employment (Louis Harris & Associates, 1998; McNeil, 1997). Disabled people consistently report that discrimination and attitudinal barriers negatively affect their self-sufficiency and participation in society (Charlton, 1998; Hahn, 1985; Oliver, 1996).

Using a Marxist analysis, Finkelstein (1980) and Oliver (1990) argue that disability was identified as a problem for medical management because of the demand of capitalist economies for unimpaired labor. Finkelstein's historical analysis proposes that disability emerged with the transformation of society from feudal to capitalist. Prior to this transition, persons with impairments worked at the lower end of the socioeconomic spectrum. With the advent of modern industrial economies, they were deemed unfit for the marketplace, barred from employment, and relegated to being problems for medical management, which often meant segregation in institutions. Oliver's analysis compares societies, arguing that the view of disability as an individual medical problem is not universal. Rather, it is a feature of societies that emphasize individualism and capitalist production.

Longmore and Goldberger (2000) argue that by casting disability as a matter of pathology, the medical perspective "individualized and privatized disability" (p. 2). This paved the way for what Albrecht and Bury (2001) refer to as the commoditization of disability goods and services. This is not without consequence. For example, economic incentives can lead rehabilitation providers to socialize clients toward some amount of ongoing dependence on their services (Scott, 1969).

they have been the victims of social oppression. This oppression, rather then personal impairments or traits, has made them unnecessarily dependent and barred them from access to the marketplace and other forms of civil participation.

Reformulating Disability as Oppression

One of the most powerful assertions to come from disability studies is that "people with disabilities are oppressed" (Charlton, 1998, p. 5). By this it is meant that disabled people are treated by society in ways that diminish their social, personal, physical, and financial well-being and are cast as members of a socially disadvantaged minority group (Charlton, 1998). Supporting the argument that disabled

> **Disabled people are treated by society in ways that diminish their social, personal, physical, and financial well-being and are cast as members of a socially disadvantaged minority group.**

Charitable organizations for persons with disabilities have also been the object of critique from disability scholars. Two points are made. First, a large number of able-bodied people work within such charities that operate as big business and inevitably generate motives of personal gain. As such, these organizations can be seen as exploiting the disabled population. Second, and more important, charitable organizations reinforce the idea that support for disabled persons is "not a social responsibility to be fulfilled by governments, but an act of kindness" (Wendell, 1996, p. 53). Public disability policies that, in effect, restrict persons from attaining self-sufficiency (e.g., encourage nursing home placement over community living and discourage entry into the labor market) have also been the target of criticism (Longmore, 1995b; Oliver, 1990; Shapiro, 1993).

In sum, disability studies scholars contradict the long-standing view that disabled persons are merely an economic drain on society because of their limitations in self-sufficiency. Rather, they argue, society economically disadvantages disabled persons. This occurs when disabled persons are barred from the marketplace, are transformed into targets of a disability industry that profits from products and services that are largely imposed, and are prevented by policies from living more self-sufficient lives.

Social Constructions of Disability

According to Longmore and Goldberger (2000), disabled persons historically have been cast as:

Victims and villains in popular culture, dependent sentimentalized children in charity fund raising, mendicants who should be allowed to beg, "unsightly disgusting objects" who should be banned from public places, potentially dependent or dangerous denizens of society,

worthy subjects of poor relief but unworthy citizens of the nation. (p. 5)

As they point out, the popular lexicon of disability has little or no place for disabled persons in the mainstream of society.

The ubiquitous misunderstanding and misconstruction of disability by society has led scholars to examine how popular cultural conceptions of disability are generated and perpetuated in art, literature, and film. Mitchell (2002) points out that although narratives freely employ the anomaly of disability as literary devices that embody and underscore other personal aberrations and social ills, they rarely address disability as either a source of personal knowledge or as a social or political injustice. Poignant recent examples are the use of physical disfigurement and mobility limitation as a metaphor for malevolence in the books and subsequent films, *Hannibal* (Lustig & Scott, 2001) and *The Red Dragon* (Davis & Ratner, 2002). Paradoxically, the personal experience of disability remains invisible, while the image of disability as negative and undesirable is reinforced by the pairing of the disability trait with personal or social ills.

The humanities approach to disability points out that disability is a multifaceted experience that has always been a part of the human condition. The humanities approach seeks to counter the assumption that amelioration of disability is necessary or even desirable. Rather, it argues for recognition of disability as a phenomenon integral to the fact that humans have bodies that are vulnerable and that age and almost invariably experience some kind of impairment. Such an approach seeks to assign disability its proper place in the human condition rather than simply treat it as an aberration.

Goffman's (1963) concept of stigma is the foundation for many elements of current arguments about societal reactions to disability. His basic argument, derived primarily from the study of persons with mental illness, is that disabled persons, by virtue of their physical or behavioral aberrations, breach cultural norms. As a result, they are assigned a spoiled identity (as bad, undesirable, dangerous, or weak) and subjected to pressure and/or efforts of others (often in the guise of medical or rehabilitation services) to minimize their deviation from norms. These social reactions serve not only to coerce disabled persons toward fitting in but also highlight and reaffirm the very social norms that have been breached. As Davis (2002) argues, disabled persons are singled out as part of a process in which individuals without impairments can be reassured they fit within a norm.

As a consequence of the stigmatizing process, Gill (2001) argues that disabled people grapple with mistaken identity, repeatedly encountering and struggling to overcome others' misconceptions of what it means to be disabled. She concludes "a core element of the experience of disability is being seen as something you are not, joined with the realization that what you are remains invisible" (Gill, 2001, p. 365). Exemplifying this argument, French (1993) notes:

> Disbelief remains a common response of able-bodied people when we attempt to convey the reality of our disabilities....when I try to convey the feelings of isolation associated with not recognizing people or not knowing what is going on around me, the usual response is "you will in time" or "it took me ages too." This type of response renders disabled people "just like everyone else"....knowing how different we really are is problematic and it is easy to become confused and to have our confidence undermined when others insist we are just the same. (p. 74)

Not surprisingly, then, negative stereo-types about disability are often internalized by the disabled individual (Fine & Asch, 1988; Gill, 1997). According to disability studies scholar Harlan Hahn (1985), one of the most pressing problems facing the political struggle of people with disabilities is developing a positive identity. An important distinction that disability scholars make is that this identity development is not an individual, but rather a social, cultural, and political process (Longmore, 1995a; Longmore, 1995b). That is, the fundamental change that needs to take place is a transformation in societal values that devalue and stigmatize disabled people in the first place. As Zola (1993a) notes, disabled persons must free themselves "from the negative loading of the concept of disability" (p. 27).

Summary

The various ways in which disability studies scholars have critiqued the traditional social and professional perspectives on disability can be summarized in the idea that disability is socially constructed. Wendell (1996) explains that the social construction of disability includes a range of social conditions from those "that straightforwardly create illnesses, injuries, and poor physical functioning to subtle cultural factors that determine standards of normality and exclude those who do not meet them from full participation in their societies" (p. 36). Taken together, the various arguments of disability studies have transformed the understanding of disability from being the inevitable and tragic consequence of impairment to being a neutral human difference. Disability is transformed into a negative condition by social definitions, attitudes, practices, and policies that devalue, exclude, and disenfranchise persons with disabilities.

🌿 Action Implications

As noted earlier, disability studies comprise a unique body of knowledge unlike others

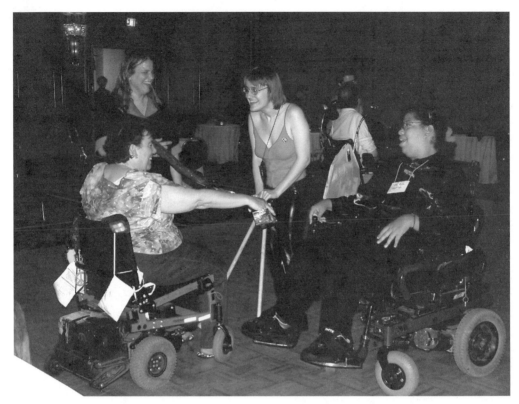

Attendees of the 2003, 16th Annual Meeting of the Society for Disability Studies, share in fellowship at the annual SDS dance. The theme "Disability and Dissent: Public Cultures, Public Spaces" explored the role of disability, dissent, and the creation of new public spaces (e.g., architectural, attitudinal, representational, and empirical) in the 21st century. (Photo courtesy of Sharon Snyder, 2003 SDS program co-director)

encountered in medicine and rehabilitation. One of the features that distinguishes these studies is the emphasis on actions that are directed not at fixing the disabled person, but rather on:

◆ Empowering persons with disabilities to engage in self-advocacy and combat discrimination

◆ Transforming social conditions that create barriers and oppression (including cultural beliefs and attitudes and public policies) (Charlton, 1998; Scotch, 2001)

Longmore (1995b) characterizes these as two phases: "The first phase sought to move disabled people from the margins of society to the mainstream by demanding that discrimination be outlawed and that access and accommodations be mandated….the second phase has asserted the necessity for self-definition…[and] repudiated nondisabled majority norms" (p. 8).

Empowerment and Civil Rights Advocacy

Charlton (1998) adopted the phrase "Nothing about us without us" as a way of urging "people with disabilities to recognize their need to control and take responsibility for their own lives and urging political-economic and cultural systems to incorporate people with disabilities into the decision-making process" (p. 17). Political activism aimed at achieving social justice and civil rights is naturally associated with the argument that disabled persons are socially oppressed (Baylies, 2002; Charlton, 1998). Activism takes on many forms, such as the kind of political advocacy in the United States that resulted in the Americans with Disabilities Act of 1990, which established civil rights for disabled persons. On the other end of the spectrum are efforts to combat movements such as eugenics and euthanasia that imply disabled persons are a negative to be avoided and that disabled persons' lives are not worth saving or maintaining. One example is Not Dead Yet, a national organization that "opposes legalized assisted suicide along with disability-based killing" (McBryde Johnson, 2003, p. 53).

> **Disabled persons are increasingly identifying themselves as members of a minority group and identifying with a disability community.**

Disability Identity, Culture, and Pride

Disability studies identifies the development of a positive identity among persons with disabilities as a key step in reversing the social construction of disability (Gill, 1997; Hahn, 1985; Zola, 1993a; Zola, 1993b). The conceptual shift in understanding disability has naturally led to changes in how disabled persons see themselves (e.g., as persons who are different but not less valuable than non-disabled persons and as members of a minority group that faces oppression). It is resulting in changes in values. For instance, Longmore (1995b) identifies the following transformation in values: "not self-sufficiency but self-determination, not independence but

> **By illuminating the hidden assumptions, biases, and practices that constitute disability, scholars are aiming to change attitudes among scholars, disciplines, professions, systems, and society at large.**

interdependence, not functional separateness but personal connection, not physical autonomy but human community" (p. 9). Disabled persons are increasingly identifying themselves as members of a minority group and identifying with a disability community (Longmore, 1995a; Longmore, 1995b; Phillips, 1990). One example of how disability is being redefined is the identification of deafness and consequent use of sign not as a handicap but as a language and culture (Shapiro, 1993).

Transforming Social Perceptions

Disability studies also seek to achieve transformations in intellectual and population conceptions of disability. Efforts to transform perceptions of the causes and nature of disability are wide-ranging in nature. By illuminating the hidden assumptions, biases, and practices that constitute disability, scholars are aiming to change attitudes among scholars, disciplines, professions, systems, and society at large.

A major contribution of disability studies comprises phenomenological accounts of disability experience. As Jeffreys (2002) notes, such accounts give voice to disability as an "authentic experience through the privileging of first-person narratives" (p. 33). Moreover, as Davis (2002) argues, such accounts underscore the variety of human experience rather than enforcing ideals of normality.

Many of these works are autobiographical texts in which disabled persons documented their own experiences. Examples are Zola's

(1982) chronicle of coming to accept his disability during a sojourn in a Dutch community for disabled persons, Williams' (1992) description of how her experiences as a child with autism placed her in a extraordinary world, Jamison's (1995) portrayal of her roller-coaster existence with manic-depressive illness, and Price's (1994) conclusion that his illness and paralysis resulted in a new and better life.

Disabled writers have asserted that living with a disability is consistent with living a fulfilling and joyful life. As Vash (1981) notes, disability can be "a positive contributor to life in its totality—a catalyst to psychological growth" (p. 124). However, as Deegan (1991) notes, it has little to do with living a life that is normative or dictated by one particular set of values.

🌿 Research

Because disability studies has incorporated concepts and methods from the humanities, different forms of scholarship (e.g., literary and art criticism) make up part of the process of inquiry and critical analysis of data. Thus, scholarship has included historical analyses such as those by Finkelstein (1980) and Longmore (1995b); philosophical works such as the one by Toombs (1992); phenomenological inquiry; and critical analysis such as the Mitchell (2002) and Snyder, Brueggeman, and Garland-Thomson (2002) discussions of literature, art, and film.

Disability studies also includes the traditional empirical traditions of the social sciences. Qualitative research in the field focuses on the "lived experience" of disability, and quantitative research is used to point toward the condition of disability. The former includes studies that range from the various ethnographic studies of disabled persons' experiences to autobiographical works. Quantitative studies are much less visible, but they do document the conditions and percep-

tions of disabled people and are part of the lexicon of the literature.

Participatory action research, which involves disabled persons as co-investigators, is an important and growing area of research (Balcazar et al., 1998). This approach has been fueled by the arguments that disabled persons' voices are absent from much research, and thus the research does not represent and, in fact, actively ignores disabled persons' experiences, perspectives, and knowledge (Kitchin, 2000; Oliver, 1992). Participatory action research seeks to respond to Oliver's call for research that is both emancipatory (i.e., seeking to change social structures) and empowering (i.e., allowing individuals to be transformed through participating in the research process).

🌿 Discussion

Because it is a new discipline, disability studies is still being defined. Disability studies today consists of a collection of scholarly approaches that participate in examining how disability comes into existence, what forces create it, how it affects people, and what it reveals about the human condition. Disability studies consists of a rapidly growing body of scholarship that has reformulated our understanding of disability.

The field is not without its own controversies. For example, Crow (1996) criticizes disability studies for having focused too exclusively on the environmental causes of disability. She differentiates the situation of disability from that of other oppressed groups based on gender, sexual orientation, or race. The latter groups are based on neutral differences, whereas impairment does produce suffering and difficulty. Crow notes many disabled persons struggle with impairment even when disabling barriers are eradicated. She recommends reinstating impairment into the study of disability and considering it at three levels:

- The objective restriction or limitation of function
- The personal experience and interpretation of the limitation
- The societal context, which can misrepresent, exclude, and discriminate

Others, such as Wendell (1996) and Jeffreys (2002), have also argued for the importance of inserting the nature and experience of impairment into disability studies discourse. Hence, whereas impairment was understandably de-emphasized both as a counterpoint to medicine's and rehabilitation's focus on impairment and society's tendency to translate impairment into tragedy, there is now a growing movement to rethink the place of impairment as a topic and concept in disability studies.

Another criticism of disability studies is that it does not represent the experience and perspectives of many disabled persons. Devlieger and Albrecht (2000) note that disability scholars are largely middle-class, white, well educated, and empowered. They argue that the ways in which these persons construe disability may well be at variance with the disability experience and perspectives of persons who do not share these demographics. Indeed, one of the important realities is that many persons with disabilities (especially in the early states of an acquired disability) may hold attitudes much more aligned with medical model or rehabilitation conceptions (i.e., they want their impairment minimized as much as possible).

These and other controversies and criticisms notwithstanding, disability studies represents a vibrant, emerging area of scholarship that will continue to transform thinking and action. Occupational therapists will need to seriously consider the critiques of rehabilitation in general, and of occupational therapy in particular, that are found in this literature.

For example, personal chronicles of disability experience sometimes include negative encounters with occupational therapy. For example, Callahan (1990), in discussing his rehabilitation experience following spinal cord injury, recalls occupational therapy, noting: "I remember having my hands harnessed for long periods of time to a rolling-pin–like apparatus that sanded a piece of wood" (p. 74). He then notes, with appropriate sarcasm: "A bright future as a finish sander stretched before me if I played my cards right" (p. 74).

The anthropologist Murphy (1990) recalls about his experience of occupational therapy:

> I thought some of the exercises ridiculous. Nonetheless, visitors to our house still scrape their feet on the doormat that I made in O.T. [My wife] is the only person who knows its origins, a sign of the care I have taken to keep secret the indignities visited upon me....(pp. 54–55)

In contrast, Robert McCrum (1998), in his account of rehabilitation and recovery from a cerebrovascular accident, recalls:

> The part of convalescence that I found most profoundly humiliating and depressing was occupational therapy....I was reduced to playing with brightly colored plastic letters of the alphabet, like a three-year-old, and passing absurdly simple recognition tests. Sitting in my wheelchair with my day-glo letter-blocks I could not escape reflecting on the irony of the situation. (p. 139)

These and other descriptions in the literature reinforce the earlier argument that disabled persons' voices and knowledge are routinely ignored in rehabilitation.

There certainly have been efforts in occupational therapy to correct many of the failures of rehabilitation noted earlier in this chapter. For example, occupational therapists have attempted to recognize and address barriers in the environment that affect persons with disabilities. However, the focus tends to be on physical barriers or social factors in the immediate environment (e.g., family, school, workplace). Therapists have not generally been involved in helping to remove broader social barriers (i.e., political and economic). These issues play out in practice and could be addressed through occupational therapists engaging in advocacy and empowerment of clients.

Disability studies systematically criticize and seek to replace the dominant paradigm of disability. As such, this body of knowledge has laid down important challenges to occupational therapy practice. It calls for occupational therapists to go beyond incremental changes in practice and, instead, to radically alter perceptions of, and practices with, disabled persons.

🌿 Summary

- Disability studies has sought to challenge and correct dominant views of disability
- It challenges standing assumptions about the causes and the very nature of disability

Interdisciplinary Base

- Disability studies has attracted scholars from a range of disciplines including:
  - Social sciences
  - Political and economic concepts
  - Gender and race studies
  - Concepts from humanities

Deconstructing and Reconstructing Conceptions of Disability

- Disability studies has:
  - Illuminated biases and fallacies in societal and professional conceptions and approaches to addressing disability
  - Offered alternative conceptions and action implications of disability

Disability as a Medical Problem Rooted in Impairment

- The medical model perspective developed by rehabilitation professionals generated a concept of disability as rooted in the disabled person's physical, emotional, sensory, or cognitive impairments
- Disability scholars have pointed out that rehabilitation perspectives:
  - Reinforce the idea that disability is the disabled person's problem
  - Cast the professional as expert on the disabled person's condition
  - Enforce a version of normalcy that pressures disabled persons to fit in by appearing and functioning as much like non-disabled persons as possible

Disability as an Economic Problem

- The development of welfare policies globally have underscored the perception that disabled persons are essentially a negative factor in the economic marketplace
- The development of rehabilitation services designed to reduce dependence on services and enhance entry into the workforce has been shaped by concern to reduce the perceived burden of disabled persons in a modern society

Reformulating Disability as Oppression

- Disability studies scholars contradict the long-standing view that disabled persons are merely an economic drain on society because of their limitations in self-sufficiency.
- Disabled persons are barred from the marketplace, transformed into targets of a disability industry that profits on products and services that are largely imposed on them, and prevented by policies from living more self-sufficient lives

Social Constructions of Disability

◆ Disabled persons historically have been misunderstood and misconstrued

◆ The humanities approach to disability:
  • Points out that disability is a multifaceted human experience that has always been a part of the human condition
  • Counters the assumption that amelioration of disability is necessary or even desirable
  • Recognizes disability as a phenomenon integral to the fact that humans have bodies that are vulnerable and that age and almost invariably experience some kind of impairment

◆ As a consequence of stigma:
  • Disabled people grapple with mistaken identity, repeatedly encountering and struggling to overcome others' misconceptions of what it means to be disabled
  • Negative stereotypes about disability are often internalized by the disabled individual

Action Implications

◆ Disability studies emphasize:
  • Empowering persons with disabilities to engage in self-advocacy and combat discrimination
  • Transforming social conditions that create barriers and oppression (including cultural beliefs and attitudes and public policies)

Research

◆ Disability studies scholarship includes:
  • Historical analyses
  • Philosophical works
  • Phenomenological inquiry
  • Critical analysis
  • Empirical traditions of the social sciences
  • Participatory action research that involves disabled persons as co-investigators as an

important and growing areas of disability studies research

Discussion

◆ Because it is a new discipline, disability studies are still being defined

◆ A criticism is that they do not represent the experience and perspectives of many disabled persons

◆ Disability studies represent a vibrant, emerging area of scholarship that will continue to transform thinking and action

References

Abberley, P. (1995). Disabling ideology in health and welfare: The case of occupational therapy. Disability and Society, 10, 221–232.

Albrecht, GL. (1992). The Disability Business: Rehabilitation in America. Newbury Park, CA: Sage Publications.

Albrecht, GL & Bury, M. (2001). The political economy of the disability marketplace. In Albrecht, GL, Seelman, K & Bury, M (eds.). Handbook of Disabilities Studies, pp 585–609. Thousand Oaks, CA: Sage Publications.

Albrecht, GL & Verbrugge, LM. (2000). The global emergence of disability. In Albrecht, GL, Fitzpatrick, R & Scrimshaw, SC (eds.). Handbook of Social Studies in Health and Medicine, pp 293–307. London: Sage Publications.

Americans with Disabilities Act of 1990. Pub. L. No. 101–336, 1991.

Asch, A & Fine, M (1988). Disability beyond stigma: Social interaction, discrimination and activism. Journal of Social Issues, 44(1), 3–22.

Balcazar, FE, Keys, CB, Kaplan, DL, et al. (1998). Participatory action research and people with disabilities: Principles and challenges. Canadian Journal of Rehabilitation, 12(2), 105–112.

Baylies, C. (2002). Disability and the notion of human development: Questions of rights and capabilities. Disability and Society, 17(7) 725–739.

Callahan, J. (1990). Don't Worry, He Won't Get Far on Foot. New York: Vintage Books.

Charlton, J. (1998). Nothing About Us Without Us. Berkeley, CA: University of California Press.

Crow, L. (1996). Renewing the social model of disability. In Barnes, C & Mercer, G (eds.). Exploring the Divide: Illness and Disability, pp 55–72. Leeds, UK: The Disability Press.

Davis, A (executive producer) & Ratner, B (director). (2002). The Red Dragon [motion picture]. United States: Universal.

Davis, L. (2002). Bodies of difference. In Snyder, SL, Brueggemann, BJ & Garland-Thompson, R (eds.). Disability Studies: Enabling the Humanities, pp 100–106. New York: The Modern Language Association of America.

Deegan, PE. (1991). Recovery: The lived experience of rehabilitation. In Marinelli, RP & Dell Orto, AE (eds.). The Psychological and Social Impact of Disability, 3rd ed. New York: Springer-Verlag.

Devlieger, PJ & Albrecht, GL (2000). Your experience is not my experience: The concept and experience of disability on Chicago's near west side. Journal of Disability Policy Studies, 11(1), 51–60.

Fine, M & Asch, M. (1988). Disability beyond stigma: Social interaction, discrimination and activism. Journal of Social Issues, 44(1), 3–19.

Finkelstein, V. (1980). Attitudes and Disabled People: Issues for Discussion. New York: World Rehabilitation Fund.

French, S. (1993). Can you see the rainbow? The roots of denial. In Swain, J, Finkelstein, V, French, S, et al. (eds.). Disabling Barriers, Enabling Environments, pp 69–77. Thousand Oaks, CA: Sage Publications.

Gill, C. (1997). Four types of integration in disability identity development. Journal of Vocational Rehabilitation, 9, 36–46.

Gill, CJ. (2001). Divided understandings: The social experience of disability. In Albrecht, GL, Seelman, K & Bury, M (eds.). Handbook of Disabilities Studies, pp 351–372. Thousand Oaks, CA: Sage.

Goffman, E. (1963). Stigma: Notes on the Management of Spoiled Identity. New York: Simon & Schuster.

Hahn, H. (1985). Disability policy and the problem of discrimination. American Behavioral Scientist, 28(3), 293–318.

Hahn, H. (1997). An agenda for citizens with disabilities: Pursuing identity and empowerment. Journal of Vocational Rehabilitation, 9, 31–37.

Jamison, KR. (1995). An Unquiet Mind: A Memoir of Moods and Madness. New York: Vintage Books.

Jeffreys, M. (2002). The visible cripple: Scars and other disfiguring displays included. In Snyder, SL, Brueggemann, BJ & Garland-Thompson, R (eds.). Disability Studies: Enabling the Humanities, pp 31–39. New York: The Modern Language Association of America.

Kitchin, R. (2000). The researched opinions on research: Disabled people and disability research. Disability and Society, 15(1), 25–47.

Linton, S. (1998). Disability studies/Not disability studies. In Linton, S. Claiming Disability: Knowledge and Identity, pp 132–156. New York: New York University Press.

Longmore, PK. (1995a). Medical decision making and people with disabilities: A clash of cultures. Journal of Law, Medicine & Ethics, 23, 82–87.

Longmore, PK. (1995b). The second phase: From disability rights to disability culture. The Disability Rag and ReSource, 16, 4–11.

Longmore, PK & Goldberger, D. (2000). The league of the physically handicapped and the Great Depression: A case study in the new disability history. [electronic version]. The Journal of American history, 87(3), 888–922.

Louis Harris & Associates. (1998). Highlights of the N.O.D./Harris 1998 Survey of Americans with Disabilities. Washington DC: National Organization on Disability.

Lustig, B. (executive producer) & Scott, R. (director). (2001). Hannibal [motion picture]. United States: MGM/Universal.

McBryde Johnson, H. (2003, February 16). Unspeakable conversations or how I spent one day as a token cripple at Princeton University. The New York Times Magazine, 152, 50–79.

McCrum, R. (1998). My Year Off: Recovering Life After a Stroke. New York: WW Norton.

McNeil, JM. (1997). Americans with Disabilities: 1994–1995. US Bureau of the Census Current Population Reports, pp 70–61. Washington, DC: US Government Printing Office.

Mitchell, D. (2002). Narrative prosthesis and the materiality of metaphor. In Snyder, SL, Brueggemann, BJ & Garland-Thompson, R (eds.). Disability Studies: Enabling the Humanities, pp

15–30. New York: The Modern Language Association of America.

Murphy, RF. (1990). The Body Silent: An Anthropologist Embarks on the Most Challenging Journey of His Life: Into the World of the Disabled. New York: WW Norton.

Nagi, SZ. (1991). Disability concepts revisited: Implications for prevention. In Pope, A & Tarlou, A (eds.). Disability in America: Toward a National Agenda for Prevention, pp 309–327. Washington, DC: National Academy Press.

Oliver, M. (1990). The Politics of Disablement. London: Macmillan.

Oliver, M. (1992). Changing the social relations of research production. Disability, Handicap and Society, 7(2), 101–114.

Oliver, M. (1996). Understanding Disability: From Theory to Practice. New York: St. Martin's Press.

Paterson, K & Hughes, B. (2000). Disabled bodies. In Hancock, P, Hughes, B, Jagger, E, et al. The Body, Culture and Society: An Introduction, pp 29–44. Buckingham: Open University Press.

Phillips, MJ. (1990). Damaged goods: Oral narratives of the experience of disability in American culture. Social Science and Medicine, 30, 849–857.

Price, R. (1994). A Whole New Life. New York: Atheneum Macmillan Press.

Rioux, MH. (1997). Disability: The place of judgment in a world of fact. Journal of Intellectual Disability Research, 41, 102–111.

Scotch, RK. (2001). From Goodwill to Civil Rights: Transforming Federal Disability Policy. 2nd ed. Philadelphia: Temple University Press.

Scott, R. (1969). The Making of Blind Men. New York: Russell Sage.

Shapiro, JP. (1993). No Pity: People with Disabilities Forging a New Civil Rights Movement. New York: Random House.

Snyder, SL, Brueggemann, BJ & Garland-Thomson, R. (eds). (2002). Disability Studies: Enabling the Humanities. New York: The Modern Language Association of America.

Stone, D. (1984). The Disabled State. Philadelphia: Temple University Press.

Toombs, K. (1992). The Meaning of Illness: A Phenomenological Account of the Different Perspectives of Physician and Patient. Dordrecht, Netherlands: Kluwer Academic Publishers.

Vash, CL. (1981). The Psychology of Disability. New York: Springer.

Wendell, S. (1996). The Rejected Body: Feminist Philosophical Reflections on Disability. New York: Routledge.

Williams, D. (1992). Nobody Nowhere. New York: Times Books.

Zola, IK. (1972). Medicine as an institution of social control. Sociological Review, 20, 487–503.

Zola, IK. (1982). Missing Pieces: A Chronicle of Living with a Disability. Philadelphia: Temple University Press.

Zola, IK (1993a). Disability statistics: What we count and what it tells us: A personal and political analysis. Journal of Disability Policy Studies, 4(2), 9–39.

Zola, IK. (1993b). Self, identity, and the naming question: Reflections on the language of disability. Social Science and Medicine, 36(2), 167–173.

Chapter 17

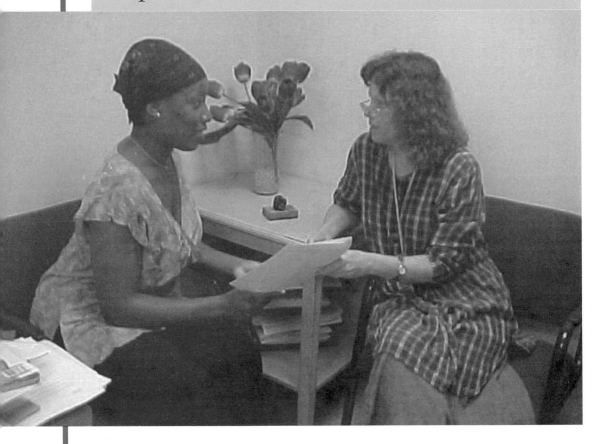

Intrapersonal and Interpersonal Concepts

In a mental health setting, an occupational therapist discusses plans for participation in group activities with a client. Being able to intervene with the client's emotionally charged challenges in interpersonal aspects of occupational participation requires therapeutic use of self. The therapist builds on knowledge from the psychodynamic tradition in understanding some of the client's difficulties in dealing with emotions and relationships. She also uses techniques from this body of knowledge to guide her interactions with the client.

Psychodynamic theories involve multiple schools of thought descended, at least in part, from Freudian psychoanalysis. They are primarily concerned with intrapersonal and interpersonal elements of motivation, affect, cognition, and behavior. This chapter, rather than attempting to capture the full range of ideas that make up psychodynamic theories, will discuss the neo- and post-Freudian ideas that have been developed. These ideas are frequently applied in psychotherapy, where the focus is on one's inner life and on encouraging people to find psychologically healthy ways to cope with everyday life, interpersonal relationships, concerns related to the self, and life crises (Wolf, 1988).

Contemporary psychodynamic thought also emphasizes understanding behavior within a cultural and interpersonal context, as opposed to Freud's focus on the libido and the transformation of infantile oral sexuality into a mature heterogeneous sexuality (Munroe, 1955; Wolberg, 1977). These more contemporary concepts are most relevant to the understanding of client behaviors in the occupational therapy context and to occupational therapists' therapeutic use of self. Throughout this chapter, the term *psychodynamic* is used to refer to the neo- and post-Freudian ideas emphasized here. It should be kept in mind that other concepts, including some at variance with those contained herein, are also included in the literature under the broad umbrella of psychodynamics. Moreover, those whose work is referenced in this chapter differ in the details of their theories. This chapter represents only those concepts and themes that are relatively consistent across the theories.

🌿 Interdisciplinary Base

As noted above, the most pervasive ideas influencing psychodynamic theory is the original work of Freud. His ideas have been widely reinterpreted and modified by later scholars. These writers were influenced by concepts from philosophy, sociology, the humanities, and psychology. They were also influenced by the social sciences that emphasize interpersonal behavior and the influence of culture on attitudes and behavior (Wolf, 1988).

🌿 Organization

Psychodynamic theorists such as Gardner (1991), Harper (1974), Munroe (1955), and Wyss (1973), whose work will be emphasized in this chapter, see interpersonal relations, cultural values, and a drive toward self-cohesion and self-actualization as key determinants of human behavior. They deemphasized the importance of biological drives while accentuating the role of the interpersonal self, society, and culture in influencing behavior. Such contemporary psychodynamic thought also presents a dynamic and holistic view of personality development while retaining a focus on how a person's history of interpersonal experiences (including early development) shape the way that a person feels, behaves, and perceives and interprets the world.

Taken together, the ideas that make up psychodynamic thought (Ford & Urban, 1963; Harper, 1974; Wolberg, 1977) emphasize:

♦ A phenomenological perspective that focuses attention on the importance of a person's inner perceptions and interpretations of events in directing future behavior

♦ The influence of culture and early interpersonal relationships on more long-standing patterns of perception, affective experience, cognitive interpretation, and behavior

♦ The centrality of achieving a loving and productive relationship with others

♦ The role of the environment in nurturing both positive and negative personal qualities

◆ An emphasis on early familial/interpersonal relationships

◆ An emphasis on achieving self-cohesion (a sense of inner regulation, psychic organization, and stability in one's inner experience)

Thus, while it is recognized that individuals have certain genetic endowments and encounter various environmental conditions, their use of, or response to, these givens are considered the most important determinants of their development (Dinkmeyer, Pew, & Dinkmeyer, 1979).

Although variously defined and emphasized by different authors (Harper, 1974; Munroe, 1955; Wyss, 1973), psychodynamic theory sees humans as endowed with fundamental needs, including:

◆ Feeling emotionally and physically secure, including having stable and predictable interpersonal relationships

◆ Feeling connected to others

◆ Satisfying biologically derived desires

◆ Maintaining a state of emotional well-being

◆ Feeling that one's talents and efforts are appreciated or admired by others

◆ Having one's feelings, perceptions, and behaviors acknowledged and accepted by others

As humans develop and seek to meet these needs, their intrapersonal characteristics interact with interpersonal influences. As a result of this process, people develop a kind of private logic (Adler, 1976) that includes certain assumptions and interpretations from which they create their own unique version of reality. This private logic also includes cer-

> **Adaptive living consists of accepting responsibility for and making choices that allow one to progress toward fulfilling personal goals and actualizing one's potentials.**

tain priorities, including an habitual pattern of acting in and responding to the world (Dinkmeyer, Pew, & Dinkmeyer, 1979). These patterns of thinking, feeling, and acting begin with smaller units learned in early development, which, over time, are formed together into larger patterns (Ford & Urban, 1963). Each person's private logic evolves from constitutional (e.g., biological characteristics that influence personality) as well as familial and other social influences.

Individuals live by their underlying private logic (i.e., the personal truths, convictions, and fictions that shape their subjective representations of reality, shape their emotions, and make sense of their actions). The consequent, taken-for-granted perspective and pattern of thinking, feeling, and behaving is nonconscious. That is, persons tend to be unaware of what assumptions guide their interpretation and action and, thus, tend to be unaware of how they organize and cope with life events (Mosak, 1979).

A psychologically healthy individual develops an altruistic and flexible interest in others guided by an honest commitment to life and to humanity (Mosak, 1979). Development of a healthy self is predicated on the person experiencing social conditions (especially in the course of early development) that nurture a sense of security and connectedness and that lead to adaptive patterns of thinking, feeling, and acting (Munroe, 1955). This involves developing the inner freedom and resources to question or adapt to the current social structure and values. It also involves coming to terms with existential realities such as mortality, accepting necessary losses associated with living, and successfully navigating social situations that often involve contradictions and difficulties (Fromm, 1947; Wyss, 1973). Accepting personal responsibility, achieving an attitude of relatedness to humanity, and facing truths about existence lead to the realization of meaning in life (Fromm, 1947). Adaptive living consists of accepting responsibility for and making choices that allow one to progress toward fulfilling personal goals and actualizing one's potentials.

 Problems and Challenges

Problems identified from the psychodynamic perspective are seen as resulting from a constricting/rigid approach or an inconsistent/unrealistic approach to life in which the individual inflexibly approaches new situations with old behavioral and cognitive patterns. Although psychodynamic theorists emphasize them differently, problems always involve degrees of anxiety and interpersonal conflict. These problems arise from:

◆ The private logic with which persons cope with life (Adler, 1976; Mosak, 1979). (This may involve: overly rigid and limiting goals and behaviors, distorted perceptions, inaccurate attitudes about one's self and capabilities, mistaken attitudes about the world and people, unrealistic goals and standards such as perfectionism, and mistaken conclusions about other people or unrealistic expectations about what will or should happen in particular situations)
◆ Feelings of inferiority that lead one to overcompensate by overemphasizing some other trait or tendency as well as overemphasis of certain behavioral responses (those which were not anxiety-provoking to the individual) at the expense of others
◆ Rigidity and compulsiveness derived from the cultural context

◆ Overreliance on a single mode of interpersonal response to the exclusion of others; e.g., seeking safety in relationships, self-reliance, or rejection of others (Munroe, 1955)

An adaptive person achieves a balance among these responses. Maladaptation occurs when a person prefers and uses one pattern exclusively while repressing the needs that relate to the unused patterns and idealizing the needs of the predominating pattern. For instance, persons who always move toward people might idealize the importance of passively acquiescing to others' wishes, thereby failing to assume responsibility for their own behavior and failing to think and act with autonomy.

Persons with such maladaptive patterns of thinking, feeling, and acting will typically:

◆ Persist in using ineffective behaviors
◆ Ignore the appropriate assertion of their own needs and desires
◆ Lack self-cohesion, as reflected in overly idealized or devalued/deprecating self-perceptions and attributions to others, or a tendency to vacillate between these two extremes
◆ Be selectively inattentive to difficult situations
◆ Have mental preoccupations that preclude addressing reality

Such tendencies can result in a constricted pattern of living, difficulty in interpersonal relationships, and ineffective coping. When a person encounters a particularly stressful situation, a major life change, or a traumatic event, these symptomatic behaviors can escalate, leading to further maladaptation.

 Action Implications

Maladaptive patterns of thinking, feeling, and acting are considered to be learned in interpersonal relationships. Consequently, therapy is viewed as a special class of interpersonal relationships in which the therapist's behavior contributes actively to the client's learning. Interaction with the therapist allows for cognitive, emotional, and behavioral re-experiencing in relation to a stable and predictable person.

Broadly speaking, psychodynamic theorists conceptualize the therapeutic relationship as a secure arena for practicing and ultimately internalizing corrective emotional experiences. Therapy is viewed as a cooperative process in which the client develops interest and investment in social relationships while learning more adaptive ways to succeed in such relationships. New ways of relating are practiced in therapy so that the client can actualize these new ways of relating with others in life. Thus, an individual's experience in therapy can then be generalized to other interpersonal situations.

The assessment process is typically open-ended and largely limited to listening rather than questioning. Conversations in the context of therapy are used by the therapist to gain insight into the client's modes of thinking, feeling, and behaving and how they influence the client's life situation. The therapist assesses the client by gathering information on the client's history and current functioning. Assessment is an ongoing process that unfolds as the therapeutic relationship unfolds (Mosak, 1979). The therapist proceeds throughout therapy to engage in detailed inquiry that serves to test hypotheses about how the client might think, feel, or act in various situations. This process enables the therapist to understand with increasing accu-

> **Therapy is viewed as a cooperative process in which the client develops interest and investment in social relationships while learning more adaptive ways of succeeding in such relationships.**

racy and empathy how the client typically thinks, feels, and acts.

The therapeutic process aims to achieve a relationship between equals in which the therapist and client identify agreed-upon goals. Therapy also aims to facilitate clients' insight and understanding (i.e., learning to recognize their private logic and response patterns and their ineffectiveness or symptoms) (Mosak, 1979). The therapist might use interpretation or explanation of the client's behavior, humor, and parables to facilitate insight. Insight is viewed as the first step to achieving change in cognitive, emotional, and behavioral patterns. Following insight, a further aim of therapy is for the client to establish new or more realistic goals for behavior and to identify new or more functional alternatives to present actions. A variety of techniques, including role-playing, role modeling by the therapist, and mutual setting of achievable goals, are used to support this aim (Dinkmeyer, Pew, & Dinkmeyer, 1979; Mosak, 1979). Therapeutic goals for clients include learning to:

◆ Assume responsibility for their actions and decisions
◆ Recognize and believe in their own hierarchy of values
◆ Develop spontaneity of feeling

Therapy, for the most part, involves a verbal exchange. The client presents information about the present and past while the therapist either reflects or interprets this information in order to help the client develop new ways of satisfying interpersonal needs. Therapists can be described as directive in their approach in terms of their willingness to make suggestions or assist the client in reinterpreting his or her environment, but psychodynamic therapists tend to vary in the degree to which they are willing to take a directive approach in the therapy. Some approaches, such as the self-psychological approaches (Gardner, 1991), focus mainly on nondirective techniques, such as empathic listening. Therapists are also cooperative in their emphasis on sharing responsibility for setting goals. While psychodynamic therapy was originally thought of as a long-term, nondirective process, more recent writers have developed approaches to applying these concepts in relatively short-term therapy (Hemmings, 2000).

In summary, some of the behaviors a therapist might demonstrate in therapy (depending on the client and the presenting problem) include:

♦ Listening to client-selected material and reflecting what has been said in a manner that conveys empathy and understanding of the client's experience (Gardner, 1991)
♦ Using Socratic questioning to help clients gain perspective or change their "private logic" (e.g., questions of clarification, questions that probe assumptions, questions that probe reason and evidence, questions about viewpoints or perspectives, and questions that probe implications and consequences)
♦ Assisting clients in drawing linkages between their current ways of relating and older ways of relating learned within their family of origin by making interpretations or pointing out areas of apparent consistency based on clients' history
♦ Facilitating emotional expression in clients with repressed emotions
♦ Responding to natural breaks in empathy, or rifts within the therapeutic relationship, in a way that allows the client to find new ways of self-assertion or self-expression in a validating environment, thus providing a

corrective emotional experience (Gardner, 1991)

 # Research

There is a substantial literature examining the outcomes of psychodynamic psychotherapy, and the evidence in support of its effectiveness is, in large part, convincing (Hemmings, 2000; Wampold, 2000). However, this literature has been somewhat controversial because the specific ingredients for effectiveness have been difficult to identify (Kopta et al., 1999). Moreover, many studies lack follow-up periods evidencing sustained positive outcomes. Most writers agree, however, on one consistent finding across studies. That is, the particular theoretical orientation of the therapist appears to be less important than the therapist's ability to establish a trusting and accepting relationship with the client (Roth & Parry, 1997).

 # Discussion

Psychodynamic thought has a wide influence on therapies that rely primarily on verbal processes. The concepts that make up this body of knowledge have been developed to a high level of sophistication. They have been developed in association with the practice of psychotherapy and influenced by a wide interdisciplinary literature. Thus, they constitute an important body of knowledge.

Occupational therapy practice has drawn upon psychodynamic and related concepts through much of its history. For example, Mosey (1970, 1986) and Bruce and Borg (1987) have presented frames of reference based on related ideas. However, because occupational therapy focuses on issues of performance and participation that require a more action-oriented therapeutic process, the use of psychodynamic concepts today is primarily to inform the therapeutic relationship with the client. That is, while therapy focuses on clients' doing, the relationship between therapist and client is an important adjunct. While psychodynamic theories do not explain the central element of the occupational therapy process, they are helpful in understanding the client's characteristics, reactions to therapy, and to the change process.

> **While psychodynamic theories do not explain the central element of the occupational therapy process, they are helpful in understanding the client's characteristics, reactions to therapy, and to the change process.**

Occupational therapists rarely encounter individuals whose sole problems are the kinds identified by psychodynamic theories. However, clients who receive occupational therapy for physical, sensory, or cognitive impairments may show some of the characteristics that are identified as problems from a psychodynamic perspective. The following are two examples. A person with a seriously impairing mental illness (e.g., psychosis) that has its basis in physiological abnormalities may also exhibit many of the maladaptive patterns described in psychodynamic theories. A person who acquires a physical disability may, under the stress of the situation, exhibit these maladaptive patterns to a degree that they interfere with the necessary coping. These problems may present as impediments to changes that individuals need to make in order to adapt to their disability.

In summary, there are a variety of approaches to psychodynamic therapy, only some of which have been summarized herein. For a more comprehensive review of the literature, the reader is referred to articles in References. Occupational therapists are not in a position (either by virtue of training or the circumstances of therapy) to engage in psychodynamically-based therapy. Nonetheless, knowledge from the psychodynamic tradition can be helpful in shaping the therapists' understanding of and style of interacting with the client. For example, an occupational therapist might observe a client having difficulty seeking supportive assistance following a traumatic injury. Knowledge of psychodynamic principles might assist the therapist in recognizing a more pervasive pattern of difficulties with assertiveness or with help seeking in that particular client. In treating a client with rigid, angry, and rejecting ways of relating, knowledge of psychodynamic theory may allow the occupational therapist to depersonalize these reactions. The therapist can recognize these behaviors as part of an underlying style of relating and understand them in the context of an interaction between the client's prior relationships and the current stressors he or she is facing. Moreover, psychodynamic theory may allow for an understanding of the importance of empathic listening as a means of communicating to the client that his or her difficulties are validated and understood.

Summary

Psychodynamic theories:

◆ Involve multiple schools of thought descended, at least in part, from Freudian psychoanalysis
◆ Are primarily concerned with intrapersonal and interpersonal elements of motivation, affect, cognition, and behavior

Interdisciplinary Base

◆ Freud's ideas have been widely reinterpreted and modified based on concepts from philosophy, sociology, humanities, psychology, and social sciences

Organization

◆ Psychodynamic theorists see interpersonal relations, cultural values, and a drive toward self-cohesion and self-actualization as key determinants of human behavior
◆ Psychodynamic thought emphasizes:
  1. A phenomenological perspective that focuses attention on the importance of a person's inner perceptions and interpretations
  2. The influence of culture and early interpersonal relationships on more long-standing patterns of perception, affective experience, cognitive interpretation, and behavior
  3. The centrality of achieving loving and productive relationships with others
  4. The role of the environment in nurturing positive and negative personal qualities
  5. Early familial/interpersonal relationships
  6. Achieving self-cohesion (a sense of inner regulation, psychic organization, and stability in one's inner experience)
◆ Psychodynamic theory sees humans as endowed with fundamental needs, including:
  1. Feeling emotionally and physically secure, including having stable and predictable interpersonal relationships
  2. Feeling connected to others
  3. Satisfying biologically derived desires
  4. Maintaining a state of emotional well-being
  5. Feeling that one's talents and efforts are appreciated or admired by others
  6. Having one's feelings, perceptions, and behaviors acknowledged and accepted by others

◆ As humans develop and seek to meet these needs, they develop a kind of private logic that includes certain assumptions and interpretations from which they create their own unique version of reality
◆ A psychologically healthy individual develops an altruistic and flexible interest in others, guided by an honest commitment to life and to humanity
◆ Adaptive living consists of accepting responsibility for and making choices that allow one to progress toward fulfilling personal goals and actualizing one's potentials

Problems and Challenges

◆ Problems identified from the psychodynamic perspective arise from:
  1. The private logic with which persons cope with life
  2. Feelings of inferiority that lead one to overcompensate by overemphasizing some other trait or tendency and overemphasizing certain behavioral responses
  3. Rigidity and compulsiveness derived from the cultural context
  4. Overreliance on a single mode of interpersonal responses to the exclusion of others
◆ Persons with such maladaptive patterns of thinking, feeling, and acting will typically:
  1. Persist in using ineffective behaviors
  2. Ignore the appropriate assertion of their own needs and desires
  3. Lack self-cohesion
  4. Be selectively inattentive to difficult situations
  5. Have mental preoccupations that preclude addressing reality
◆ Such tendencies can result in a constricted pattern of living, difficulty in

interpersonal relationships, and ineffective coping

Action Implications

◆ Psychodynamic theorists conceptualize the therapeutic relationship as a secure and sacred arena for experiencing, practicing, and ultimately internalizing corrective emotional experiences

◆ Therapy is a cooperative process in which the client develops interest and investment in social relationships while learning more adaptive ways to succeed in such relationships

◆ The assessment process is an informal one in which conversations in the context of therapy are used by the therapist to gain insight into the client's private logic and how it influences the client's lifestyle

◆ The therapist assesses the client by gathering information on the client's history and on current functioning

◆ Therapeutic goals include the client's learning to:
  1. Assume responsibility for his or her actions and decisions
  2. Recognize and believe in his or her own hierarchy of values
  3. Develop spontaneity of feeling

◆ Therapy involves a verbal exchange in which the client presents information about the present and past, and the therapist interprets this information in order to help the client develop new ways of satisfying interpersonal needs

Research

◆ There is a substantial literature examining the outcomes of psychotherapy, which emphasize the importance of developing a trusting relationship with the client

Discussion

◆ Psychodynamic thought has a wide influence on therapies that rely primarily on verbal process

◆ In occupational therapy, psychodynamic concepts inform the therapeutic relationship with the client

References

Adler, A. (1976). Individual psychology and crime. Journal of Individual Psychology, 32, 131–144.

Bruce, MA & Borg, B. (1987). Frames of reference in psychosocial occupational therapy. Thorofare, NJ: Slack.

Dinkmeyer, DC, Pew, WL & Dinkmeyer, DC, Jr. (1979). Adlerian Counseling and Psychotherapy. Monterey, CA: Brooks/Cole.

Ford, DH & Urban, HB. (1963). Systems of Psychotherapy: A Comparative Study. New York: Wiley.

Fromm, E. (1947). Man for Himself. New York: Holt, Rinehart, & Winston.

Gardner, JR. (1991). The application of self-psychology to brief psychotherapy. Psychoanalytic Psychology, 8, 477–500.

Harper, RA. (1974). Psychoanalysis and Psychotherapy: 36 Systems. New York: Jason Aaronson.

Hemmings, A. (2000). A systematic review of the effectiveness of brief psychological therapies in primary health care. Families, Systems & Health, 18, 279–313.

Kopta, SM, Lueger, RJ, Saunders, SM, et al. (1999). Individual psychotherapy outcome and process research: Challenges leading to greater turmoil or a positive transition? Annual Review of Psychology, 50, 441–469.

Mosak, HH. (1979). Adlerian psychotherapy. In Corsini RJ (ed.). Current Psychotherapies, 2nd ed, pp 44–94). Itasca, IL: FE Peacock.

Mosey, AC. (1970). Three Frames of Reference for Mental Health. Thorofare, NJ: Slack.

Mosey, AC. (1986). Psychosocial Components of Occupational Therapy. New York: Raven Press.

Munroe, RA. (1955). Schools of Psychoanalytic Thought. New York: Holt, Rinehart, & Winston.

Roth, AD & Parry, G. (1997). The implications of psychotherapy research for clinical practice and service development: Lessons and limitations. Journal of Mental Health, 6, 367–380.

Wampold, BE. (2000). Outcomes of individual counseling and psychotherapy: Empirical evidence addressing two fundamental questions. In Brown, SD & Lent, RW (eds.). Handbook of Counseling Psychology, 3rd ed, pp 711–73). New York: John Wiley.

Wolberg, LR. (1977). The Techniques of Psychotherapy, 3rd ed. New York: Grune & Stratton.

Wolf, ES. (1988). Treating the Self: Elements of Clinical Self Psychology. New York: The Guilford Press.

Wyss, D. (1973). Psychoanalytic Schools from the Beginning to the Present. New York: Jason Aaronson.

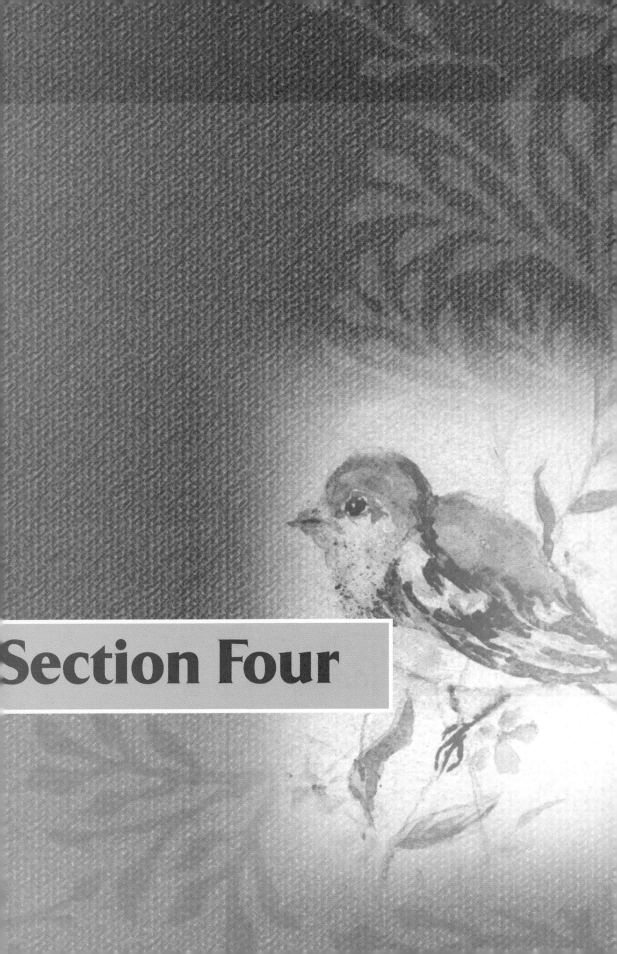

Section Four

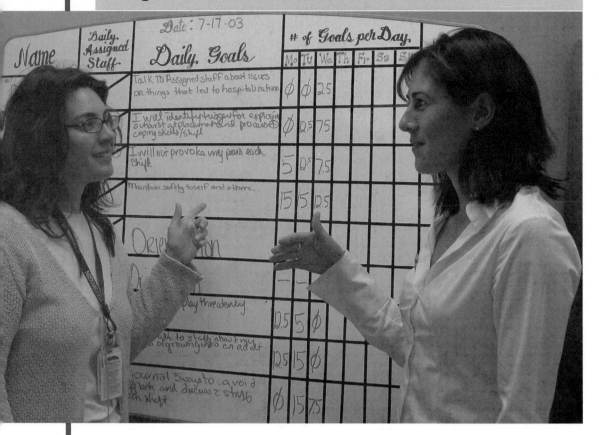

Chapter 18

Professional Identity and Competence

When an occupational therapy student begins her first field-work experience, she has two primary challenges. The first is to begin presenting herself to clients and peers as a particular kind of professional: an occupational therapist. The second is to know what to do to work with the clients to whom she is assigned. These dual challenges involve enacting identity and competence as an occupational therapist.

This text began with the argument that the field's conceptual foundations provide occupational therapists with professional identity and competence. The intervening chapters considered the nature of knowledge in occupational therapy focusing on:

♦ The historical development of the field's paradigm
♦ The nature and status of the field's conceptual practice models
♦ The kind of related knowledge that supports the field's practice
♦ In this chapter, I consider how these elements of the conceptual foundations translate into practitioners' identity and competence.

Professional Identity

Professional identity is grounded in the paradigm that binds members of the profession together and gives them both a sense of themselves and a collective public identity. Each occupational therapist's professional identity reflects a unique set of personal experiences. Nonetheless, the coherence of the profession requires that all therapists participate in a common identity that reflects a shared paradigm.

Historical Challenges to Professional Identity in Occupational Therapy

As we saw in Chapter 3, occupational therapy's identity has changed with transformations in its paradigm. The profession was founded on a paradigm that embraced the vision of occupation as a domain of human life and as a therapeutic tool. During this era, the identity of the profession was organized around a mission of supporting the occupational well-being of clients and the use of occupation as a means of enabling persons to adapt to the challenges posed by disability. During the subsequent mechanistic paradigm era, the field adopted a view of therapy as the use of activities to remediate underlying impairments. This shift resulted in a loss of the original identity of the field, coupled with a lack of clarity about the definition and nature of occupational therapy. Individual therapists experienced this identity confusion as discomfort and frustration in not being able to explain (to themselves, much less others) what occupational therapy was.

Because they lacked a clear professional identity, occupational therapists at times adopted a professional image shaped by other professions (O'Shea, 1977) or allowed their role to be defined by their work setting or specialty (e.g., hand therapy) (Barris, 1984). Therapists sometimes assumed roles as generic workers that did not reflect any unique occupational therapy perspectives or skills (Harrison, 2003). Therapists not only accepted these alternative ways of viewing themselves but also engaged in practice that reflected them. For example, therapists adopted techniques of other disciplines as central (sometimes defining) components of their practice (e.g., the use of pure exercise and physical agents in physical rehabilitation or the use of verbal psychotherapy in mental health settings [Barris, 1984]).

The problem of professional identity was one of the primary reasons for returning to a focus on occupation as the core of the field's paradigm. As discussed in Chapter 4, the contemporary paradigm identifies occupational therapy as:

♦ Uniquely concerned with the role of occupation in human life and well-being
♦ Focused on solving problems that occur with personal impairments and/or environmental factors that prevent or threaten participation in life occupations
♦ A practice that uses occupational engagement as a therapeutic agent

This paradigm incorporates concepts of impairment from the second paradigm and calls attention to how biological, psychosocial, and environmental factors together influence occupational adaptation. It recognizes that therapy can involve strategies of:

◆ Reducing physical, cognitive, and emotional impairments and/or their interference with occupational performance
◆ Enabling clients to make lifestyle decisions, set priorities, negotiate roles with others, and advocate for themselves in order to pursue the kind of occupational lives they want
◆ Changing and adapting the physical and sociocultural environment to remove physical and social barriers and to create opportunities that enhance occupational participation

The clear focus of the field's contemporary paradigm on occupation is an important step in the development of a professional identity. However, these ideas alone are not enough to allow practitioners to develop competence in doing occupationally focused practice.

In fact, while publications that articulate the occupational nature of humans and justify the therapeutic use of occupation currently abound, this vision is not consistently realized in practice (Fisher, 1998). As Christiansen (1999, p. 556) argues, "a full and genuine appreciation of the power of occupation to enable health and well-being has not yet made its way across the landscape of the profession."

The professional identity occupational therapists derive from the field's paradigm helps to define the nature of their practice. Nonetheless, practitioners need more to be able to practice. They require sound conceptual practice models.

Professional Competence

Thinking and acting with competence requires the use of the field's conceptual practice models. But just how do therapists employ these models in practice? In this section we will consider what is involved.

Naming and Framing Problems

Professional decision-making and action begin with a process of naming and framing client problems (Schon, 1983). In practice, the problems that therapists and clients encounter are not immediately apparent. Rather, each client is ordinarily faced with ambiguous and complex circumstances. Converting these circumstances into a recognizable problem requires that practitioners support their clients to make sense of an uncertain and indeterminate situation. In order to identify a problem that can be addressed in therapy, the therapist and client must transform complexity and uncertainty into something that can be understood and acted upon.

Importantly, identifying the nature of a problem serves not only to clarify what is wrong but also to specify what needs to be changed or altered. Consequently, therapists work with their clients to both name the problem (giving it a certain character) and frame what needs to change.

> **Professional decision-making and action begin with a process of naming and framing client problems.**

The theory provided by conceptual practice models facilitates the process of identifying and solving problems. Theory enables therapists to name problems by providing a conceptual language and the underlying explanations that go with that language. So, for example, therapists employing the human occupation, sensory integration, biomechanical, or motor control models might recognize a client who is experiencing such problems as:

◆ A poor sense of personal causation
◆ Dyspraxia
◆ Limited range of motion
◆ Low muscle tone

The concepts of the theory in these models not only provide a language for giving identity to the problem but also offer explanations for the source and consequence of these problems. For instance, the model of human occupation indicates that a poor sense of personal causation (reflected in a lack of belief in capacity and a sense of inefficacy) can be the result of experiencing a loss/lack of abilities coupled with failure in performance. It also indicates that a poor sense of personal causation can lead persons to avoid doing things that might maintain or increase ability, thus disadvantaging the client further. The biomechanical model might offer an understanding of how changes in the structure of joints associated with disease processes limit range of motion. It also provides an understanding of how limited range might affect performance of daily life occupations.

In this way, the model's language can take the client's experience of feeling unmotivated or having difficulty moving and translate it into something more completely understood. Moreover, it gives the therapist and the client ways to pinpoint and clarify the implications of various aspects of the client's circumstances.

When professionals name and frame problems, they map theory onto the actual features of the client's situation. Mapping theory onto the real world and transforming theoretical knowledge into practical action are complex processes. Therapists must first make a judgment about which theories are most appropriate to formulate the nature of the client's problems and their action implications. In addition, therapists must close the inevitable gap between abstract theoretical concepts and the concrete phenomena that are part of each client's unique situation (Mattingly, 1988; Rogers, 1983).

Conceptual practice models provide technology that facilitates the process of mapping theoretical concepts onto client circumstances. The various assessments developed for use with each model and the case examples that illustrate how the concepts can be applied to clients are important resources that make this practical work possible. Assessments provide a concrete means of translating concepts to the real world. For example, the goniometer (which measures the degrees of available motion about the axis of a joint) gives expression to the biomechanical concept range of motion. Similarly, the Sensory Integration and Praxis Test (see Chapter 12) operationalizes concepts from the sensory integration model.

Deciding a Course of Action

Once a problem to be addressed in therapy is named and framed, a course of action must be decided upon. This means that the therapist must have an idea of how the problem is going to be solved. The inherent organization of models can facilitate therapist decision-making concerning how to address identified problems.

The theory in each model serves as a guide for deciding action because it addresses both the nature of problems that interfere with occupation and how therapy achieves change related to those problems. Take, for instance, the motor control model.

> **When professionals name and frame problems, they map theory onto the actual features of the client's situation.**

According to this model, difficulties in occupational performance are a function of the task being done, the person's characteristics (including impairments), and the conditions in the environment (see Chapter 11). According to this model, limitations in performance are a function of the confluence of impaired movement capacity, environmental conditions, and the task being done. The model also specifies that change in performance can be achieved by modifying any single element or a combination of these elements. Thus, a therapist using this model can systematically proceed to remediate the client's impairment and alter environmental and task conditions.

In addition to the theory they provide, models also offer case examples, protocols of intervention, and other kinds of technology that serve as means and exemplars for deciding a course of action. Even though models vary in the extent to which such resources have been developed, therapists will generally find a range of resources for each model.

Using the theory and other resources associated with a model requires therapists to have thorough understanding of and to be aware of the literature associated with each model. In order for therapists to actively employ a model as a way of seeing and solving client problems, they must have a good working knowledge of that model.

Therapists' Responsibilities in Using the Field's Conceptual Foundations

The profession provides a paradigm and conceptual practice models that serve as primary resources for occupational therapy practice. The responsibility of the occupational therapist includes:

◆ Being aware of the paradigm of the field and translating its vision of occupational therapy into one's practice approach
◆ Selecting and using models appropriate to one's practice

◆ Selecting and using related knowledge appropriate to one's practice

The following sections consider each of these elements.

Establishing a Practice Approach

As discussed in Section One and earlier in this chapter, the field's paradigm provides an orientation to the nature of occupational therapy. The themes of the paradigm are very broad. Consequently, occupational therapists must always examine their own practice situation to decide how occupational therapy can best contribute to addressing client needs in that situation.

For example, an occupational therapist working in a school system would focus on the child's occupational roles of student and friend that are enacted in that context. Moreover, the kinds of occupations that will be used as therapy would likely be the classroom and playground occupations that are readily available. On the other hand, an occupational therapist working in home health care might focus on the family, self-care, and homemaking occupations of the client and use occupations from that context as therapy. In a vocational rehabilitation program, the therapist might focus primarily on the worker role and use industrial tasks as the therapeutic medium.

No matter what the setting, the key elements of defining one's practice involve:

◆ Concern for the client's occupational well-being
◆ Addressing client problems in terms of their impact on the client's occupational life
◆ Using occupations as the primary therapeutic medium

When a therapist has considered carefully how these three core themes of the paradigm can best be reflected given client needs and the practice setting, the stage has been set for defining the components and processes of one's practice.

Selecting and Using Conceptual Practice Models

Therapists ordinarily choose a subset of the field's models to guide their practice. The collective resources provided by conceptual practice models were examined in Section Two and overviewed in Chapter 13. One must know the field's models and the approaches they provide in order to effectively select the models most appropriate to be used in one's practice.

Therapists must carefully select from the field's models those that are most suited for seeing and explaining the problems of their clients. Consider, for example, a client who has suffered a spinal cord injury, is currently in rehabilitation, and appears depressed and unmotivated. The biomechanical model would serve as a way of understanding the specific effects of the spinal lesion on muscle enervation and the consequent loss of active and passive range of motion, strength, and endurance. This model also provides a way to consider how these impairments will impact on the movement capacity of the individual in occupational tasks.

This one aspect of the client's situation is made more understandable and is framed as a particular kind of problem when seen through the biomechanical model. It is important to note that the biomechanical model is silent on the emotional or motivational dimension of the client's situation. Hence, there is a need for more than one model if one wishes to name and frame other problems experienced by the client.

For instance, the model of human occu-

> **Therapists must carefully select from the field's models those that are most suited for seeing and explaining the problems of their clients.**

pation could be used to address the client's motivational status. This model would be concerned with how the spinal cord injury has affected the client's personal causation (sense of competence), interests, and values. This model orients the therapist to construct a picture of the client's intense feelings of loss of capacity and control, fears about the future, disruption of ability to participate in and enjoy old interests, and the disintegration of long-term life goals. These factors, viewed together, provide a way to name the client's unmotivated status as disruption of volition.

The two models together provide ways of conceptualizing the impact of spinal cord injury more holistically, and they allow the therapist to see in more depth the nature of two very different aspects of the client's circumstances. The biomechanical and human occupation models provide a way to name the musculoskeletal and motivational problems and to frame their meaning for function (e.g., limited movement affecting functional tasks and disrupted volition affecting motivation).

Other circumstances may call for different models. The sensory integration model may be used to make sense of the clumsiness of a schoolchild. The cognitive-perceptual model may shed light on the memory and problem-solving difficulties of the victim of a stroke. In each case, a problem is named and framed by the model of practice.

Each model of practice frames a problem in occupation and provides the therapist with a perspective for enhancing the occupational functioning of the individual. The models provide rationales for how occupation can be used as a therapeutic agent. Thus, they serve as a means by which the therapist operationalizes the professional identity provided by the field's paradigm.

Therapists should select and use those models that, together, provide a holistic picture of the biological, psychosocial, and environmental circumstances that influence a person's occupational functioning. It is usually not possible to create an adequate picture with a single model of practice; therefore, the therapist will often use two or more models in tandem.

The effectiveness of strategies suggested by one model can be enhanced through insights provided by another model. If we consider the earlier example of combining the biomechanical model and the model of human occupation, we see that intervention goals derived from both models may be met together. For example, if a person with spinal cord injury participates in a therapeutic occupation that has meaning because of a connection to a life role, biomechanical goals may be enhanced (since a client may feel less fatigue and exert more effort in a meaningful activity). Volitional goals may be realized simultaneously (a sense of possibilities for competence and a regeneration of interest and meaning may emerge from the activity). By combining models, therapists can achieve a more holistic and efficacious approach.

Selecting and Using Related Knowledge

While the paradigm and models of occupational therapy provide the most basic knowledge used in practice, there are always situations in which practitioners must draw on knowledge outside the field. In this instance, therapists employ related knowledge. For example, consider the type of client discussed above.

In providing services to a client with spinal cord injury, a therapist may employ a range of information from outside the field. Consider the field of disability studies discussed in Chapter 16. The person who acquires a spinal cord injury enters a new experience and social status as a disabled person. The occupational therapist working with this client should be aware of concepts from disability studies and use these concepts at appropriate points. Similarly, if the therapist recognizes the client struggling with emotional coping or interpersonal processes, the psychodynamic model may provide useful concepts.

When employing related knowledge it is important that therapists:

◆ Select appropriate and relevant related knowledge to complement their conceptual practice models
◆ Derive their identities and the main elements of their practice from the paradigm and practice models, not from the related knowledge

In this way, related knowledge assures that therapists have the full range of knowledge necessary for practice while functioning within the parameters of their professional role.

Conclusion

The conceptual foundations of occupational therapy provide the fundamental resources to provide the identity and competence of practitioners. In the end, therapists must select from and actively use this knowledge in order to define their role and to organize their practice. The conceptual foundations are the practitioner's most basic tools for being an occupational therapist.

References

Barris, R. (1984). Toward an image of one's own: Sources of variation in the role of occupational therapists in psychosocial practice. The Occupational Therapy Journal of Research, 4(1), 3–23.

Christiansen, C. (1999). Defining lives: Occupation as identity: An essay on competence, coherence, and the creation of meaning: American Journal of Occupational Therapy, 53, 547–558.

Harrison, D. (2003). The case for generic working in mental health occupational therapy. British Journal of Occupational Therapy, 66(3), 110–112.

Fisher, AG. (1998). Uniting practice and theory in an occupational framework. American Journal of Occupational Therapy, 54(7), 509–521.

Mattingly, C. (1988). Perspectives on clinical reasoning for occupational therapy. In Roberson, S (ed.). In Focus: Skills for Assessment and Treatment, pp 81–88. Rockville, MD: American Occupational Therapy Association.

O'Shea, BJ. (1977). Pawn or protagonist: Interactional perspective of professional identity. Canadian Journal of Occupational Therapy, 44, 101–108.

Rogers, JC. (1983). Clinical reasoning: The ethics, science, and art. American Journal of Occupational Therapy, 37(9), 601–616.

Schon, D. (1983). The Reflective Practitioner: How Professionals Think in Action. New York: Basic Books.

Chapter 19

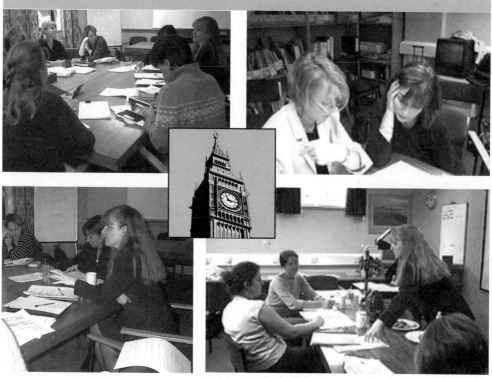

Future Directions for the Development of Occupational Therapy's Conceptual Foundations

Under auspices of the United Kingdom Center of Outcomes Research and Education (UKCORE), practitioners and academics have partnered to bridge a gap that often exists between scholarship and practice. Through seminars, study groups, case conferences, and other activities, they work together to integrate a conceptual practice model into occupational therapy services. Moreover, they collaborate to assure that the needs and circumstances of practice shape theory development and research. All participants take on the role of scholar-practitioners sharing responsibility for developing and applying a conceptual practice model.

There is no universally accepted answer to the question of how a profession should organize and develop its knowledge. However, the scenario just described exemplifies an important direction that scholarship must take for the future development of occupational therapy. This final chapter revisits some of the most basic themes of this text, considering why and how they suggest such an approach to generating and applying the conceptual foundations of the field.

The first premise of this text is that occupational therapy's conceptual foundations can be distinguished into:

◆ A paradigm that reflects the most basic themes, viewpoint, and values of the profession
◆ Conceptual practice models that articulate and apply the field's theory underlying practice
◆ A collection of related knowledge employed in practice but not generated by the field

Occupational therapy is responsible for the development of its own paradigm and conceptual practice models. Therefore, it is important to consider how efforts in the field further these two important aspects of its conceptual foundations.

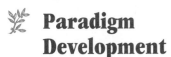

Paradigm Development

The paradigm supplies identity to the profession as a whole and, therefore, its themes are broad. The paradigm is developed as members of the field articulate and share their vision of occupational therapy. Moreover, the paradigm is also shaped by various sociopolitical and historical forces. We saw evidence of this process in examining the transformations that have taken place in occupational therapy's paradigm. In the end, the paradigm is shaped primarily by dialogue both within occupational therapy

and between the field and the various professional, scientific, economic, political, and societal trends that influence health care. As noted in Chapter 1, this dialogue includes a range of activities, from the stories that therapists tell about practice to the articles and books that are written in the field.

Occupational therapy's first paradigm was the deliverance of many interacting forces. It was grounded in European moral treatment concepts that were first brought to North America in the 19th century. These moral treatment concepts were integrated with concepts from new leaders of a practice movement that became occupational therapy in North America at the beginning of the 20th century. By mid-century this occupational paradigm was being replaced with a mechanistic perspective derived from medicine. Reilly (1962) first recognized that this paradigm change had severed occupational therapy from its original grounding in the concern for occupation in human life. She initiated the move to return the field's attention to occupation, arguing that occupational therapy should develop its own knowledge base independent of medicine. Reilly (1962) proposed that the proper scholarly focus for occupational therapy was on occupation and its relationship to human adaptation. The idea of organizing the field around the concept of occupation was controversial when Reilly proposed it in 1962, but increasingly over the following decades other scholars in the field embraced it. As discussed in Chapter 4, occupation is universally accepted now as the thematic focus of the field's paradigm.

Occupational Science

Occupational therapy's newfound enthusiasm for the importance of occupation to human life and well-being is also reflected in the development of occupational science. When originally proposed, occupational science was defined as "the scientific discipline that provides explanations of the human as an occupational being" (Clark et al., 1991, p. 300). Proponents of occupational science distinguish between the profession of occupational therapy and occupational science (Zemke and Clark, 1996). The latter is proposed as new discipline, separate from but supporting the applied science of occupational therapy. Consequently, occupational science was envisioned to be more like sociology or biology, which are not directly concerned with matters of practical application (Zemke & Clark, 1996).

Nonetheless, proponents of occupational science asserted that this new academic discipline would naturally benefit occupational therapy since it would generate knowledge useful to the field (Zemke & Clark, 1996). As Zemke and Clark note, "Occupational science is apt to create changes in the way that therapists perceive and approach their work because of what they will have learned about occupation from occupational scientists" (p. vii).

Occupational science clearly has its roots in Reilly's exhortation to focus on occupation. Nonetheless, its emphasis on creating a basic understanding of occupation without immediate concern for application differs from Reilly's assertion (1969) that occupational therapy scholarship should "generate ideas in research relevant to our field and to develop them as soon as possible within a clinic" (p. 299). For this reason, Mosey (1992) recommended partitioning occupational science from occupational therapy. She noted that such a division would allow the former to establish itself as a nonapplied discipline while the profession of occupational therapy would be freed to pursue applied scientific inquiry to advance practice. Disagreeing with Mosey, proponents of occupational science (Clark et al., 1993) argued for a more symbiotic relationship between the discipline and the profession. They observed that most occupational science researchers would be occupational

therapists, and consequently their research on occupation would be "more directly targeted toward practice considerations" (Clark et al., 1993, p. 185).

Mosey countered that this blurring of distinctions between the discipline of occupational science and the profession of occupational therapy would detract from both. She argued that if occupational science was in service to the profession, it would be unlikely to be accepted by established disciplines (Mosey, 1993). She also argued that occupational therapy should not concern itself and devote its resources to support occupational science because it was in critical need of developing its applied science. Mosey noted (1993): "No science-based profession can survive and thrive without engaging in applied scientific inquiry focused on developing theoretically based, safe, effective, and efficient sets of guidelines for action" (p. 752). Occupational therapy must, she reasoned, focus its energies and resources on generating knowledge for practice if it is to continue to be valued by society.

Nearly a decade and a half after its introduction, occupational science has evolved as a movement clearly based in occupational therapy. Contrary to Mosey's recommendation, those who describe themselves as doing occupational science are members of the profession of occupational therapy. Journals, articles, and books that describe occupational science are almost exclusively by occupational therapy scholars. Clearly, then, occupational science has not developed as a separate discipline but rather as a movement within occupational therapy.

In some cases, authors have included applied work as part of occupation science (Clark, 1993; Zemke & Clark, 1996). However, authors primarily continue to describe occupation science as an effort to generate more basic knowledge about occupation (Wilcock, 2001). Moreover, proponents of occupational science continue to emphasize how knowledge generated about occupation will positively impact occupational therapy practice (Carlson & Dunlea, 1995; Clark, 1993; Clark et al., 1993; Wilcock, 2001). In response to such claims, critics have raised questions about whether occupation science will really inform practice (Forsyth, 2001a; Forsyth, 2001b; Summerfield-Mann, 2001). Certainly, it is worth asking whether the study of occupation will contribute to the practice of occupational therapy.

It is likely, as suggested by occupational science proponents (Zemke & Clark, 1996), that the study of occupation will enhance occupational therapists' appreciation of the role of occupation in life and health. This appears to be what Wilcock (2001) meant when she noted that while occupation science does not "provide a prescriptive programme of therapy" (p. 60), it does provide a way of thinking about practice. The question remains, however, about whether this approach to informing practice is sufficient.

The Theory-Practice Gap

While the concept of occupation has clearly become the central focus in the field's literature today, it is not universally reflected in practice (Fisher, 1998). As Christiansen (1999) observes, "a full and genuine appreciation of the power of occupation to enable health and well-being has not yet made its way across the landscape of the profession" (p. 556). Similarly, Wood (1998) argues that knowledge about occupation is "sadly inert among clinicians who feel ill prepared to face complex life issues, who believe that they lack the expertise to construct more robust interventions, who feel at a loss for words in expressing the full value of their profession, and who thereby ostensibly fail to apply its published

research and scholarship to align practice with current thought" (p. 408). As reflected in the observations of these writers, it is a common observation of academicians that practice simply lags behind scholarship about occupation. However, this observation would appear to contradict the assertion of occupation science that increased scholarship about occupation will naturally inform practice. Instead, there appears to be an ongoing gap between concepts and practice in occupational therapy.

Writers in a number of fields argue that such a gap between academic knowledge and practice is due to how academicians produce knowledge. For example, MacKinnon (1991) argues that academics tend to assume "a relationship between theory and practice that places theory prior to practice, both methodologically and normatively, as if theory is a terrain unto itself" (p. 13). Such a view places theory in a privileged position of dictating what should go on in practice. The divide between theory and practice exists because knowledge generated to answer basic questions about the nature of some phenomena is not the same knowledge required to solve problems in practice (Boyer, 1990; Higgs & Titchen, 2001; Schon, 1983).

In the occupational therapy context, this argument can be taken to mean that findings and theories about occupation do not directly shed light on what might or should be done in occupational therapy practice. There is an important gap between understanding occupation and the challenge of identifying how occupations can be used as therapy in a specific context with particular clients.

Observations about the role of occupation in human life do not tell a practitioner what to do when the client with cerebral

> **Findings and theories about occupation do not directly shed light on what might or should be done in occupational therapy practice.**

palsy, a stroke, spinal cord injury, or schizophrenia arrives with all of his or her life challenges. Occupational therapy practice requires knowledge that directly addresses client support for achievement in occupational participation. If the field wishes to have occupation-based practice, it must generate knowledge specifically about doing occupation-based practice.

Developing Knowledge for Practice

I argued in Chapter 2 that conceptual practice models reflect the particular theoretical, practical, and scientific concerns of occupational therapy. As shown in Figure 19-1, theory within models is organized to simultaneously explain:

◆ The workings of some aspect of occupation

◆ The nature of related occupational problems

◆ The dynamics of the therapeutic process that address those problems

Within models, this theory is translated into a technology for practice that includes specific tools and strategies for conducting therapy. Finally, research within models yields empirical support for the theory and for the efficacy of applications that emanate from the theory. Consequently, the research based on conceptual practice models includes basic and applied aims.

Basic research is ordinarily thought of as testing explanations offered by a theory. Such research examines whether the concepts and

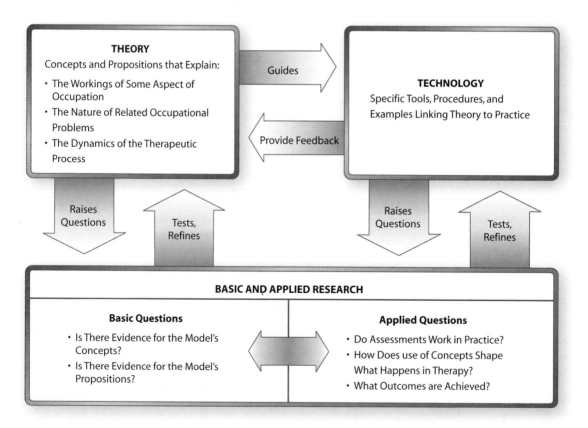

Figure 19-1. Knowledge Development within a Conceptual Practice Model.

propositions of the theory are supported by evidence. Basic research is guided by the following two questions:

◆ Is there evidence for the model's concepts?
◆ Is there evidence for the model's propositions about relations between concepts?

These questions are concerned with improving the accuracy and adequacy of the explanations offered in the model's theory. Findings from such questions either increase our confidence in the theory or indicate the need to alter, eliminate, or add concepts and propositions.

Applied research examines the practical results of using theory to solve problems. Such studies ordinarily address the following broad questions:

◆ Do assessments based on a model provide dependable and useful information when applied in practice?
◆ When the model's concepts are operationalized in practice, how do they shape what occurs in therapy?
◆ What outcomes are achieved from therapy based on the model?

Importantly, when practical applications of theory are shown to work, they provide evidence not only about occupational therapy practice but also about the viability of the model's theory. In other words, if the theory can be used to predict, understand, and control processes in practice, then one can be more confident of the explanations the theory provides.

While one can distinguish basic from applied research purposes, these two research aims are naturally integrated in studies of models. Studies that examine models typically incorporate both basic and applied research aims. Moreover, when studies are undertaken within the framework of a conceptual practice model, they tend to have both applied and basic relevance, no matter what their primary aim.

For instance, studies that seek primarily to examine the dependability of an assessment tool provide evidence about underlying concepts they are designed to measure. Furthermore, such studies often result in changing or elaborating the concepts within a theory. For example, research on the Sensory Integration and Praxis Tests has shed light on the nature of sensory processing (Bundy, Lane, & Murray, 2002).

In similar fashion, studies that have had as their primary or sole purpose the testing or development of theory have contributed to applied concerns. For example, some research based on the model of human occupation has examined the nature of occupational narratives and how they are shaped over time (Helfrich, Kielhofner, & Mattingly, 1994; Jonsson, Josephsson, & Kielhofner, 2000; Jonsson, Josephsson, & Kielhofner, 2001; Jonsson, Kielhofner, & Borell, 1997). These studies, which were primarily concerned with examining occupational identity and its development, have direct implications for how therapists might best support clients to change and develop their narratives in therapy. Thus, while the main aim of the research was basic, the findings have immediate applied relevance. Moreover, because the studies were conducted within the framework of a model designed for clinical utility, the findings from the studies were readily integrated into the technology for application. In this case, the methods of analyzing narratives developed for research have been adapted for use in assessment (Kielhofner et al., 1998), and strategies for applying the ideas in intervention have been examined (Goldstein, Kielhofner, & Paul-Ward, in press; Helfrich & Kielhofner, 1994).

Therefore, as shown in Figure 19-1, basic and applied research overlap and interact within a model. Conceptual practice models naturally integrate theoretical, practical, and scientific concerns in the field, creating cohesion and dialogue between these activities. In occupational therapy, where theorizing is primarily in the service of practice, theoretical and practical concerns must be synergistic. Consequently, the most efficient and effective way for the field to develop its conceptual foundations will be to advance conceptual practice models.

> **The most efficient and effective way for the field to develop its conceptual foundations will be to advance conceptual practice models.**

Developing Models Through a Scholarship of Practice

The previous discussion indicated that conceptual practice models naturally integrate theory, research, and practice. It is important to consider how the work of developing models should be undertaken. Typically, the development of theory and conduct of research have been activities reserved for those in academic roles while application of the theory and research has been left up to practitioners. Finally, clients who receive services are often passive recipients of those services.

This situation serves to perpetuate the divide between theory and research on the one hand and practice on the other. As I noted in Chapter 3, the scholarship of practice emphasizes that knowledge development in occupational therapy should grow out of

> **The scholarship of practice emphasizes that knowledge development in occupational therapy should grow out of collaboration between those in academic and practice roles and should also include and empower occupational therapy clients.**

collaboration between those in academic and practice roles and should also include and empower occupational therapy clients. Consequently, the development of conceptual practice models requires an active dialogue in which theory informs practice and practice informs theory.

Thus, we can conclude this text with the ideal represented at the beginning of this chapter. The development of occupational therapy's conceptual foundations will best be served through efforts in which theorists, researchers, practitioners, and clients enter into partnership to refine conceptual practice models and the services that emanate from them.

References

Boyer, E. (1990). Scholarship Reconsidered: Priorities of the Professoriate. Princeton, NJ: The Carnegie Foundation for the Advancement of Teaching.

Bundy, AC, Lane, SJ & Murray, EA. (2002). Sensory Integration: Theory and Practice, 2nd ed. Philadelphia: FA Davis.

Carlson, M & Dunlea, A. (1995). Further thoughts on the pitfalls of partition: A response to Mosey. American Journal of Occupational Therapy, 49, 73–81.

Christiansen, C. (1999). Defining lives: Occupation as identity: An essay on competence, coherence and the creation of meaning. American Journal of Occupational Therapy, 53(6), 547–558.

Clark, F. (1993). Occupation embedded in a real life: Interweaving occupational science and occupational therapy. American Journal of Occupational Therapy, 47(12), 1067–1078.

Clark, F, Parham, D, Carlson, M, et al. (1991). Occupational science: Academic innovation in the service of occupational therapy's future. American Journal of Occupational Therapy, 45, 300–310.

Clark, F, Zemke, R, Frank, G, et al. (1993). Dangers inherent in the partition of occupational therapy and occupational science. American Journal of Occupational Therapy, 47(2), 184–187.

Fisher, AG. (1998). Uniting practice and theory in an occupational framework. American Journal of Occupational Therapy, 54(7), 509–521.

Forsyth, K. (2001a). Occupational science as a selected research priority [Letter to the editor]. British Journal of Occupational Therapy, 64(8), 420.

Forsyth, K. (2001b). Supporting occupational therapy [Letter to the editor]. British Journal of Occupational Therapy, 64(9), 464–466.

Goldstein, K, Kielhofner, G & Paul-Ward, A. (in press). Occupational narratives and the therapeutic process. The Australian Occupational Therapy Journal.

Helfrich, C & Kielhofner, G. (1994). Volitional narratives and the meaning of occupational therapy. American Journal of Occupational Therapy, 48(4), 319–326.

Helfrich, C, Kielhofner, G & Mattingly, C. (1994). Volition as narrative: An understanding of motivation in chronic illness. American Journal of Occupational Therapy, 48(4), 311–317.

Higgs, J & Titchen, A. (eds.). (2001). Practice Knowledge and Expertise in the Health Professions. London: Butterworth Heinemann.

Jonsson, H, Josephsson, S & Kielhofner, G. (2000). Evolving narratives in the course of retirement: A longitudinal study. American Journal of Occupational Therapy, 54(5), 463–470.

Jonsson, H, Josephsson, S & Kielhofner, G. (2001). Narratives and experience in an occupational transition: A longitudinal study of the retirement process. American Journal of Occupational Therapy, 55(4), 424–432.

Jonsson, H, Kielhofner, G & Borell, L. (1997). Anticipating retirement: The formation of narratives concerning an occupational transition. American Journal of Occupational Therapy, 51(1), 49–56.

Kielhofner, G, Mallinson, T, Crawford, C, et al. (1998). A User's Guide to the Occupational Performance History Interview-II (OPHI-II) (version 2.0). Chicago: Model of Human Occupation Clearinghouse, Department of Occupational Therapy, College of Applied Health Sciences, University of Illinois at Chicago.

MacKinnon, C. (1991). From practice to theory, or what is a white women anyway? Yale Journal of Law and Feminism, 4(13), 13–22.

Mosey, AC. (1992). Partition of occupational science and occupational therapy. American Journal of Occupational Therapy, 46(9), 851–853.

Mosey, AC. (1993). Partition of occupational science and occupational therapy: Sorting out some issues. American Journal of Occupational Therapy, 47(8), 751–754.

Reilly, M. (1962). Occupational therapy can be one of the great ideas of 20th century medicine. American Journal of Occupational Therapy, 16(1), 1–9.

Reilly, M (1969). The educational process. American Journal of Occupational Therapy, 23(4), 299–307.

Schon, D. (1983). The Reflective Practitioner. New York: Basic Books.

Summerfield-Mann, L. (2001). Supporting conceptual models of practice [Letter to the editor]. British Journal of Occupational Therapy, 64(9), 463–464.

Wilcock, AA. (2001). Occupational science: The key to broadening horizons. British Journal of Occupational Therapy, 4(2), 56–61.

Wood, W. (1998). It is jump time for occupational therapy. American Journal of Occupational Therapy, 52, 403–411.

Zemke, R & Clark, F. (1996). Occupational Science: The Evolving Discipline. Philadelphia: FA Davis.

Index